Essential Pathophysiology for Nursing and Healthcare Students

Praise for this book

"Essential Pathophysiology for Nursing and Healthcare Students *is a book that should be kept no further than an arm's reach away. The book is easy to navigate and easy to understand. Each chapter has handy diagrams to support the text and the self-assessment questions at the end of each chapter help the reader to review their learning. Any nursing and healthcare student will find that this book is essential in helping them comprehend and learn about the systems and mechanisms of the human body in health and ill health. This book would also be a good read for anybody working with or teaching students as a refresher on pathophysiology.*"

Rebecca Bailey-McHale, Lecturer,
Faculty of Health and Social Care,
University of Chester, UK

Essential Pathophysiology for Nursing and Healthcare Students

Ann Richards and Sharon Edwards

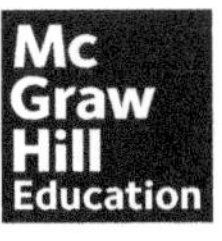

Open University Press

Open University Press
McGraw-Hill Education
McGraw-Hill House
Shoppenhangers Road
Maidenhead
Berkshire
England
SL6 2QL

email: enquiries@openup.co.uk
world wide web: www.openup.co.uk

and Two Penn Plaza, New York, NY 10121-2289, USA

First published 2014

A catalogue record of this book is available from the British Library

ISBN-13: 9780335238323
ISBN-10: 0335238327
eISBN: 9780335238347

Library of Congress Cataloging-in-Publication Data
CIP data applied for

Contents

Figures

Preface

ORGANISATION AND CONTENT

Our approach in this book is to attempt to deal with the problem of how students, teachers and clinicians cope with the expanding knowledge related to pathophysiology and its link to normal anatomy and physiology. To do this we have compressed the data into simplified bullet points. The disorders included in the book can affect patients in any healthcare setting and therefore, the information can be a useful resource for healthcare professionals in any setting. However, the primary focus of this book is to develop understanding in relation to the body's transition from normal biological functioning to diseased pathophysiological states.

Each chapter contains a short introduction to set the scene for the contents. The main body of the text of all chapters includes an anatomy and physiology section, which highlights the aspects we felt to be of special interest, as it was not possible to cover all aspects. This is followed by pathophysiology, which discusses a number of diseases developed using a logical format that begins with an introductory paragraph, aetiology, pathology, clinical features, investigations, treatment and drug therapies. At the end of each chapter there is a set of self-assessment questions to help students plan their learning.

The book is organised in a way that the first six chapters focus on the healthcare professional's ability to comprehend cellular and tissue responses to injury, which determines the development of many common diseases presented in chapters 7 to 16.

Chapters 1 to 6 consider aspects of cellular physiology and the understanding of molecular, cellular and tissue level interactions. Cells live in a microenvironment with neighbouring molecules, which communicate with each other and provide the basis for comparison with and understanding of all alterations in anatomy and physiology brought about by disease. In this section is the consideration of total body processes such as fluid and electrolyte balance, acid base balance, normal and altered immune system and cancer. This section is central as it gives a study of the main concepts of pathophysiology, which form the underlying processes of disease.

Chapters 7 to 16 provide a systems approach to understanding disease within body systems.

FEATURES TO PROMOTE LEARNING

While reading through this book, consider the system at the cellular biological level and consider the cause of the condition(s) using chapter 1. This is to help you understand your practice in more depth and detail, linking the interventions used in the treatment of disease. At the cellular level damage due to injury can be reversed, either by normal body healing methods or treatment therapies. However, the body cannot heal if treatment and interventions are not instigated to reverse or slow down cellular damage; the processes mentioned in chapter 1 can lead disease, acute or chronic illness or to cellular death. Once cellular death occurs the end result may be failure of the organ and death.

Case studies

The inclusion of case studies is to embed into your practice the need for timely and prompt interventions, and at the same time help to contextualise knowledge and understanding of integrating theory into clinical practice. In each chapter the case studies provide real life application of concepts, and to help link the clinical features observed in patients to the aetiology and pathology, supported by making frequent references to chapter 1. This cross-checking will help organise your thoughts around making links between the preclinical (before disease) to the clinical (the point of the emergence of clinical feature). It is recommended to study the sample patients, facilitating the important aspect of putting it all together. Whatever your area of clinical practice the engagement with the case studies can serve to increase your confidence and capability to respond appropriately in a variety of care situations and settings, and enable sound clinical moment-to-moment decision-making skills.

In addition, it is important to remember the patients represented in the case studies should be considered with care and compassion. Through these case studies you demonstrate the humanness of caring practices, which needs to be included in and at the forefront of what all healthcare professionals do.

Self-assessment questions

Self-assessment questions appear at the end of each chapter to facilitate with the identification of healthcare practitioners' own learning so far, and to continue to build on this knowledge as you go through each chapter.

Practice points

Practice points are incorporated through all of the chapters to help healthcare professionals think about the underlying disease processes in relation to interventions and treatment.

1 Introduction to pathophysiology and some important definitions

Sharon Edwards

INTRODUCTION TO PATHOPHYSIOLOGY

Pathophysiology is the study of the changes that occur in cells, tissues and organs when altered by disease and/or injury and the effects these have on normal body function. As a foundation of understanding pathophysiology healthcare professionals need knowledge and understanding of cellular biology as well as anatomy and physiology and the organ systems of the body. The study of cellular biology, changes in the cellular environment and immunity are the most important bridges between determining the preclinical to the clinical condition observed in clinical practice situations.

The overriding primary focus of this book is to relate normal body function to the pathological changes that occur and can lead to disease processes. This can lead to developing understanding in relation to the body's transition from normal biological functioning to diseased pathophysiological states. From this understanding, healthcare professionals can learn to recognise and categorise the different aetiologies, pathologies and clinical features of disease. This interpretation leads to further investigations, treatment and interventions, the possibility of drug therapies and therapeutic evaluation.

Aetiology

- Aetiology is the study of the cause(s) of disease and/or injury
- The causes of disease can be either:
  - Endogenous originating from within the body
  - Exogenous coming from outside the body
- Diseases can be of unknown cause e.g. idiopathic
- Some conditions are caused by the effects of treatments and called iatrogenic.
- Nosocomial denotes a new disorder, not the patient's original condition e.g. hospital-acquired infection

- Risk factors exist which include dietary, occupational or lifestyle conditions e.g. smoking
- Predisposing factors make an individual more susceptible to disease
- In some instances disease prevention is highlighted for healthcare professionals to consider and incorporate if appropriate.

In pathophysiology there are some diseases such as pneumonia, which easily identify a specific cause or aetiology and the infection to some extent follows a standardised disease process. However, other diseases such as multiple sclerosis or arthritis follow pathological changes that are not so easy to define and the cause is less clear. The aetiology of conditions such as type 2 diabetes mellitus and atherosclerosis are due to several interacting factors.

Pathology

- Pathology is the scientific study of disease
- It includes the study of structural alterations in cells, tissues and organs that help to identify the cause of disease.

The pathology of a disease can identify the process of cell, tissue and organ damage, helping to identify the cause of disease.

Clinical features

- The aetiology and pathogenesis of disease leads to clinical features and include the signs and symptoms of disease
- A symptom is an indication that a disease is present and is what the patient usually complains of
- A sign is what the clinician or healthcare practitioner is looking or feeling for. The clinical features of a disease are often accompanied by structural or functional changes that can be investigated.

The pathophysiology of some conditions identify similar clinical features to describe them such as indigestion and angina; the same descriptions of chest pain appear in both conditions and it is difficult at times to tell them apart (differential diagnosis). In addition, some conditions have the same clinical features such as diarrhoea and vomiting, which occur in a number of conditions with the same and even multiple symptoms that frequently occur together.

Investigations

- Proper investigation of disease is required to ensure prompt and accurate diagnosis to allow treatment to be instigated. This usually involves:

  - A clinical history and examination
  - A range of diagnostic interventions may be required such as:
    - X-ray
    - Laboratory investigations:
      - Microbiology
      - Immunology
      - Biochemistry
      - Haematology
      - Histopathology
      - Genetics
- Investigations are valuable in determining a disease or to identify any improvement or deterioration in diseased state and patients' condition. This is achieved using assessment to ensure optimum care is delivered. This involves:
  - A patient history using pertinent questions and recognising verbal and non-verbal cues to elicit clinical features
  - Physical examination using critical thinking skills to prioritise and guide interventions and treatment
  - The use of both subjective and objective findings obtained during the assessment, such as:
    - Monitoring (vital signs, electrocardiography, Glasgow Coma Scale (GCS))
    - Observation (skin colour, skin temperature, patient's ability to self-care e.g. nails, shaving, verbal response)
    - Measurement (blood results, arterial blood gases)
    - Interpretation (putting it all together)
    - Prompt response (instigate actions)
  - These are to provide the basis for possible actions to ensure early improvement with better outcomes or in the event of further deterioration
- Investigations, once undertaken, need to be interpreted. The role of the healthcare practitioner is to be able to:
  - Recognise physiological deterioration and communicate this to the wider clinical team, as
    - Expert collaboration to support the care of patients whose condition is at risk of deteriorating is essential
    - Healthcare practitioners need to be able to communicate their concerns succinctly and efficiently regarding the relevant features of a patient's condition in any given situation
  - Implement sound clinical decision-making to inform interventions and treatment
  - Prevent an adverse event.

It is important to identify how interacting factors such as the aetiology, pathology and the development of clinical features relate to each other. As a healthcare professional an understanding of and an appreciation for this idea can revolutionise your understandings. The connecting of these activities determines treatment and drug therapies that may be required. Early diagnosis and treatment determine patient outcomes and therapeutic evaluation will govern whether treatment was successful. For additional terminology used in pathophysiology see Table 1.1.

Pathophysiology includes the complex element of suffering emphasising the fact that individuals do become ill and experience disease. In addition, it needs to be remembered that 'health' and 'illness' are not viewed the same in any two individuals, as patients and their own conception of health and illness is very different. Therefore, the use of the word health should be treated with caution, in the same way the individual's conception of disease and illness is subjective and based on personal beliefs and how illness and disease are understood and experienced.

Related term	**Definition**
Health	Can be defined as the absence of clinical features associated with any disease or 'a state of physical, mental and social well-being and not merely the absence of disease' (WHO)
Pathogenesis	Pattern of tissue changes associated with the development of disease or how the causative agents act to produce the clinical and pathological changes characteristic of a specific disease. The effects of the disease on a person are referred to as morbidity. The mortality of a disease describes the possibility of causing death. Some conditions have a rapid onset known to be acute, others have a more gradual onset over a longer period of time and are termed as chronic
Epidemiology	The study of how diseases spread in populations in relation to their aetiology. It includes the prevalence of disease in a population affected at a specific time. The incidence is the number of new cases. Some diseases are notifiable such as some infectious diseases. Epidemiology is influenced by certain socioeconomic factors such as poverty and overcrowding

Table 1.1 Other terms and definitions related to pathophysiology

Pathogens	These are the micro-organisms that cause infection, in many cases antibiotics are available to treat the pathogen
Idiopathic	Diseases with no identifiable cause
Iatrogenic	Diseases and/or injury as a result of medical intervention(s)
Nosocomial	Diseases acquired as a consequence of being in a hospital environment
Diagnosis	Naming or identification of disease
Differential diagnosis	Two or more diseases with similar presentation and clinical features
Prognosis	Expected outcome of disease, which varies between different diseases and is influenced by interventions and treatment
Acute disease	Sudden appearance of signs and symptoms lasting a short time
Chronic disease	Develops more slowly lasting a long time or a lifetime
Relapse	Occurs when the symptoms of a disease returns after a period of apparent recovery or remission
Remissions	Periods of good health with a reduction or disappearance of clinical symptoms or they diminish significantly
Exacerbations	Periods when clinical manifestations become worse or more severe
Sequelae	Any abnormal conditions that follow and are the result of a disease, treatment or injury

Table 1.1 Continued

In addition, individuals with the same disease may experience different outcomes. Conversely, patients can have concomitant but unrelated disease processes, indicating the co-existence of two or more diseases.

With this in mind, the healthcare professional needs to approach pathophysiology with an open and tolerant mind, in parallel with an understanding that in-depth knowledge and understanding of the scientific processes and principles of pathophysiology alone will not give all the answers.

The language of pathophysiology can be complex and healthcare professionals can find it difficult to learn the terminology. Most of the words used are based on either Greek or Latin. There are some common meanings that can help you to understand the meaning when combined with another either at the beginning (prefix) or at the end (suffix).

Prefix	Meaning	Example
anti-	Against, opposing	Antiemetic (against vomiting)
arthr-	Joint	Arthritis (inflammation of the joints)
bi-	Two, double	Bifocal (two types of lenses)
de-	Down, from	Dehydrated (reduced water content)
dia-	Between, through, apart, across	Diaphragm (breathing muscle across chest)
dis-	Apart from, free from	Discomfort
em-	In	Empyaemia (pus in the lung cavity)
epi-	Upon, on, over	Epidermis (outer layer of the skin)
glyc-	Sugar or sweet	Glycaemia (blood sugar)
haem-	Blood	Haemoglobin (blood protein)
hemi-	Half	Hemicolectomy (half the bowel removed)
hyper-	Excessive, above	Hyperglycaemia (high blood sugar)
hypo-	Under, deficient	Hypothyroidism (underactive thyroid gland)
in-, im-	In, into, within	Injection (pushing fluid into) Implant (insert into)
inter-	Between	Intercostal muscles (between ribs)
micro-	Small	Micro-organisms (small organisms)
multi-	Many	Multi-system organ failure (MSOF)
osteo-	Bone	Osteoarthritis (bone, joint swelling)
neo-	New, recent	Neonatal (new born)
pan-	All, entire	Panacea (cure all)
per-	Through, excessive	Permeable (may pass through)
poly-	Many, much, excessive	Polycystic ovaries (many cysts on the ovaries)
post-	After, behind	Postoperative (after surgery)
pre-	Before, in front of	Preoperative (before surgery)

Table 1.2 Prefixes to help explain pathophysiology

semi-	Half	Semiconscious (half conscious)
sub-	Under, beneath	Subcutaneous (under the skin)
trans-	Across, through	Transurethral (cut across the urethra)
rhin-	Nose	Rhinitis (nose inflammation)
sepsis	Infection	Septacaemia (infection in the blood)

(Modified from Austrin and Austrin, 1995)

Table 1.2 Continued

Prefix	Related organ
adeno-	Gland
adreno-	Adrenal gland
angio-	Blood vessel
arterio-	Artery
arthro-	Joint
bronchi-/broncho-	Bronchus
cardio-	Heart
cerebri-/cerebro	Cerebrum of the brain
colpo-	Vagina
costo-	Ribs
cysti-/cysto-	Bladder
duodeno-	Duodenum of intestine
encephalo-	Brain
entero-	Gastric, stomach
hepato-	Liver
histo-	Tissue
hyster-	Uterus
ile-/ilo-	Ileum of the intestine
jejuno-	Jejunum of the intestine
laryngo-	Larynx
lympho-	Lymphatic system
meningo-	Membranes covering the brain and spinal cord
myelo	Bone marrow or spinal cord
myo-	Muscle

Table 1.3 Prefixes used in pathophysiology to depict organs affected by disease

nephro-	Kidney
neuro-	Nerves or nervous system
oophoro-	Ovary
orchio-/orchido-	Testis or testes
osseo-/ossi-/oste-/ osteo-	Bone or bones
pharyngo	Pharynx
phlebo-	Vein or veins
pleuro-	Pleura or rib
pneuma-/pneumo-	Lungs or respiration
pulmo-	Lungs
pyelo-	Pelvis of the kidney
salpingo-	Fallopian tube

(Modified from Austrin and Austrin, 1995)

Table 1.3 Continued

Suffix	Meaning	Example
-ac, -al, -ic	Relating to	Cardiac (relating to the heart) Neural (relating to nerves) Haemorrhagic (relating to bleeding)
-aemia	Blood condition	Leukaemia (cancer of the blood)
-emesis	Vomit	Haematemesis (vomiting blood)
-esis, -ia, -iasis, -ism, -ity, -osis, -sis, -tion, -y	State or condition	Paresis (partial paralysis) Anaesthesia (loss of sensation) Psoriasis (skin condition) Priapism (persistant erection) Acidity (excess acid) Narcosis (drugged state) Inhalation (state of inhalation) Therapy (treatment condition)
-ent, -er, -or	Person or agent	Recipient (a person who receives) Examiner (a person who examines) Donor (a person who receives)
-gram, -graphy	Recording, written record	Electrocardiogram (recording of heart electrical activity) Mammogram (X-Ray of the breast)

Table 1.4 Suffixes to help explain pathophysiology

-graph	Instrument that records	Echocardiogram (record of sound)
-ible, -ile	Capable, able	Flexible bronchoscopy (capable of bending) Contractile (able to open)
-itis	Inflammation	Meningitis (inflammation of the meninges of the brain)
-logy	Science, study of	Biology (science of life) Histology (study of tissues)
-oma	Tumour, growth	Carcinoma (malignant growth) Sarcoma (cancerous tumour)
-penia	Lack of, deficiency of	Leukopenia (deficiency of white blood cells)
-phobia	Abnormal fear or intolerance	Acrophobia (fear of heights)
-plasty	Surgical shaping or formation	Angioplasty (reshaping of arteries)
-pnea	Breathing	Apnoea (absence of breathing) Dyspnoea (difficulty in breathing)
-ptosis	Prolapse, downward, displacement	Proctoptosis (prolapse of the anus) Nephroptosis (prolapse of the kidney)
-rrhage, -rrhagia	Excessive flow	Haemorrhage (excessive bleeding) Metrorrhagia (abnormal periods)
-stomy	Surgical opening	Colostomy (colon to the surface of the abdomen) Gastrostomy (into the stomach)
-scopy	Act of examining	Microscopy (observing minute objects under a microscope) Cystoscopy (examination of the bladder)
-tomy	Cutting, incision	Phlebotomy (incision into the vein)

(Modified from Austrin and Austrin, 1995)

Table 1.4 Continued

REFERENCE

Austrin, M.G. and Austrin, H.R. (1995) *Learning Medical Terminology: A Worktext* 8th edn, St Louis: Mosby Lifeline.

2 Cellular biology

Ann Richards and Sharon Edwards

CELLS

All body functions depend on cells, thus cellular biology is integral to the understanding of disease (McCance and Huether, 2010).

The function of cells

Cellular function is specialised, some cells perform one kind of function, whereas others will perform different functions, these include:

Movement

- This can occur due to cells being able to generate forces to produce motion
  - Muscles which include contractile cells that allow movement of limbs e.g. skeletal muscles, organs to contract and stretch e.g. heart and lungs and the digestive system
  - Blood vessels can constrict and dilate due to contraction of smooth muscle.

Conductivity

- Cells can respond to an electrical stimulus, called an electrical potential, which is initiated by nervous and cardiac cells
- Cells are electrically charged with electricity and there is a difference between two points in living cells, for example the inside of the cell is negative and the outside is positive, the difference is the resting membrane potential
- Cells can change the resting membrane potential in response to electrochemical stimuli known as an action potential
- Depolarisation is when a cell is stimulated the cell becomes more permeable to sodium, and sodium moves into the cell

  - To generate an action potential resulting in depolarisation a threshold potential has to be reached
  - Once reached the cell requires no further stimulation to continue depolarisation
  - During the action potential a cell cannot respond to another stimulus:
    - A phase when calcium enters the cell, a period known as absolute refractory phase (Marieb, 2012)
    - Normal cellular levels of calcium are returned to normal by the calcium pump in the cell membrane
- Repolarisation is the returning of the cell to its resting membrane potential:
  - Membrane permeability to sodium decreases and increases to potassium
  - The sodium/potassium pump returns cellular concentration back to normal.

Metabolic absorption

Cells utilise nutrients obtained from their surroundings e.g. carbohydrates, proteins, fats, minerals, vitamins and water and expel the waste products.

Transport and intake and output of a cell takes place by different processes depending on the features of the element to be transported. These include passive and active transport:

- Passive transport requires no energy for movement of solutes such as sodium and potassium dissolved in a solution or water to take place, and include:
  - Diffusion:
    - Solutes move from a high concentration to a low
    - Known as the concentration gradient
    - The rate is influenced by the differences in electrical potential across the membrane
  - Filtration
    - Solutes and water move from a high pressure to a low pressure
    - Determined by hydrostatic pressure (HP)
    - In the vascular system HP is the blood pressure generated in vessels by the contraction of the heart
  - Osmosis
    - Is the movement of water from a low solute concentration to a high, which dilutes the high concentration of a substance

        - Osmolality controls the distribution and movement of water between body cells, normal is 280–294 mOsm/kg used to determine hydration
        - Tonicity describes the effective osmolality of a solution and is important to consider when correcting fluid imbalances:
            - Isotonic solution has normal osmolality e.g. 285 mOsm/kg for example 5% dextrose and 0.9% normal saline
            - Hypotonic solution has a lower than normal osmolality and is a dilute solution
            - Hypertonic solution has a high osmolality of more than 285 mOsm/kg for example 20% dextrose solution
- Mediated transport
    - Facilitated diffusion where a transporter protein binds with a specific solute and facilitates its movement across a membrane e.g. insulin facilitates the movement of glucose into cells
- Active transport
    - This requires the use of adenosine triphosphate (ATP) as molecules are moved against a diffusion gradient for example:
        - The sodium/potassium ATP dependent pump regulates levels of sodium and potassium inside cells
        - The calcium ATP dependent pump regulates calcium in the cell cytoplasm regulating muscle contraction and relaxation cycles
- Vesicular transport
    - Large particles, small molecules and fluids are transported across plasma and intracellular membranes, this is used for:
        - Exocytosis – the movement of substances from the intracellular to the extracellular space
        - Endocytosis – the movement of substances across the plasma membrane into the cell from the extracellular environment.

Secretion

- Certain cells can draw in nutrients and produce new substances that are required elsewhere for example:
    - Adrenal glands which produce steroid hormones e.g. aldosterone, cortisol; sex hormones e.g. testosterone (men) and oestrogens (women); and stress hormone e.g. epinephrine and norepinephrine
    - Testes produce sperm
    - Ovaries release eggs.

Excretion

- All cells can rid themselves of waste products, derived from the metabolic processes the cells were designed for
- Lysosomes in cells use enzymes to break down or digest waste products and excrete them from the cells.

Cellular respiration or metabolism

- Cells utilise oxygen, which combines with nutrients to produce energy in the form of ATP
- This occurs in the mitochondria where cellular respiration takes place.

Reproduction

- The majority of cells are able to divide and reproduce themselves accurately
- Nerve cells are incapable of division
- Most cells reproduce by mitosis:
  - Mitosis is reproduction asexually and is undertaken by most human cells, the cells finish up as exact copies of the parent cells each with 23 pairs of chromosomes. Mitosis is divided into stages:
    - Interphase – a resting period before and after a cell divides, getting ready for replication, the deoxyribonucleic acid (DNA) copies itself. 4 phases:
      - Prophase – each chromosome splits into two chromatids
      - Metaphase – the 2 chromatids arrange themselves around the centre of the cell
      - Anaphase – the chromatids separate and 1 chromatid from each chromosome moves from the centre to either side of the cell
      - Telophase – 46 chromosomes on each side of the cell, the cell membrane narrows in the centre dividing into 2 cells
- Meiosis is the process by which cells end up with one each of the 23 chromosomes e.g. spermatozoa and ova reproduce in this way
  - Meiosis is divided into stages and they have the same name, and referred to as either I or II.

Communication

- Cells are bound together by an extracellular matrix, a glue-like substance; but through it the diffusion of nutrients, wastes and other solutes are allowed to move from cell to cell, from cells to blood and vice versa

- The extracellular matrix joins cells together to form tissues that work together and communicate with each other. If communication between cells alters it can affect disease onset. Cells communicate in 3 ways:
  - By producing protein channels
  - Through the use of receptor sites
  - By secretion of chemicals that signal cells, which can be some distance away; this is the most common way
- If deprived of appropriate signals, most cells undergo a form of cell suicide referred to as programmed cell death or apoptosis (Watson, 2005).

CELLULAR COMPONENTS

There are 2 major components to a cell (Figure 2.1): the outer membrane called the plasma membrane, and a fluid centre called cytoplasm in which all the organs, referred to as organelles, reside within the cell.

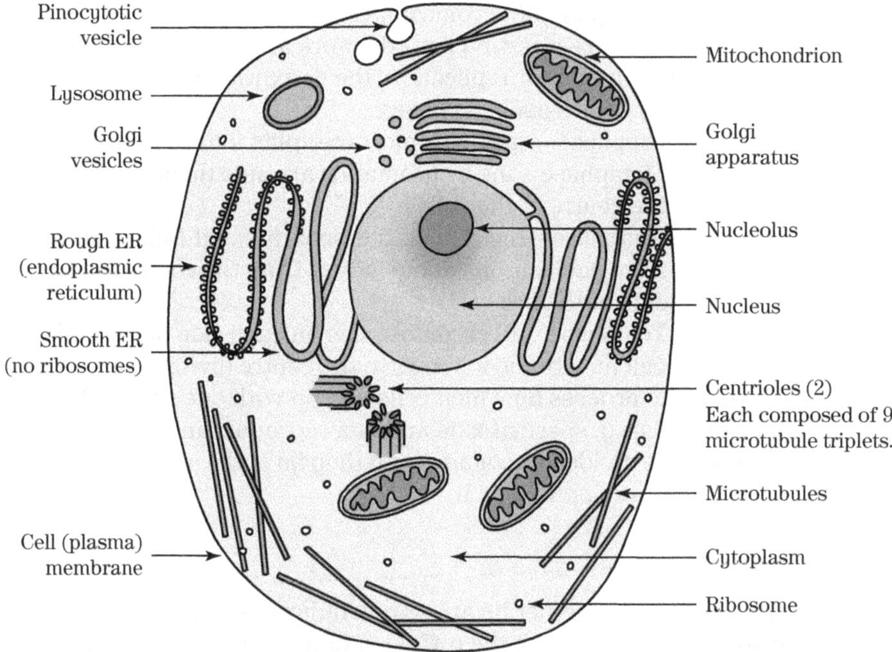

Figure 2.1 The cell and its components

Plasma membrane

- The plasma membrane is integral to the function of a cell as it controls what enters and what exits the cell:
    - Potassium and sodium levels in the cell are maintained by the sodium/potassium pump in the plasma membrane
    - Calcium levels are kept at functional levels, and excess is pumped out by the calcium pump
- It can exclude various molecules due to a selective transport system within its membrane.

Plasma membrane receptors

- The plasma membrane contains protein receptors which are capable of recognising and binding with smaller molecules called ligands, which include:
    - Hormones
    - Neuro-receptors
    - Antigens implicated in allergic reactions
    - Components of the immune system e.g. complement, a group of 20 plasma proteins that when activated destroy foreign substances in the body
    - Lipoproteins
    - Infectious agents such bacteria, viruses and parasites which can stimulate the immune system and inflammatory process
    - Drugs e.g. antibiotics, opiates, chemotherapies
    - Metabolites
- Understanding of protein receptor sites on plasma membranes and the binding of the particular ligand have provided a basis for understanding disease
- Plasma membrane receptors determine which ligands a cell will bind with and how the cell will respond.

Cytoplasmic organelles

These are the functioning units of a cell and the structures contained within it are surrounded by cytoplasm.

Nucleus

- Located in the centre of the cell
- Control centre of the cell, it controls:
    - Cellular division and genetic information
    - Instructions needed to build all the body's proteins, the kind and amount

- Contains nucleoli:
  - There are one or two nucleoli per nucleus, but there may be more
  - Contains DNA that issues genetic instructions for the synthesising of ribosomal RNA (rRNA).

Ribosomes

- Provide sites for protein synthesis
- Attach themselves to the endoplasmic reticulum.

Endoplasmic reticulum

- Circulate proteins and lipids to other organelles
- These provide a source of energy for the functioning of other organelles within the cytoplasm and are used to construct and repair their membranes
- There are two types:
  - Rough endoplasmic reticulum, as ribosomes are attached to it
  - Smooth endoplasmic reticulum:
    - Contains no ribosomes
    - Contains enzymes required to remove toxic substances from the cell
    - Works closely and communicates with the Golgi complex, lysosomes and peroxisomes, that help to breakdown long-chain fatty acids.

Golgi complex

Is involved in the removal of waste products from the cell, directing them to the plasma membrane for excretion.

Lysosomes

- Are the cell's digestive system
- Use enzymes to break down waste products so they do not cause internal damage to the cell
- If lysosomes become damaged they release toxic enzymes into the cell cytoplasm, causing breakdown of the cell from within
- Lysosome abnormality is implicated in cellular injury and death
- Peroxisomes are similar to lysosomes but use oxygen to remove hydrogen ions and produce hydrogen peroxide, if it is allowed to escape it can be destructive to cells.

Mitochondria

- Mitochondria have a specific role in cellular energy metabolism
- Glucose breakdown takes place in 3 stages:

  - Glycolysis
  - Krebs cycle
  - Electron transport chain
- At all stages these processes produce energy in the form of ATP
- There are additional pathways for lipids and amino acids.

Cytoskeleton

- Gives the cell its shape; a network of protein filaments
- Provides movement so the substances within the cell can be moved around
- Microtubes add strength to the cell's structure.

Centrioles

- Centrioles consist of 9 bundles or microtubules, arranged to form a hollow tube
  - They are involved in cell division
  - Cells that do not contain centrioles cannot divide e.g. central nervous system.

TISSUES

Cells of the same structure adhere together to form tissues; to form tissues cells have to exhibit intercellular recognition. There are generally considered to be 4 types of tissue.

Epithelial tissue

Covers most internal and external surfaces of the body.

- Functions
  - Protection
  - Absorption
  - Secretion
  - Excretion
- Some contain microvilli and cilia
- 3 different types
  - Simple epithelium
  - Stratified epithelium
  - Pseudostratified epithelium
- 3 basic cell shapes
  - Squamous are flat and thin

    - Cubiodal are square in appearance
    - Columnar are oblong in appearance
- The types and shapes of cell form the different types of tissues; these are explained in the following way:
    - Simple squamous epithelium allows rapid diffusion to take place through the thin tissue
        - Lines major body cavities and organs e.g. heart, kidney and lungs
        - Oxygen and carbon dioxide exchange takes place through the air sacs of the lungs
        - Nutrients and gases pass through from cells into and out of the capillaries
    - Simple cupoidal epithelium
        - Lines tubes and ducts of glands e.g. salivary glands, pancreas
        - Forms the walls of kidney tubules and covers the surface of the ovaries
    - Simple columnar epithelium cells are fitted closely together and contain goblet cells which produce mucus:
        - Lines the total length of the gastrointestinal tract (GIT) (see chapter 11)
        - Lines all body cavities and contain mucous membranes (see chapter 5)
    - Stratified squamous epithelium is strong, thick and hardy:
        - Usually found at the edge in areas that is subjected to friction and cells are constantly being replaced:
            - Cuboidal or columnar epithelial tissue are found close to the basement membrane and lines places most at risk of every day damage e.g. interior of the mouth, tongue, oesophagus, outer surface of the skin and vagina
        - Contains stratified cuboidal and columnar epithelial tissue which is fairly rare, found only in the ducts of large glands
        - Transitional epithelium
            - Highly specialised stratified squamous epithelium
            - Forms the linings of few organs and structures all of which are found in the urinary system
    - Glandular epithelium consists of cells that make and secrete a variety of products:
        - Exocrine gland epithelium contains ducts and produces sweat, enzymes of the liver and pancreas
        - Endocrine gland epithelium has no ducts and secretes directly into the blood stream, produces and secretes hormones, glands include thyroid, adrenal and pituitary gland (see chapter 13).

Connective tissues

Connective tissue is concerned with connecting parts of the body together. It is the most widely distributed tissue in the body and occurs where epithelial cells cluster to form organs

- Function
  - Binding of various tissues and organs together
  - Supporting organs in their position in the body
  - Serving as storage sites for excess nutrients
- Characterised by an extracellular matrix composed of ground substance, which fills the space between the cells and contains the fibres, which varies in consistency:
  - Collagenous (white) are strong fibres
  - Elastic (yellow) are fibres that are able to stretch and recoil, found in the:
    - Lungs
    - Arteries
    - Trachea
    - Vocal cords
  - Reticular are fibres that form the soft skeleton of soft organs such as the spleen
- The characteristics of connective tissue determine types and functions of organs:
  - Loose connective tissue, there are 4 types:
    - Areolar tissue:
      - Surrounds organs and cushions and protects it such as the heart and kidney
      - Holds internal organs together
      - Provides a reservoir for water and salts
      - Other cells obtain nutrients and release waste into it
    - Adipose tissue or fat
      - Forms the deep layers of the skin known as the subcutaneous layer
      - Insulates and protects the body from extreme heat and cold
      - Acts as an energy store
    - Reticular connective tissue supports lymphocytes in the lymph nodes, spleen and bone marrow
    - Blood transports many life-sustaining substances around the body, and is considered a connective tissue as it is comprised of blood cells surrounded by blood plasma
  - Dense connective tissue
    - Tendons attach skeletal muscles to bone

    - Ligaments connect bones to other bones at joints
- Cartilage is found in a few places in the body:
    - Covers the ends of bones where they form joints
    - Tip of nose
    - Parts of the larynx
    - Trachea
    - Attaches ribs to the sternum
    - Fibrocartilage:
        - Forms discs between the vertebrae of the spinal cord
        - In the external ear
- Bone – is hard and provides:
    - Protection
    - Support
    - Muscle attachment.

Muscle tissues

Composed of myocytes, which are involved in contraction and movement (see chapter 12).

- 3 types
    - Skeletal muscles – attached to bones and involved in movement, they are controlled voluntarily
    - Cardiac muscle – found in the heart and acts as a pump, works involuntarily (some muscles can be both voluntary and involuntary e.g. the respiratory muscles)
    - Smooth muscle – found in the walls of hollow organs, causes movement in the hollow organ
        - GIT – peristalsis
        - Uterus – to contract during labour
        - Urinary bladder – a reservoir for urine
        - Blood vessels – vasoconstriction and dilatation.

Nervous tissue

Highly specialised tissue called neurons, which can receive and initiate electrical impulses and control body processes (see chapter 10).

- Neurons are different from other cells
- Impulses pass from neuron to neuron or from neuron to muscle across synapses or junctions
- Synapses are points of contact between neurons
- They use chemical messengers called neurotransmitters
- If damaged they cannot repair or be replaced.

ALTERED CELLULAR BIOLOGY

Altered cellular biology can be a result of trauma or injury, hypoxia, ageing, cellular death and healing processes. Cells can heal, adapt to injuries, change as a result, or may incur adaptations to the cells that can either be to maintain a normal physiological state or become abnormal and lead to disease or death. Some injuries may be reversible others irreversible.

Cellular injury

Most diseases begin with cell injury and occur if a cell is unable to maintain homeostasis.

Aetiology

Injury can be induced by a wide variety of physiological variables. Most causes can be grouped into the following categories.

Nutritional imbalances

- Cells require nutrients to function properly, if too little or excessive amounts are consumed then cell development and normal functioning can be effected
- Proteins are required for all body processes
- Glucose:
  - In excess over long periods of time can lead to obesity and type 2 diabetes, atherosclerosis
  - Deficiencies can lead to protein energy malnutrition
- Lipid deficiencies can lead to an excess of ketone bodies, loss of water, dehydration and thirst. If severe, can cause a metabolic acidosis and death
- Vitamin and minerals are important in maintaining normal cell functions and deficiencies can lead to disease and disorders.

Hypoxia

- Is a lack of sufficient oxygen for cells and is the most common cause of cellular injury
- Impinges on aerobic respiration and is an important and common cause of cell injury and death
- Causes of hypoxia
  - Inadequate oxygenation of the blood:
    - Renal failure
    - Hypothermia

        - Tight compression bandages/casts
        - Compartment syndrome
        - Shock, heart failure
        - Respiratory failure
        - Deep vein thrombosis
    - Loss of oxygen-carrying capacity of the blood:
        - Carbon monoxide and cyanide poisoning
        - Anaemia
    - Decrease in oxygen in the air.

Physical processes

- Trauma
- Asphyxia – a failure of cells to receive or use oxygen
- Extremes of temperature:
    - Hypothermia is very dangerous to cells
        - If prolonged can lead to irreversible damage
        - Therapeutic hypothermia is used in surgery and neurological injury
    - Hyperthermia has 3 types:
        - Heat cramps usually the result of vigorous exercise
        - Heat exhaustion progression of heat cramp, loss of salt and water leads to hypovolaemia and collapse, a common injury
        - Heat stroke is a life-threatening condition, body temperature rises as a result of thermoregulatory failure (hypothalamus), widespread vasodilation, decrease in circulating volume
    - Hyperpyrexia (sepsis) a very high temperature due to infection in the blood stream, can be as high as 41°C
- Radiation from the environment and other sources e.g. radiotherapy
- Noise has the potential to inflict harm to cells:
    - One loud noise can lead to inner ear damage
    - Damage can be an accumulation of exposure to noise over time e.g. in the workplace
    - Age deteriorates cells of the ear leading to hear impairment
- Drowning – a reduced oxygen delivery to tissues
- Electric shock
- Sudden changes in atmospheric pressure transmitted by air or water:
    - Blast injuries such as an explosion or water blast

- High altitudes as at high altitudes there is a reduction in available oxygen
- Decompression sickness due to deep sea diving.

Chemicals and drugs

- Virtually any chemical agent may cause injury:
  - Glucose or salt in extreme concentration
  - Oxygen in sufficiently high concentrations is also toxic
  - Pollutants such as insecticides
  - Asbestos
  - Therapeutic drugs, heroin, cocaine, methamphetamine
  - Lead, mercury
  - Gases such as:
    - Carbon monoxide
    - Ethanol.

Microbiologic agents

- Micro-organisms survive and reproduce in the human body, where they can injure cells and tissues
- Range from:
  - Sub-microscopic viruses
  - Bacteria
  - Fungi
  - Parasites such as tape worms.

Immunologic reactions

- Cellular membranes are injured by components of the immune and inflammatory response
- Anaphylactic reactions
- Autoimmune diseases and self-antigens.

Genetic defects

- Genetic factors can alter the plasma membrane structure, shape, receptors, or transport mechanisms:
  - May be conspicuous as in Down syndrome
  - May be subtle such as a single amino acid substitution in the haemoglobin S of sickle cell anaemia.

Pathology

The pathology of cellular damage can involve a number of processes all of which are not mutually exclusive, for example one can lead to the other or vice versa. These involve the stress response, hypoxia, the immune system and changes in atmospheric pressure.

Tissue injury: the role of stress

- Increased sympathetic nervous system arousal
  - Adrenaline/noradrenaline and baroreceptor activation bring up blood pressure
  - Cortisol release in long term stress stimulates the breakdown of fats and proteins as a source of energy
  - Aldosterone release stimulates reabsorption of salt and water to increase blood pressure
  - Angiotensin II stimulates the release of anti-diuretic hormone and noradrenaline
  - Cytokines IL-1 stimulates inflammation and the immune response
- Continued exposure leads to:
  - Raised blood pressure
  - Reduced cardiac function
  - Reduced wound healing
  - Reduced immune system response to infection.

Hypoxia

Hypoxic injury is not mutually exclusive, as it can lead to the release of inflammatory mediators causing interstitial swelling and oedema further cutting off blood supply (Edwards, 2003a). Hypoxia results in:

- Anaerobic metabolism/lactic acid production (Edwards, 2003a)
  - As oxygen levels fall in the cell, there is a rapid shift from aerobic to anaerobic metabolism
  - Anaerobic glycolysis leads to the accumulation of lactic acid, and a reduction in ATP for cellular work
  - Anaerobic metabolism in the electron transport chain leads to cellular membrane disruption and eventually the formation of oxygen free radicals and nitric oxide (NO):
    - Generally results from an absence of oxygen in the electron transport chain (ETC)
    - When oxygen is diminished in the ETC (the final stage of glucose breakdown), electrons build up as carriers, and are unable to pass on their electrons to the next
    - In excess they can become potent ions and form nitric oxide (NO), a potent vasodilator

    - NO can accumulate in large amounts:
      - Preventing DNA repair as repair enzymes bind to NO
      - Preventing release of iron stores – inhibition of ATP synthesis in the ETC
      - Inhibition of glycolysis
      - The mitochondria can lose membrane potential and halt ATP production altogether
- Cellular membrane disruption
  - This leads to electrolyte disturbances, as a result of the reduction in ATP from anaerobic metabolism
  - Without sufficient supplies of ATP the plasma membrane of the cell can no longer maintain normal ionic gradients across the cell membranes
  - In the absence of ATP the sodium potassium pump can no longer function
  - This changes the ionic concentration of potassium and sodium
  - Potassium leaks into the extracellular space and sodium followed by water will move into the cell
  - Cellular oedema and an increased intracellular osmotic pressure occurs
  - The cell may eventually burst
  - This may effect the conduction of electrical impulses to the skin and muscles
    - These impulses require the movement of sodium and potassium ions in and out of the cell to produce an action potential
  - These changes are reversible if oxygen is restored, allowing muscle, blood vessel cells to contract normally
- The role of calcium
  - The calcium pump is dysfunctional because of a lack of ATP, calcium accumulates in the cell
  - The increase in calcium in the mitochondria causes structural derangement of the organelles
  - Calcium may be the hallmark of irreversible cellular injury and eventually cell death
- The role of lysosomes
  - An important cell structure containing enzymes which break down cell waste
  - The lysosome membrane is quite stable, but becomes fragile when the cell is injured or deprived of oxygen
  - Lysosomal membrane instability is made worse by the lack of ATP and the cell starts to use its own structural phospholipids as a nutrient source

- Eventually the lysosome membrane becomes more permeable and may rupture
- This allows the release of lysosome enzymes resulting in self-digestion of the cell
- The use of steroids is thought to help stabilise the lysosome membrane and prevent lysosomal-enzyme damage to the cell.

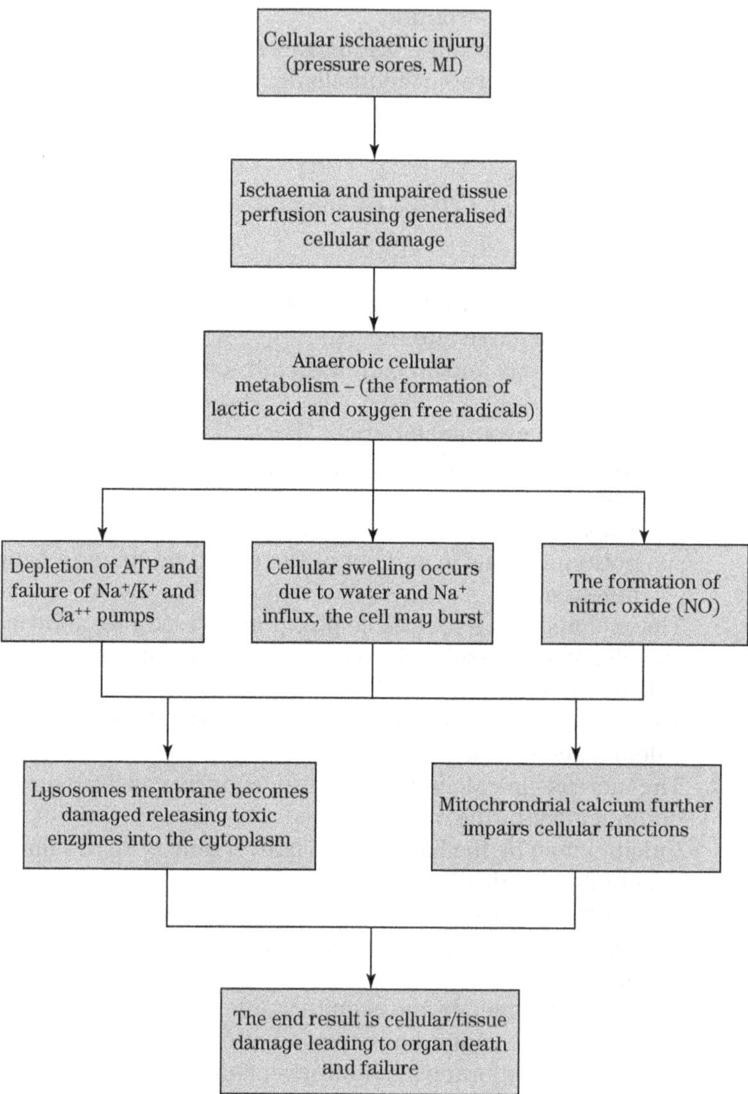

Figure 2.2 Cellular hypoxia

Physical agents, chemicals, immunological response and microbes

Stimulation of the inflammatory immune response (IIR) leads to swelling and oedema, which can, if severe, lead to reduced blood supply to the area and hypoxia (Edwards, 2003b).

- The IR is stimulated in many conditions e.g. leg ulcers, surgical procedures, trauma
- The inflammatory response (IR) ends with repair to damaged cells and tissues
- Activation of the IR is part of the innate immune system and represents a major physiological event in the body
- Following the damage, the damaged endothelium releases mediators
- The inflammatory response includes the following:
  - The most important mediators are
  - Histamine
  - Kinins
  - Prostaglandins
  - Complement
  - Cytokines
  - The release of these mediators is intended to:
  - Protect the body from invading micro-organisms
  - Limit the extent of blood loss and injury
- Promote rapid healing of involved tissues
- The mediators act as a signalling system (chemotaxis) to attract nutrients, fluids, clotting factors and neutrophils and macrophages to the damaged site
- In addition, the mediators cause a localised increase in:
  - Capillary permeability
  - Vasodilation to increase blood supply
  - The release of interleukin 1 (IL-1) from macrophages, which causes a small rise in temperature
- Endothelial damage (Edwards, 2002)
  - Is a major contributor to the activation of the IIR
  - It is not just an inert barrier between the flowing blood and the substructure of the blood vessels and tissue
  - But an active metabolic organ responsible for anticoagulation and always accompanies injury
  - Stimulation of the clotting cascade prevents excessive blood loss and isolates the injured site
- Poisons may alter membrane permeability or the integrity of an enzyme – putting the whole organism at risk
- Infectious agents have potential to cause damage to cells if they can:

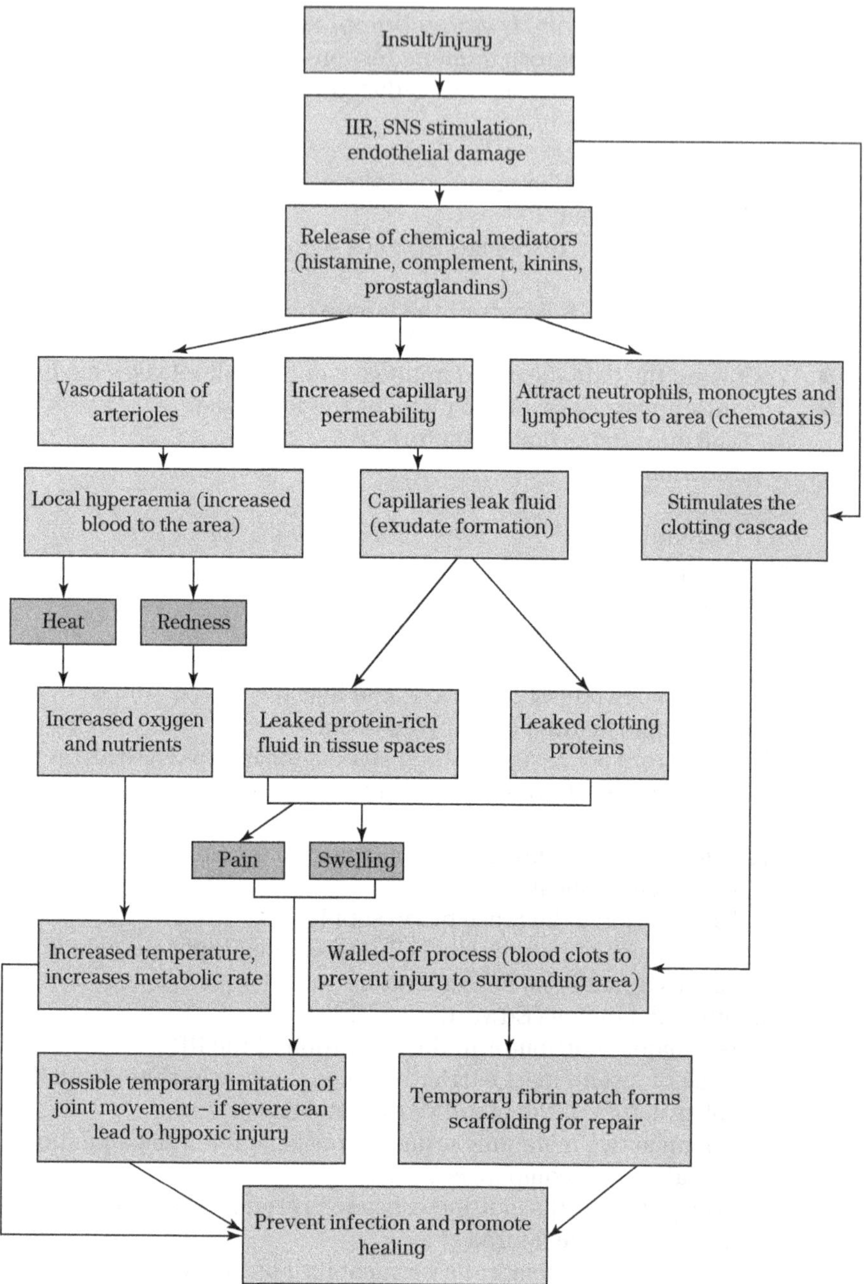

Figure 2.3 The inflammatory response

- Invade and destroy cells e.g. viruses
- Produce toxins that damage cells
- Produce damaging hypersensitivity reactions.

(See Figure 2.3.)

Practice point

There is a link between hypoxic cell damage the inflammatory immune response, oedema and the conditions observed in clinical practice e.g. pressure ulcer, myocardial infarction and wounds.

Sudden changes in atmospheric pressure

- Any sudden changes in atmospheric pressure can damage cells
- Usually transmitted by air or water:
  - Blast injury:
    - A sudden blast of air increasing pressure in the thorax, followed by a sudden decrease of air reducing pressure in the thorax
    - The sudden change may collapse the thorax, rupture internal solid organs, and lead to widespread haemorrhage
  - A decrease in atmospheric pressure
    - This occurs at high altitudes above 15,000 feet
    - The higher the altitude there is a decrease in available oxygen
    - This can lead to hypoxic injury and high altitude pulmonary oedema (McCance and Huether, 2010)
  - An increase in atmospheric pressure
    - This is experienced during deep sea diving, by returning to the surface too quickly and not allowing time for the increase in atmospheric pressure to reduce slowly, decompression sickness
    - The gases (nitrogen and oxygen) in the blood bubble out of the circulation forming air emboli
    - Oxygen is re-dissolved back into the blood quickly, the nitrogen bubbles persist and block blood vessels
    - This is experienced during deep sea diving, by returning to the surface too quickly and not allowing time for the increase in atmospheric pressure to reduce slowly leading to decompression sickness.

Clinical features

Cells can adapt to their environment to protect themselves from injury, but it is not always possible for cells to adapt quickly enough in some acute conditions, and injury can produce cellular adaptations that can be fundamental to many disease states, especially chronic illness/disease.

Atrophy

- Cells decrease in size
- If atrophy occurs in sufficient numbers the organ shrinks
- Cell function is diminished
- Can affect any organ
- Most common in skeletal muscle, ear and brain, myocytes of the heart, CNS neurones, secondary sex organs
- Causes include
  - Decrease in workload
  - Use
  - Blood supply
  - Nutrition
  - Hormonal secretion and nervous stimulation
- There is a decrease in the size/number of endoplastic reticulum, mitochondria, myofibrils.

(See Figure 2.4.)

Hypertrophy

- There is no increase in the number of cells
- Individual cells increase in size and the organ will increase in size

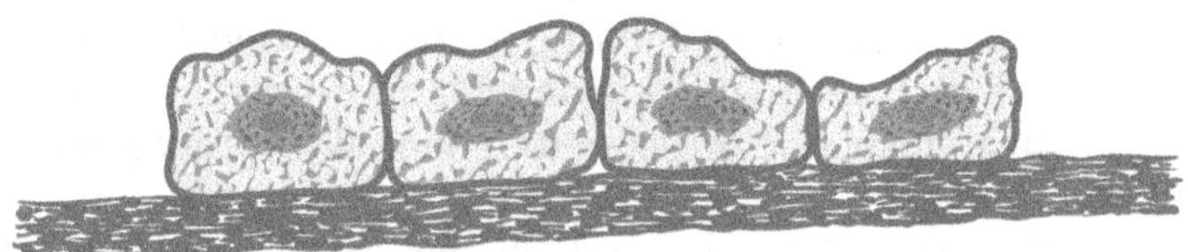

Figure. 2.4 Atrophy
(McCance and Huether, 2010)

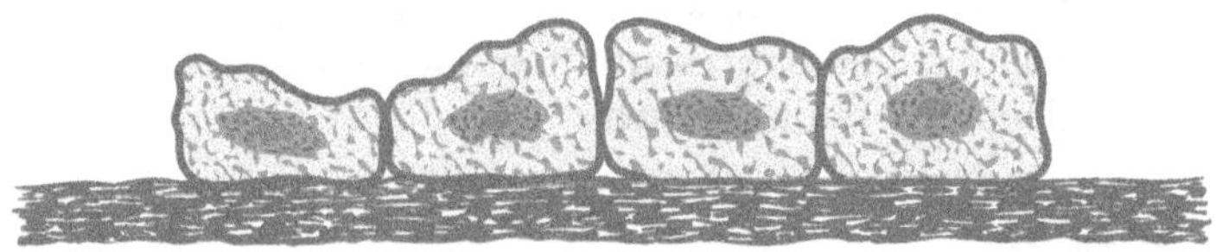

Figure 2.5 Hypertrophy
(McCance and Huether, 2010)

- After the removal of one kidney, the other kidney size increases, adapting to the extra workload by increasing in size
- Increase in functional work demand on the tissue
- Seen in cells that can not easily divide e.g. skeletal and cardiac muscle.

Hypertrophy can be compensatory initially before de-compensation (failure) occurs.

(See Figure 2.5.)

Hyperplasia

- Is an increase in the number of cells due to an increase in cell division – regeneration of the skin
- Compensatory hyperplasia e.g. regeneration of the liver, after removal of up to 70%, regeneration can occur in 2 weeks
- Callus or thickening of the skin is an example of hyperplasia
- Hormonal hyperplasia – oestrogen dependent organs
- Pathological hyperplasia – often oestrogen dependent, over secretion of oestrogen leads to endometrial hyperplasia.

(See Figure 2.6.)

Hypertrophy and hyperplasia

- These can often occur together
- Increased cell mass through hypertrophy of hyperplasia can be physiological:
  - Thyroid increases in size and activity in pregnancy due to thyroid-stimulating hormone (TSH) (hyperplasia)
  - Skeletal muscle fibres increase in size (hypertrophy) in response to exercise
  - May occur in response to disease states:
    - Low serum calcium means the parathyroids increase in size
    - Narrow aortic valve leads to enlargement of muscle cells in the left ventricle

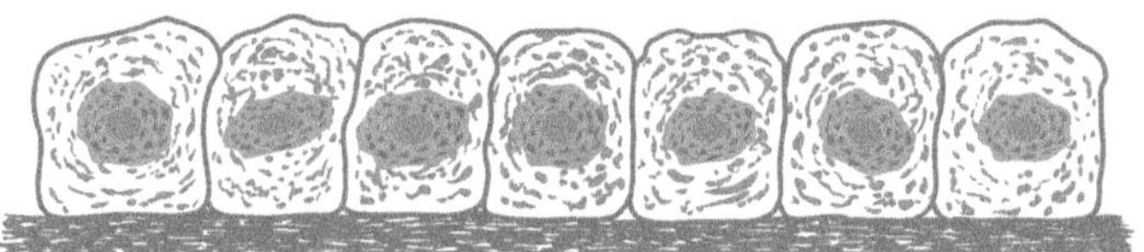

Figure 2.6 Hyperplasia

(McCance and Huether, 2010)

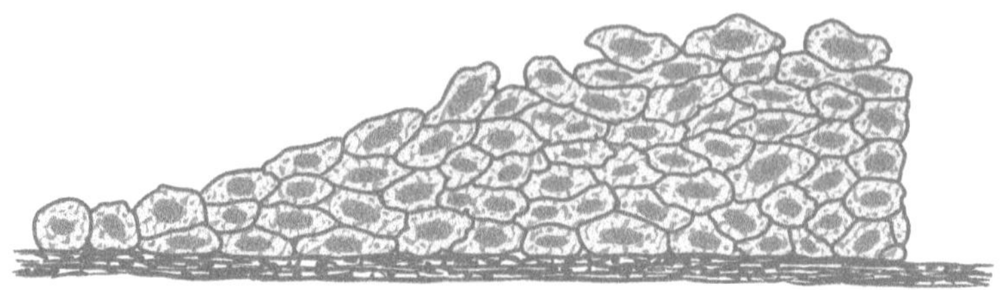

Figure 2.7 Dysplasia
(McCance and Huether, 2010)

- Obstruction of colon leads to increased size of smooth muscle cells proximal to the obstruction
- Following removal of stimulus to hyperplasia or hypertrophy the tissue reverts to normal.

Dysplasia

- Abnormal changes in size, shape and organisation of mature cells
- Related to hyperplasia and may be called atypical hyperplasia
- Frequently seen in the epithelial cells of the cervix and respiratory tract
- May be associated with neoplastic growths, which is abnormal tissue that grows by cellular division that occurs more rapidly than normal, and continues to grow after the stimulus that initiated the new growth cease, and can become cancerous.

(See Figure 2.7.)

Metaplasia

- The reversible replacement of one cell type by another, sometimes less differentiated cell type
- Most commonly occurs in epithelial tissues

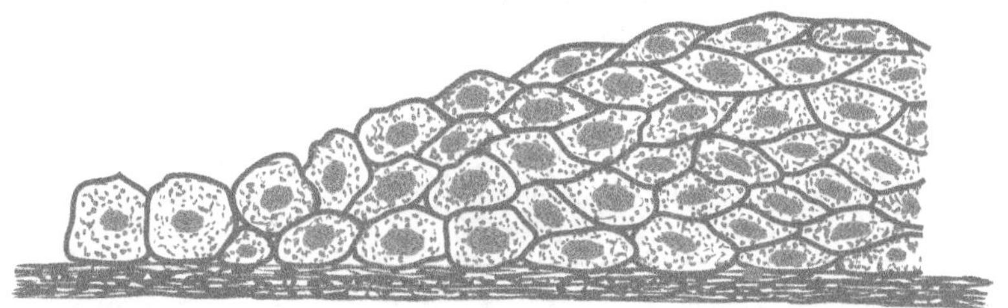

Figure 2.8 Metaplasia
(McCance and Huether, 2010)

- Ciliated columnar epithelial cells of the respiratory tract may become replaced by stratified squamous epithelial cells in the bronchial lining e.g. from smoking.
- Can be reversed if the stimulus is removed (such as stopping smoking).

(See Figure 2.8.)

Investigations

A number of investigations can be undertaken (Ahmed *et al*, 2007), but these are not always conclusive:

- Past medical history
- Clinical examination
- Radiographic examination:
  - MRI scan
  - Ventilation perfusion scan
  - X-ray
  - Computer tomography scan (CT scan)
  - Cardiac angiography
- Examination using sound waves:
  - Echocardiography
  - Doppler
- Pathological laboratory investigations:
  - Biochemistry – investigate the biochemical changes that occur in disease
  - Haematology – studies into the disorders of blood cells
  - Histopathology – the identification of changes in body tissues to diagnose disease
  - Immunology – studying the body's immune response in health and disease
  - Microbiology – concerned with the detection and identification of micro-organisms
  - Clinical genetics – focuses on the identification of genetic abnormalities.

Treatment

- Following hypoxic cell injury, stimulation of the inflammatory response
  - Administer oxygen to ensure oxygen supply and demand are maintained to prevent imbalance
  - Prevention of a low circulating volume and administration of fluids, blood (Edwards, 2002)

- The observations of shock (Edwards, 2001)
- Relieve pain – analgesia
- Aid healing and prevent further tissue damage
- Treatment of the conditions generally focus on haemodynamic and localised abnormalities which determines interventions
- Prevention of cellular death necrosis and apoptosis
    - Necrosis is the result of sudden or severe injury – indicates irreversible cell injury, 5 main types indicating the mechanism or cause of cellular injury
        - Coagulative necrosis – kidneys, heart, adrenal glands due to hypoxia or severe ischaemia from chemical injury
        - Liquefactive necrosis – ischaemic injury to neurones, bacterial infection
        - Caseous necrosis – is a combination of coagulative and liquefactive necrosis, frequently results from tuberculosis
        - Fat necrosis – occurs in the breast, pancreas and other abdominal structures
        - Gangrenous necrosis – refers to death of tissue from severe hypoxic injury, with cellular necrosis and bacterial infection
    - Apoptosis is programmed cell death; cells need to die, so that new cells can be renewed, ageing is thought to be a form of apoptosis.

CONCLUSION

Cellular, chemical involvement and activation of neuro-hormones are the true culprits in death and disability associated with tissue injury. Research is now looking at the release of mediators following cell and tissue injury. Following cell damage the body initiates physiological processes, necessary for healing and survival. These processes demonstrate the interconnections between cellular elements, their secretion, the immune system and the nervous system. These processes need to be recognised and understood as if ignored they can lead to irreversible cell and tissue death and possible loss of organ function or limb.

SELF-ASSESSMENT QUESTIONS

1. Provide an outline of the functions of the cell, plasma membrane and cellular components.
2. Describe the 4 different types of tissue.

3. Identify the causes of cellular and tissue injury.
4. Explain how cells adapt to injury and the effects these can have.
5. Describe the general investigations and treatments commonly used for cellular and tissue injury.

REFERENCES

Ahmed, N., Dawson, M., Smith, C. and Wood, E. (2007) *Biology of Disease*, Abingdon: Taylor & Francis Group.

Edwards, S. (2001) Shock: types, classifications and explorations of their physiological effects, *Emergency Nurse*, 9(2), 29–38.

Edwards, S. (2002) Physiological insult/injury: pathophysiology and consequences, *British Journal of Nursing*, 11(4), 263–274.

Edwards, S. (2003a) Cellular pathophysiology, Part 2: responses following hypoxia, *Professional Nurse*, 18(11), 636–639.

Edwards, S. (2003b) Cellular pathophysiology, Part 1: changes following tissue injury, *Professional Nurse*, 18(10), 562–565.

McCance, K.L. and Huether, S.E. (2010) *Pathophysiology: The Biologic Basis for Disease in Adults and Children*, 6th edn, Missouri: Mosby Elsevier.

Marieb, E. (2012) *Essentials of Human Anatomy and Physiology*, 9th edn, San Francisco, CA: Benjamin Cummings.

Watson, R. (2005) Cell structure and function, growth and development, in S.E. Montague, R. Watson and R.A. Herbert (eds) *Physiology for Nursing Practice*, 3rd edn, Edinburgh: Elsevier.

3 Genes and environment

Ann Richards

Human disease used to be thought to be either genetically determined, almost entirely environmentally determined or the result of both nature and nurture in combination. Nowadays it is realised that even diseases such as microbial infections that were thought to be entirely due to the environment are partly determined by our genetic makeup and immunological response. Take the common cold as an example – not everyone in a household may catch the cold and some will have more severe and long lasting symptoms than others. Thus, we are coming to believe that nature, i.e. genetics, has a major role to play in most diseases.

GENETIC DISEASES

Chromosomal abnormalities are responsible for approximately half of miscarriages in the first three months of pregnancy and many more foetuses are likely to be lost because of gene mutations.

Humans have a complement of 46 chromosomes made up of 23 pairs. This is known as the human karyotype. The chromosomes carry all our genetic material and 22 of these pairs are austosomal, the remaining pair being sex chromosomes (XX for female and XY for male). The normal male karyotype is shown in Figure 3.1.

Throughout childhood disorders that have a genetic origin are common but many diseases that occur later in life are multifactorial and result from polygenic inheritance together with environmental impact e.g. hypertension, type 2 diabetes.

- Hereditary disorders are derived from one's parents and are familial
- Congenital means present at birth and so includes disorders that are not familial e.g. foetal alcohol syndrome
- Not all genetic diseases are congenital as they may present in later life e.g. Huntingdon's disease

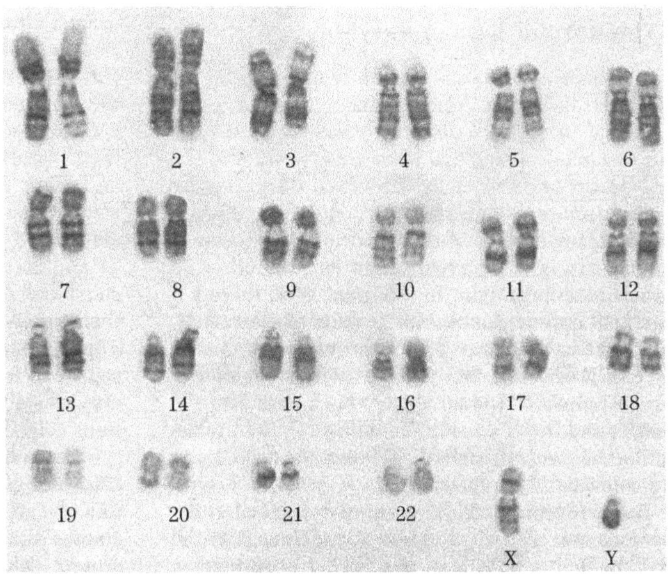

Figure 3.1 The normal human karyotype

- Many of the commonest diseases are multifactorial and are a complex mix of multiple gene transmission combined with environmental factors.

Single gene defects

These are due to a defect in a single gene. As a child receives 1 gene from each parent it depends whether the gene in question is dominant or recessive.

Autosomal dominant diseases

- If it is a dominant gene it means that it will always be expressed and the child will have the disease even though the gene from 1 parent is normal
- These diseases are autosomal dominant and include familial hypercholesterolaemia, Huntingdon's disease and polycystic kidney disease
- When an affected person marries an unaffected person then the child from this union has a 1 in 2 chance of having the disease
- Sometimes these diseases arise because of a new mutation i.e. the person does not have a parent with the disease.

Autosomal dominant transmission is shown in Figure 3.2.

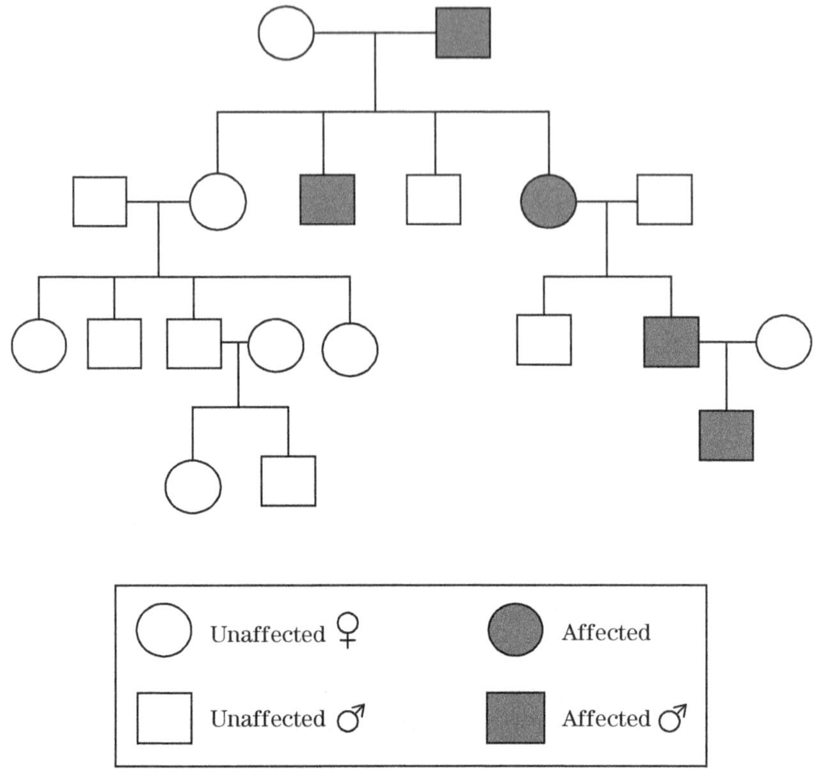

Figure 3.2 Autosomal dominant transmission

Autosomal recessive diseases

- If the gene carrying the disorder is recessive, this means that if the child has a normal copy of the gene from the other parent it will not have the disease but will still carry the other affected gene and could pass it on when it reproduces
- To actually have the disease the child would need 2 copies of the defective gene i.e. 1 from each parent
- These diseases may skip generations (remaining hidden) and appear again
- The parents do not usually have the disease but brothers and sisters may. Each child has a 1 in 4 chance of being affected
- These disorders include sickle cell anaemia, cystic fibrosis and galactosaemia.

Autosomal recessive transmission is shown in Figure 3.3.

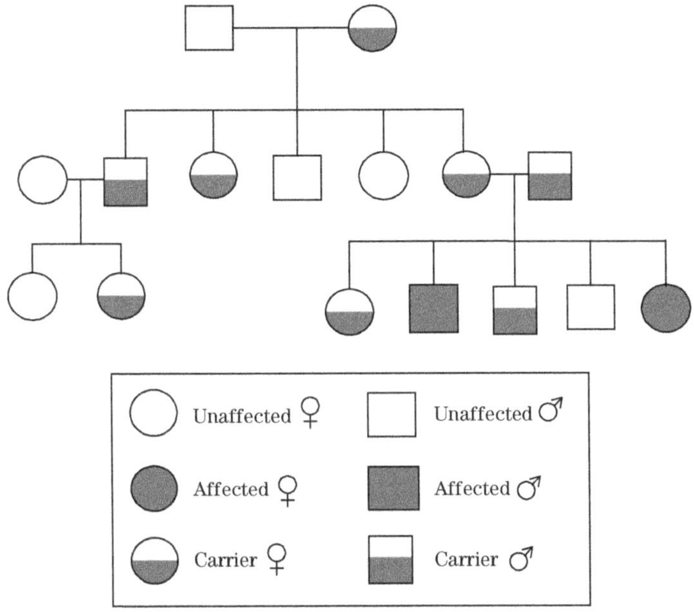

Figure 3.3 Autosomal recessive transmission

X-linked diseases

- Other diseases are carried on the X-chromosome and are known as X-linked
- A woman has 2 X chromosomes and a man has 1 X and 1 Y chromosome i.e. the Y chromosome confers masculinity
- If a disease is carried on the X chromosome it can be recessive but will still present in a male child if he has that X chromosome as he only has this one X chromosome
- If the child is female and gets one X chromosome carrying the gene and 1 normal X chromosome, the disease will not be present as the gene is recessive. The female child in this case however, would be a carrier and could pass the bad X chromosome on to her children
- Examples of such diseases are haemophilia, colour blindness and Duchenne muscular dystrophy.

The transmission of haemophilia is shown in chapter 7.

Multifactorial inheritance

- Many of our physiological characteristics are transmitted this way. Several genes are involved in producing the characteristic i.e. it is polygenic. Examples are hair colour, weight, height and blood pressure

- If a trait is multifactorial it results from the additive effect of 2 or more genes together with environmental influences. Thus how tall we are does not just depend on the genes we receive but also the diet we receive when young. High blood pressure may be partly the result of genes from our parents but smoking, exercise and diet also play a large part in its development
- Diseases transmitted this way include type 2 diabetes mellitus, gout, coronary heart disease, schizophrenia and bipolar disorder.

Chromosomal abnormalities

There are more chromosomal abnormalities than is normally believed and about 1 in 200 newborn babies have some form of chromosomal abnormality.

Some abnormalities are numerical and may be due to the presence of an extra chromosome. An example here is Down syndrome – trisomy 21 – this means that there are 3 copies of chromosome 21 where normally there are only 2. The person has a total of 47 chromosomes, not 46 as is normal.

- There may be the absence of a chromosome, excess chromosomes or abnormal rearrangements of chromosomes
- Loss of a chromosome is usually more severe than gain
- There may be an extra chromosome e.g. trisomy 21 or just part of a chromosome
- An imbalance of sex chromosomes is tolerated more than an imbalance of autosomes and may be detected at puberty or when infertility becomes a problem
- Most chromosomal abnormalities are new and the parents have a normal number of chromosomes. The problem arises in the cell division process (meiosis) and defects are commoner in older parents.

Trisomy 21 (Down syndrome)

This is the commonest chromosomal disorder and maternal age has a strong impact on its occurrence.

In women under 20 years the rate is about 1 in 1550 pregnancies. In women over 45 years it is about 1 in 25. In about 95% of cases the extra chromosome is maternal and not from the father. This results from a meiotic defect in the ovum.

Prenatal screening is now used to identify Down syndrome allowing the pregnancy to be terminated if this is what the mother decides.

Characteristics of Down syndrome include:

- A flat facial profile and protruding tongue
- Single palmar crease
- Cardiac malformations (in about 40% of cases)
- Learning difficulties
- Increased risk of acute leukaemia and susceptibility to infections.

Sex chromosomes

Many abnormal karyotypes involving the sex chromosomes are compatible with life.

- An extra Y chromosome in a man (XYY) may not even be detected although it may lead to antisocial behaviour
- An extra X chromosome (XXY) in a man is Kleinfelter syndrome and the man is infertile. Intelligence may be near normal
- The presence of just 1 X chromosome (XO) in a woman is Turner syndrome and growth is retarded. There is a short, webbed neck with a low hairline at the back of the head. The chest is broad and there may be other congenital malformations such as horseshoe kidney. The girl is infertile and usually does not menstruate.

ENVIRONMENTAL DISEASES

The environment has a part to play in all disease that is not completely genetic in origin. It has already been pointed out that the environment has an impact on some inherited diseases and that much disease results as a combination of the genes we are given and the environment in which we live.

The following are some important environmental influences that play a large part in some disease processes.

Environmental pollution

This could be any contaminant so it may be cholera bacteria in drinking water for example or may be air pollution due to heavy industry.

Air pollution

Since the industrial revolution this has been a problem. Burning coal results in the release of toxic chemicals into the air. Smog is the accumulation of particles in the atmosphere and is now rare in England as clean air policies have taken over.

- Air pollutants can affect a variety of body systems but mostly have an impact on the respiratory system. Many pollutants lead to chronic obstructive pulmonary disease. Examples include tobacco smoke, coal dust, asbestos and silicone
- Coal workers pneumoconiosis due to the inhalation of coal dust in the mines has resulted in much chronic bronchitis and emphysema in this country
- Asbestosis is a disease linked to working with asbestos (now illegal)
- Asbestos is not only linked to inflammation and fibrosis of lung tissue but is also linked to bronchial carcinoma and mesothelioma.

Chemical agents

Exposure to such chemicals includes drugs and medicines taken therapeutically – they may produce adverse drug reactions

This category also includes poisons, alcohol and overdoses of medication.

- There are many dangerous chemicals in the home for example cleaning fluids and bleach
- The metabolism of drugs occurs at differing rates according to the genetic makeup of an individual and the efficiency of the enzymes involved
- Many drugs are dangerous when taken above the recommended daily dose – an example here is paracetamol which is very safe at therapeutic doses but can cause acute liver failure if the dose is increased as in cases of paracetamol overdose.

Physical agents

Included in this category are ionising radiation, electrical injury, mechanical trauma and thermal injury such as burns.

NUTRITIONAL DISEASES

Our diet not only needs to provide enough energy for our daily activities but also amino acids and essential fatty acids needed as building blocks for protein production in order that growth and cellular replacement can occur. Micronutrients such as vitamins and minerals are needed in very small amounts for body functioning for example in enzyme systems. Calcium and phosphorous are needed for bone formation.

- In primary malnutrition, 1 or more of these vital components of our diet is lacking. Even in Britain today this is possible, partly due to lack of education or extreme poverty. It is also possible in eating disorders such as anorexia nervosa

- In secondary malnutrition, the diet is not lacking but there is malabsorption of one or more of these nutrients
- Obesity is also a nutritional disease and is becoming increasingly common in the developed world as calories consumed do not fall but exercise does. Obesity is linked to many other disorders such as coronary heart disease, type 2 diabetes and some cancers.

AGEING AND DISEASE

- The ageing process is irreversible but the effects of ageing vary widely from person to person and are not totally dependent on chronological age. Different organs may show signs of ageing in various orders and at different times and some of these changes will be determined by our genetic makeup
- With more understanding of healthy living and increased medical care, the average lifespan is increasing. This means that the elderly form a greater proportion of the population and of those needing our care
- On average, women live longer than men
- Most diseases are commoner in old age and some tissues such as the brain and the myocardium cannot regenerate
- The immune system weakens meaning that infections are more difficult to eliminate. The heart is less strong and so heart failure is more likely to occur
- Most cancers have an increased incidence in the elderly as there may be a build up of mutations within the nuclear DNA. Most cancers are due to an accumulation of factors and as we get older we have been exposed to more of these factors. By the age of about 85 years approximately 30% of adults will have developed cancer. This is not just the case in humans but is also common in other animals as they age too
- There are hormonal changes with ageing such as the menopause in women and a gradual decrease in testosterone by men
- After the menopause in women, osteoporosis becomes commoner. The bone mass is decreased and calcium is lost. This leads to an increase in fractures (chapter 12)
- Ageing of the skin is accelerated by exposure to sunlight and the weather. The skin becomes dry and appears wrinkled as the collagen fibres are no longer flexible
- Cellular proliferation slows down and this leads to the skin becoming thinner. Sensory reception is decreased and so injury may not be so easily felt

- Vulnerability to disease is increased by the ageing process. This is true for some diseases more than others. Common examples are type 2 diabetes, osteoarthritis, cataracts, stroke and Alzheimer's disease.

CONCLUSION

This chapter has taken a brief look at the effect of our genes and the environment on disease processes. It must be considered only as an introduction to a very complex subject area but should aid your understanding of how both nature and nurture play a part in life processes. The chapter ends with a brief look at the effects of ageing on the body and our health.

SELF-ASSESSMENT QUESTIONS

1. Briefly describe the impact of genes and environment of disease.
2. What does 'multifactorial' mean when describing the causation of disease?
3. Name a disorder that is carried on the X chromosome.
4. If a disease is 'autosomal recessive' what does this mean in terms of its heritability?
5. Describe two lung diseases that are caused by the environment a person lives/works in.
6. Explain why most diseases are commoner as we get older.

FURTHER READING

Gould B.E. and Dyer R. (2010) *Pathophysiology for the Health Professions,* 4th edn, Philadelphia: Saunders, Elsevier.

Tobias E.S., Connor M. and Ferguson Smith M. (2011) *Essential Medical Genetics,* 6th edn, Oxford: Wiley-Blackwell.

4 The environment of the cell

Sharon Edwards

HEALTHY FLUID AND ELECTROLYTE BALANCE

The body consists of two major fluid compartments: extracellular fluid (ECF) and intracellular fluid (ICF). The ECF compartment is sub-divided into the plasma and the interstitial fluid (ISF) compartments (Doherty and Buggy, 2012). The compartments contain certain electrolytes and non-electrolytes. A combination of these and other factors maintain a constant equilibrium between body fluid compartments.

Body fluids

The main component of all body fluids is water.

- Fluid intake – is around 2–2.5 litres (L) of water per day obtained in drinking and from food
- Fluid output – mainly lost through the kidneys, faeces, skin and respiratory tract.

Body water content

- 60% of body weight – approximately 42 L in a 70 kg man
- 50% for women, less water due to increase in body fat
- 73% for infants
- 45% is a typical value for the elderly.

Fluid compartments of the body

- Water in the body is contained within 2 main fluid compartments:
  - Two thirds are intracellular fluid (ICF) – contained within cells (approx. 28 L, or around 40% of body weight)
  - Extracellular fluid (ECF) volume – is fluid outside of the cells (approx. 14 L, or around 20% of body weight), and further divided into:

    - Interstitial fluid (ISF) – the space between the ICF and ECF (11 L, 80% of ECF)
    - Plasma volume (3 L, 20% of ECF)
- A small amount is contained as transcellular fluid, which is anatomically separate and not available for water and solute exchange (Kaye and Riopelle, 2009), but during disease and illness transcellular fluid is made at the expense of ECF volume. This includes:
    - Synovial fluid between joints
    - Gastrointestinal secretion
    - Cerebral spinal fluid (CSF)
    - Intraocular fluid – aqueous fluid in the eye.

Movement of fluids among compartments

Several factors contribute to and maintain the differences in solute composition between the ECF and ICF. In order to pass between the ECF and ICF, a solute must cross the plasma membrane; it does so in a number of ways:

- Diffusion is the passive movement of solutes from an area high concentration to an area of low concentration e.g. the exchange of oxygen and carbon dioxide. It depends on:
    - Membrane permeability
    - The solutes' electrical charge
    - The pressure gradient around the membrane
- Active transport – the movement of solutes against a diffusion gradient, requires ATP e.g. the sodium potassium pump in the plasma membrane of cells
- Facilitated diffusion – the movement of solutes using a medium e.g. insulin is needed to facilitate glucose into cells
- Osmosis – the movement of water towards a high solute concentration e.g. if ECF sodium is high, water will move towards the high concentration to dilute it
- Filtration – the movement of water and solutes from a high pressure to a low pressure e.g. glomerular filtration rate (GFR) requires a high pressure in the renal artery for fluid to move into the renal tubules
- Capillary dynamics – the blood in the capillaries is under pressure, and fluid leaks out of the capillaries into the interstitial space to allow nutrients to enter the cell. Counteracting forces determine the fluid moving from the plasma to the interstitial space and vice versa, two forces govern the movement of fluid across the wall of a capillary (Figure 4.1):
    - The hydrostatic pressure (HP) gradient is the difference between the HP of fluid inside the capillary and the HP of fluid outside the capillary, determined in the capillary by the blood pressure:

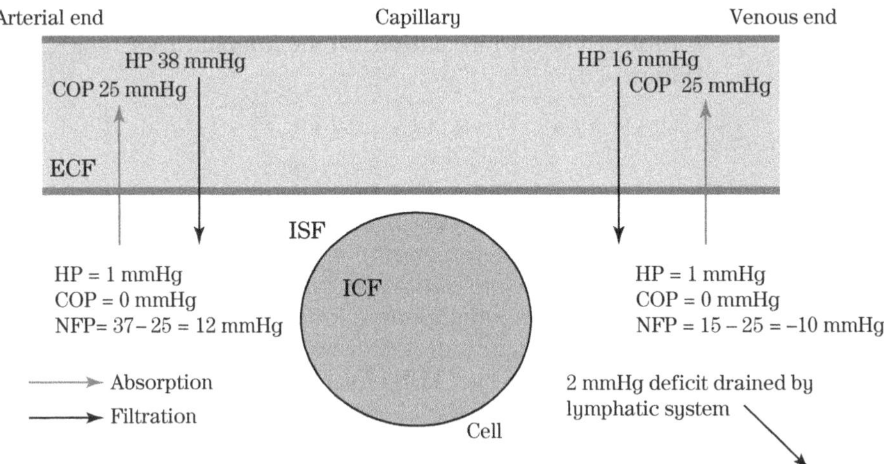

Figure 4.1 Normal capillary dynamics

  - When HP is higher water tends to move from the side with the higher HP to the lower, driving water out of the capillaries
  - The HP in the capillary varies, because the pressure of blood declines continually as blood flows from the arteriolar end of the capillary to the venous end
  - There is no variation in HP outside the capillary
- Osmotic pressure (OP) gradient is the difference between the OP of fluid inside the capillary and the OP of fluid outside the capillary
  - When an OP gradient exists, water tends to flow from the side where the osmotic pressure is higher
  - This is determined by the protein concentration between the plasma and the ISF because it creates a difference in osmotic pressure between the inside and outside of capillaries
  - The osmotic pressure exerted by proteins is directed inward and drives water into the capillaries
- Net filtration pressure (NFP) is the direction of water flow across the wall of a capillary e.g. the difference between the HP and the OP.

$$NFP = HP - OP$$

  - When the NFP is positive, the HP gradient is greater than the OP gradient, and fluid flows outward (filtration); when it is negative the OP gradient is greater than the HP gradient, and fluid flows inward (absorption)

- The majority of the fluid filtered out of the ESF into the ISF is returned to the circulation, by the lymphatic system (Figure 4.1).

Water balance

- Regulation of water intake:
  - Too little water (dehydration):
    - Determined by the osmolarity of blood (the amount of solutes is increased in relation to water), monitored by osmoreceptors located in the hypothalamus, increased excitation of these receptors in dehydration will stimulate the release of antidiuretic hormone (ADH) from the pituitary gland
    - Net effect of ADH in the blood supply to the kidneys is opening of the aquaporins in the renal tubules and water will pass back into the ECF and circulation
    - Activation of osmoreceptors will stimulate the thirst mechanism
- Regulation of water output
  - Too much water (a long cool drink):
    - Determined by the osmolarity of blood (the amount of solutes is reduced in relation to water), monitored by osmoreceptors, reduced excitation of these receptors e.g. overload of intravenous fluid will reduce the release of ADH from the pituitary gland
    - Net effect of a reduced ADH in the blood results in closure of aquaporins in the renal tubules and excess water is passed out in the urine
  - Insensible water loss – approximately 500 ml per day in health, increases in conditions such as pyrexia or asthma.

Composition of body fluids

Electrolytes and non-electrolytes are found in the blood stream. These are important for maintaining the human body's delicate fluid and metabolic requirements. Alteration in the level of any individual electrolyte and non-electrolyte effects the homeostatic environment of the cell, causing a variety of effects on the body.

Sodium

Sodium (Na^+) is the major cation (an atom that loses electrons, acquires a mainly positive charge) of ECF, and determines plasma osmolarity. It has a major role in the movement of water and electrolytes between body fluid compartments. The normal is between 136–145 mmol/l. Adults require around

2–4 grams of sodium per day, but it is more usual that intake is higher at around 6–10 grams/day in the form of table salt. Sodium is essential for:

- Nerve impulse transmission
- Muscle contraction
- Movement of glucose, insulin and amino acids.

Regulation of sodium balance

Sodium is regulated in a number of ways:

- Aldosterone – this is released in response to a reduced blood pressure (BP) (see Chapter 8), Na^+, increase in potassium (K^+) and stress:
  - Stimulates the release of the renin, angiotensin, aldosterone system (Figure 4.2)
  - Renin release is converted to angiotensin I by angiotensinogens
  - Angiotensin 1 is converted into angiotensin II by the angiotensin converting enzyme (ACE), which circulates to the adrenal gland and aldosterone is released
  - Net effect is the re-absorption of sodium and the return of water back into the ECF
  - Potassium is excreted in exchange
- Baroreceptors are in the arch of the aorta and maintain BP and blood volume (see chapter 8):
  - When BP is increased pressure on the receptors sends sensory messages to the brain stem and motor output dilates blood vessels to bring down BP
  - When BP is reduced pressure on the receptors decreases sensory input to the brain stem and motor output vasoconstricts blood vessels to bring BP up
  - Sends nervous impulses to the kidneys to dilate blood vessels via the SNS to increase GFR and sodium is lost
- ADH – the reabsorption of water dilutes electrolytes influencing balance
- Atrial natriuretic factor/peptide (ANF/P) is released by cells of the atria of the heart when stretched by an increase in BP and is a potent diuretic excreting salt and water and vasodilator to reduce BP.

Potassium

Potassium (K^+) is the major intracellular cation, the normal value is between 3.6–5.0 mmol/L. An increase in potassium will stimulate an increase excretion in urine, in renal failure ECF K^+ levels increase, and if not treated death will ensue. A reduction in ECF K^+ will cause reabsorption in the renal tubules to maintain homeostasis. Potassium is essential for:

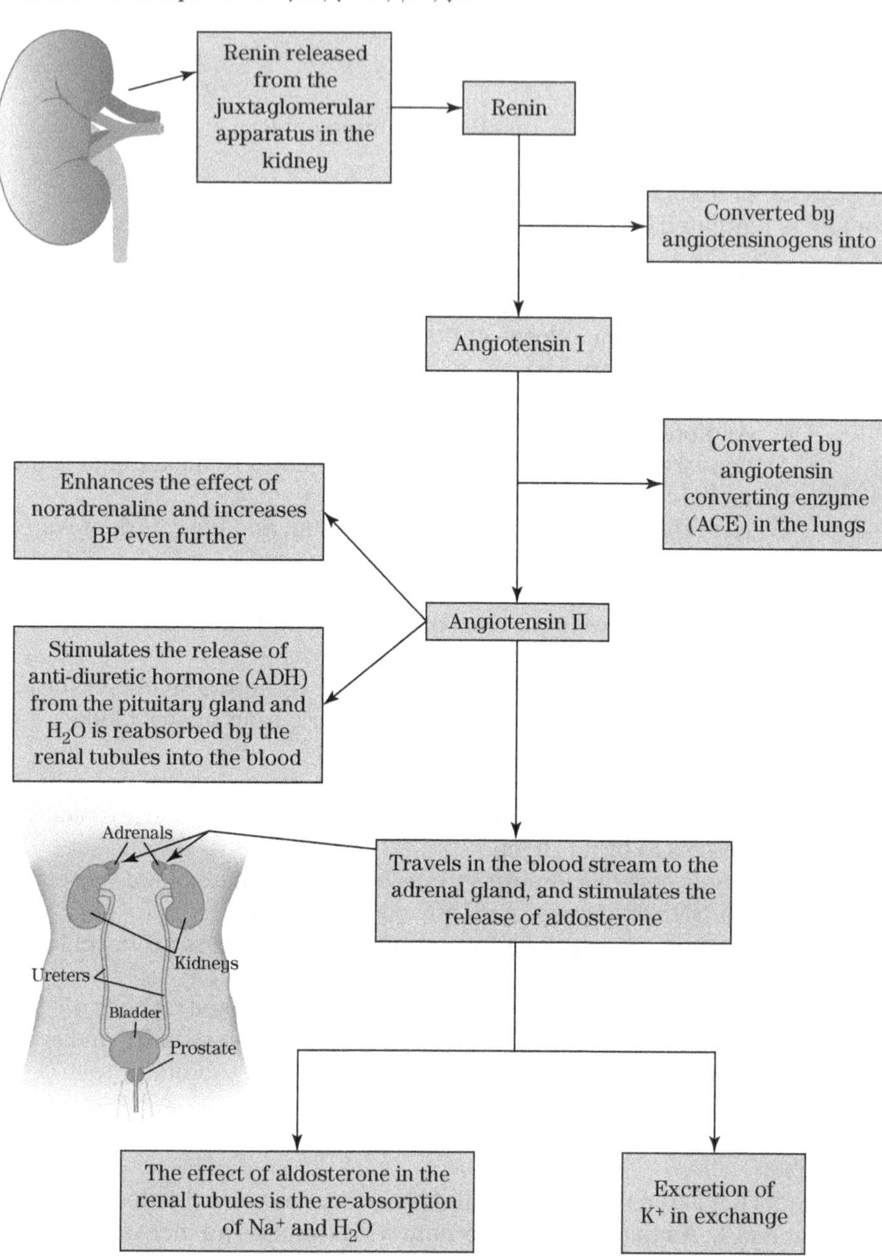

Figure 4.2 The renin-angiotensin-aldosterone (RAA) system

- Muscle contractions
- Transmission and conduction of nerve impulses
- Maintenance of normal cardiac rhythm – ECG changes if potassium is increased or reduced (Figure 4.3a, b)
- Skeletal and smooth muscle contraction resting membrane potential.

Regulation of potassium balance

Potassium is regulated in a number of ways:

- In the corticol collecting ducts of the kidneys
  - 90% of K^+ is reabsorbed
  - 10% is however lost regardless

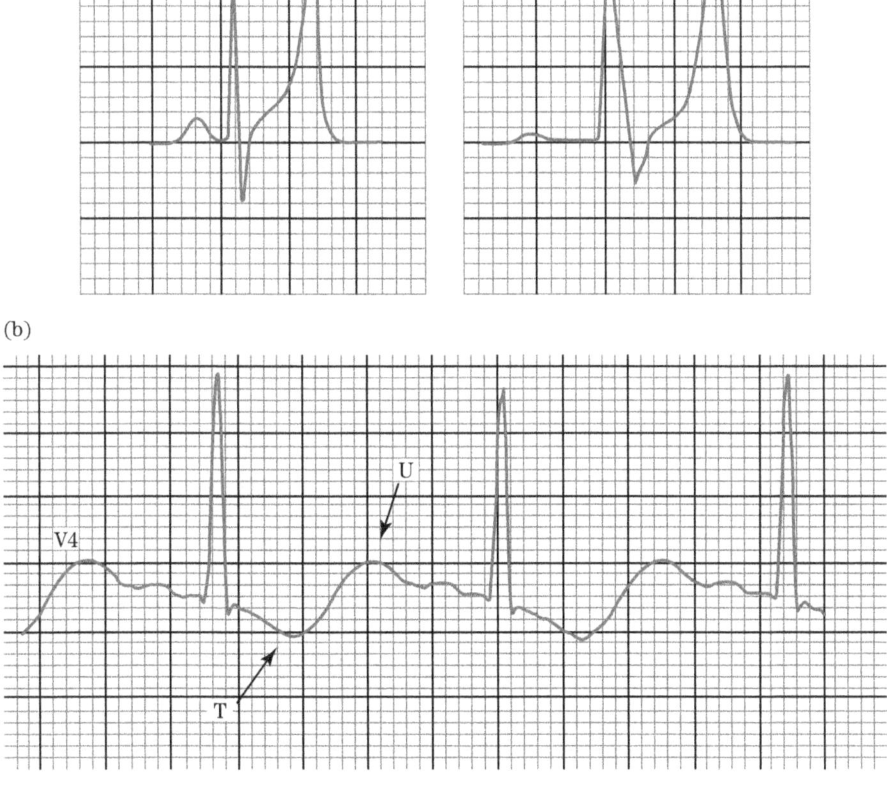

Figure 4.3 a) Changes in ECG rhythm in hyperkalaemia; b) Hypokalaemia

- By plasma concentration of K^+
  - If plasma concentration of K^+ is increased excess is excreted and Na^+ reabsorbed in exchange
  - If plasma concentration of K^+ is reduced renal cells will conserve K^+ and excretion is minimal
- Aldosterone
  - Adrenal cells are sensitive to K^+, if ECF concentration increases even slightly it stimulates the release aldosterone (see above).

Chloride

- Chloride (Cl^-) is an anion or negatively charged ion, it is usually paired with sodium a cation or positively charged ion because opposites attract, the normal value is between 95–105 mmol/L
- The movement of chloride throughout the body facilitates the movement of sodium, thus allowing fluid accumulations to be controlled
- Chloride is secreted by the stomach mucosa as hydrochloric acid and used to assist digestion
- Balance is maintained by the kidney
- Function includes maintaining acid-base balance as chloride is involved in the removal of oxygen and carbon dioxide from haemoglobin (Hb) in red blood cells, known as the chloride shift.

Bicarbonate

- The greatest proportion of carbon dioxide in the blood is in the form of bicarbonate (HCO_3^-). The red blood cells act as a factory for manufacturing bicarbonate
- Bicarbonate plays a crucial role in acid base balance and as such the normal value is usually measured in arterial blood
- The normal value is 22–28 mmol/L
- Bicarbonate is the conjugate base to carbon dioxide and water (hydrogen ions):
  - The carbon dioxide-bicarbonate system is a buffer pair to carbon dioxide as the buffer acid and bicarbonate as the buffer base
  - Bicarbonate balance is controlled by the kidney, which may increase or decrease the excretion of bicarbonate as components of physiological control mechanisms
  - The carbon dioxide-bicarbonate system acts as a buffer to completely restore the blood pH to normal.

Calcium

- Calcium is the most abundant mineral in the human body
- The body does not make calcium; it must absorb it every day in the diet (Edwards, 2005)
- The bones and teeth contain more than 99% of the body's calcium, where it functions to support their structure
- The remaining 1% is in the serum and exists in two forms:
  - Ionised or free calcium (found in foods, and the only type the body can use)
  - Bound to albumin – which accounts for about half of the serum calcium.

Serum levels of free calcium are 4.5–5.5 mmol/L, and total serum calcium including bound and free is 8.5–10 mmol/L.

Calcium is a necessary ion for many fundamental metabolic processes:

- The normal transmission of nerve impulses – it flows into nerve cells and stimulates the release of molecules (neurotransmitters)
- Muscle contraction
- Healthy blood pressure
- The initiation of coagulation
- Bone mineralisation
- Plasma membrane potential
- Regulation of various hormones and enzymes
- For the absorption of calcium from the intestine vitamin D is required.

Phosphorus

- Phosphorus is a primary anion or negative charged ion in intracellular fluid
- If enough calcium is ingested then enough phosphorus is likely, as both electrolytes are present in many of the same foods
- The normal level is around 2.5–4.5 mmol/L, but can be lower in a fasting patient, with a result between 0.8–1.4 mmol/L and needed for:
  - Formation of stored energy in cells (ATP)
  - Assistance with the formation of bones and teeth
  - Interaction with Hb to promote oxygen release to tissues
  - White blood cell activation
  - Metabolises fats, carbohydrates and proteins.

Regulation of calcium and phosphate balance

Calcium and phosphate balance is undertaken in 2 ways:

- Parathyroid hormone (PTH)

- In response to a reduction in blood calcium levels which stimulates the parathyroid gland to release PTH and increases plasma calcium levels by:
  - Stimulating the release of calcium from bones
  - Small intestine re-absorption is enhanced
  - Kidneys calcium re-absorption is increased in the renal tubules
- Calcitonin
  - Released by the thyroid gland in response to an increase in blood calcium levels
  - Increase in excretion by the kidneys.

Magnesium

- Magnesium is a mineral and must be absorbed through dietary intake
- It is the most abundant intracellular positive ion, but around 1% of total body magnesium is extracellular
- The recommended daily amount is around between 280–350 mg/day, 53–55% in bones, and 27% in muscles
- The normal level is 0.7–1.0 mmol/L.

Magnesium is involved in:

- Enzyme reactions resulting in ATP production
- Ensuring there is the right amount of excitability in nerves and muscle cells including the heart
- Energy metabolism
  - Glycolysis
  - Helps to regulate blood sugar
  - Protein synthesis
- Promoting normal blood pressure
- Myocardial contractility – influences the movement of ions across cells e.g. sodium and potassium
- Cell division and replication
- Protein biosynthesis
- PTH increases renal tubular reabsorption of magnesium.

Homeostasis is maintained by the kidney and is determined by the plasma concentration.

Non-electrolytes

- Glucose
  - The final product of carbohydrate digestion and the chief source of energy in human metabolism

  - The principle sugar of the blood
  - Insulin is required for the use of glucose
  - The normal fasting level in venous blood is between 3.6–5.8 mmol/L
- Lipids
  - Substance extracted from animal (saturated fats) or vegetable cells (unsaturated fats, which are either monounsaturated or polyunsaturated)
  - Triglycerides composed of fatty acids and glycerol
  - Phospholipids are modified triglycerides and used by cells to build their membranes
- Creatinine
  - A waste product of metabolism, excreted in the urine
  - The normal level is around 55–150 mmol/L
- Urea
  - The chief end product of nitrogen metabolism
  - Excreted in urine
  - The normal level is around 2.5–6.5 mmol/L
- Albumin
  - Present in plasma, the amount is determined by protein in diet
  - Determines the oncotic pressure (colloid osmotic pressure) in blood, as it is created by the presence in fluid of large molecules, such as plasma proteins, that are prevented from moving through the capillary membrane
  - Such molecules draw water towards them
  - Works opposite hydrostatic pressure to maintain circulating volume and homeostasis
  - The normal level is between 36–46 g/L.

A complex interplay occurs between fluid compartments and the electrolytes and non-electrolytes in the body. The HCPs role in relation to assessment and monitoring of fluid and electrolyte balance is well established. HCPs require effective knowledge and observational skills. When the activity of the fluid compartments and electrolytes become disrupted, or when homeostatic mechanisms, which maintain them within normal limits, malfunction and can no longer maintain a balance, disturbances occur.

ACID BASE BALANCE

The main function of acid base balance is to maintain arterial blood pH; the normal level is 7.4. This is undertaken in a number of ways by the lungs, which dispose of carbonic acid as carbon dioxide (CO_2), and the kidneys excrete other acids generated by cellular metabolism such as phosphoric, uric and lactic acids, and ketone bodies. A good understanding of these processes is essential to better place HCPs to manage any resulting problems logically and effectively (Edwards, 2008).

Dalton's Law of Partial Pressures (PP)

Dalton's law of PP is that each gas in a mixture of gases exerts its own pressure as if all the other gases were not present. PP of a gas is determined by atmospheric pressure:

- Atmospheric pressure
  - is 101 kPa,
  - 21% of air is oxygen
- Contents of air:
  - Nitrogen 78.6% of air
  - Oxygen (O_2) 20.9% of air
  - Carbon dioxide (CO_2) 0.04% of air
  - Water vapour 0.5%
- Partial pressure of oxygen in atmospheric air is:

$$\frac{21}{100} \times 101 \text{ kPa} = 21.2 \text{ kPa}$$

  - Gas will move from an area of high PP to an area of lower PP until an equilibrium is reached
  - Constant consumption of oxygen and production of carbon dioxide in the alveoli means that there is a PP gradient both in the lungs and at tissue level.

Composition of alveolar air

- The gaseous makeup of the atmosphere is quite different from that in the alveoli:
  - O_2 is 14%
  - CO_2 is 6%
  - Nitrogen is 80%
- Alveolar air contains much more carbon dioxide and water vapour and much less oxygen due to:
  - Gas exchanges occurring in the lungs
  - Humidification of air by the conducting passages
  - The mixing of alveolar gas that occurs with each breath.

Internal and external respiration

External respiration

- The movement of oxygen and carbon dioxide across the respiratory membrane from lungs to blood, influenced by:
  - Partial pressure gradients and gas solubility
  - Structural characteristics of the respiratory membrane
  - Functional aspects, such as the matching of alveolar ventilation and pulmonary blood perfusion.

Internal respiration

- Gaseous exchange between the systemic capillaries and the tissue cells

External and internal respiration take place by simple diffusion driven by the partial pressure gradients of oxygen and carbon dioxide that exist on the opposite sides of the exchange membranes.

The role of blood

Blood transports O_2 and CO_2 and so plays a significant role in maintaining blood pH, as the rate at which Hb reversibly binds or release O_2 is regulated by PO_2, temperature, blood pH and PCO_2.

Oxygen transport

- Blood carries oxygen (O_2) in 2 ways:
  - 3% dissolved in plasma
  - 97% bound in haemoglobin (oxyhaemoglobin HbO_2) within the red blood cells
- Haemoglobin
  - Is made up of protein, globin, bound to iron containing pigment – haem
  - The oxygen diffuses into the blood and binds with the haemoglobin–oxyhaemoglobin – HbO_2
- Association of oxygen and haemoglobin
  - It is an S shaped curve with a steep slope between 1.5 kPa and 7 kPa which plateaus between 9.5 and 18 kPa (Figure 4.4)
  - The relationship between the amount of O_2 bound to Hb (oxygen saturation) and the PO_2 of the blood is not linear because of the above

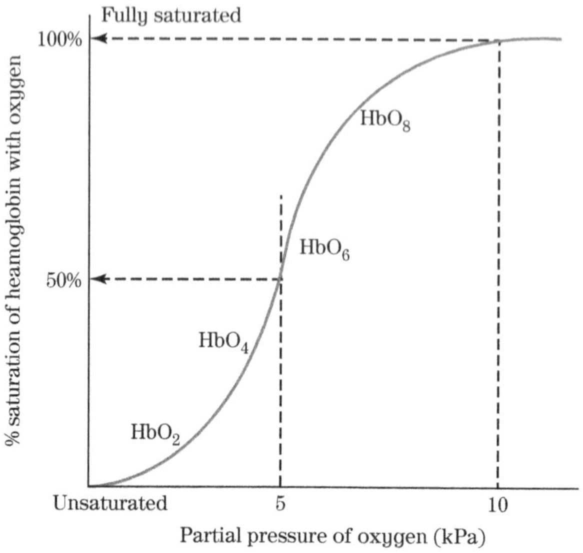

Figure 4.4 The oxygen disassociation curve

- Each haemoglobin molecule can combine with 4 molecules of O_2
- After the first molecule binds – haemoglobin molecule changes shape
- Haemoglobin more readily take up 2 more – uptake of fourth is further facilitated
- All 4 are bound – fully saturated
- 1, 2, 3 – partially saturated
- The unloading of 1 oxygen molecule enhances the unloading of the next, and so on

- Influence of temperature, H^+, PCO_2 on haemoglobin release
  - All of these factors influence haemoglobin saturation by modifying its structure and thereby its affinity for oxygen
  - An increase in these factors decreases Hb's affinity for O_2 and causes the oxygen-haemoglobin dissociation curve to shift to the right – enhancing oxygen unloading from the blood
  - An increasing H^+ and declining blood pH (acidosis) weakens the haemoglobin-oxygen bond – Bohr effect, leads to oxygen unloading being accelerated where it is needed most
  - A decrease in these factors increases haemoglobin's affinity for oxygen and shifts the dissociation curve to the left – decreasing the amount of O_2 available

- Impairments of oxygen transport:
  - Anaemic hypoxia
  - Ischaemic (stagnant) hypoxia
  - Histotoxic hypoxia
  - Hypoxaemic hypoxia.

The Bohr effect occurs when conditions within the body are normal; the bond between Hb and O_2 is stable. O_2 binding affinity of Hb is inversely related to acidity and concentration of CO_2. In certain conditions the Hb–O_2 bond is either weakened or strengthened:

- Weakened in acidosis, high temperatures and reduced pH–oxygen unloading is accelerated where it is most needed
- Strengthened in alkalosis, low temperatures and increased pH–oxygen unloading is slowed down and the O_2 remains attached to the Hb.

Carbon dioxide transport

- Blood carries carbon dioxide (CO_2) in 3 ways:
  - 7% dissolved in plasma
  - 20–30% bound to haemoglobin in red blood cells (carbaminohaemoglobin $HbCO_2$)
    - Rapidly dissociates from Hb in the lungs where the PCO_2 of alveolar air is lower than in the blood
    - Deoxygenated Hb combines more readily with CO_2–the Haldane effect
    - 60–70% of CO_2 is converted to bicarbonate ions and transported in plasma
  - Diffuses into RBC and combines with water to produce carbonic acid (H_2CO_3)
  - This is unstable and quickly dissociates into hydrogen ions and bicarbonate ions
  - This does occur in plasma but is much faster in the RBC due to the presence of carbonic anhydrase – an enzyme that reversibly catalyses the conversion of carbon dioxide and water to carbonic acid
  - Hydrogen ions released bind to Hb to produce the Bohr effect. Thus oxygen release is triggered by carbon dioxide loading
  - The bicarbonate ions diffuse quickly from the RBCs and into the plasma where they are carried to the lungs
  - To counteract this rapid movement of negative ions from the RBC chloride ions move from the plasma into the erythrocyte (the chloride shift).

The Haldane effect is when carbon dioxide transported in blood is affected by oxygenation of the blood.

- The lower the PO_2 and the Hb saturation with oxygen, the more carbon dioxide can be carried in blood
- Reflects the ability of reduced Hb to form carbaminohaemoglobin and to buffer H^+
- The Haldane effect encourages CO_2 exchange in both tissues and lungs.

The role of the lungs

Changes in respiratory rate or depth can produce changes in blood pH. For example, slow, shallow breathing increases CO_2 levels in the blood and blood pH drops; or rapid, deep breathing removes excessive amounts of CO_2 from the blood, and increases blood pH. These changes in respiratory ventilation can provide a fast acting technique to adjust blood pH (and PCO_2) when it is disturbed by illness or disease.

Pulmonary ventilation

- Inspiration
  - Required to remove carbonic acid (H_2CO_3) as CO_2
  - Negative pressure 101 kPa reduces in the pleura – air will move from a high to a low pressure
  - As moves through the passages air is warmed and increases expansion of the lungs
- Expiration
  - This is a passive process
- Influences on pulmonary ventilation
  - Resistance by the airways
  - Compliance – the ability to expand and recoil the lungs, determined by the presence of surfactant, which aids recoil of the lungs, if reduced tension stops and the alveoli stick together
  - Tidal volume (TV) × respiratory rate (RR) = Minute volume (MV)
  - Dead space – this needs to be cleared before adequate ventilation can take place.

Alveolar ventilation

- Gaseous exchange in the body
  - Partial pressures, Dalton's law
- External and internal respiration
- Carbon dioxide and blood pH
- Bicarbonate ions in the plasma act as an alkaline reserve and form part of the carbonic acid – bicarbonate buffer system of the blood

- If the hydrogen ion concentration of the blood starts to rise, excess H^+ is removed by combining with HCO_3^- to form carbonic acid
- If HCO_3^- concentration falls, carbonic acid dissociates, releasing hydrogen ions and lowering pH again
- Changes in respiratory rate and depth can produce dramatic changes in blood pH
- Respiratory ventilation can provided a fast acting system to adjust blood pH.

Metabolic aspects of acid base balance

The body contains a number of chemical buffers that act to resist changes in pH when a strong acid or base is added, achieved by biding to hydrogen ions (H^+) whenever the pH drops and releasing them when pH rises.

The bicarbonate buffer system

- The carbonic acid – bicarbonate buffer system consists of the following reaction:

$$CO_2 + H_2O \leftrightarrow H_2CO_3 \leftrightarrow H^+ + HCO_3^-$$

- This reaction is freely reversible; changing the concentrations of any participant will affect the concentrations of all the other parts
- Its primary role is to prevent pH changes caused by organic acids and fixed acids in the ECF, for example:
  - If there is an increase in CO_2 as in conditions such as COPD – respiratory acid is buffered by bicarbonate and so HCO_3^- is reduced
  - If there is an increase in H^+ as in conditions such as renal failure or diabetic keto acidosis – the metabolic acid is buffered by bicarbonate and so HCO_3^- is reduced
  - If there is a reduction in H^+ as in conditions such as severe vomiting – there is an increase in alkaline which is buffered by H^+ and therefore HCO_3^- is increased.

The phosphate buffer system

- Is similar to the carbonic acid–bicarbonate buffer system, the components are dihydrogen phosphate $\left(H_2PO_4^-\right)$ that acts as a weak acid, and monohydrogen phosphate $\left(H_2PO_4^-\right)$ acts as a weak base

$$H_2PO_4^- = H^+ + HPO_4^{2-}$$

- This buffer system plays only a supporting role in the regulation of pH, because the concentration of HCO_3^- far exceeds that of HPO_4^{2-}

- The phosphate buffer system plays an important role in buffering pH in the ICF
- Also important in excreting Na^+ and reabsorbing HPO_4^{2-} (in the kidneys) for use as a buffer in metabolic and respiratory acidosis to maintain pH.

The protein buffer system

- This process is slow and dependent on the ability of amino acids to respond to alterations in pH by accepting or releasing H^+
  - When the pH of the ECF decreases cells pump H^+ out of the ECF and into the ICF, where they can be buffered by intracellular proteins
  - When the pH of the ECF rises, exchange pumps in cell membranes exchange H^+ in the ICF for K^+ in the ECF
- This buffer system helps prevent drastic alterations in pH when the plasma PCO_2 is rising or falling (Edwards, 2008).

The role of the kidneys

- The ultimate acid base regulatory organs are the kidneys, which act slowly to compensate for acid base imbalances resulting from variations in diet, metabolism or from disease states.
- The most important renal mechanisms for regulating acid base balance of the blood involve:
  - Excreting bicarbonate ions and conserving (reabsorbing) H^+, as in an alkalosis
  - Excreting H^+ and reclaiming HCO_3^-, conserving (reabsorbing) bicarbonate ions, as in an acidosis (the dominant process in the nephrons).

Neurological control

- The higher centres control the rhythm and depth of breathing to further regulate acid base balance (see chapter 10)
- Rhythm is controlled by respiratory centres:
  - Controlled ultimately by nervous stimuli
  - Under autonomic and somatic nervous control
  - Suppressed by drugs
- Depth is influenced by:
  - Hering-Breuer reflex prevents overstretching of the lungs
  - An increase in arterial PCO_2
  - A reduction in arterial PO_2
  - Arterial pH.

The acid base balance of the body is maintained by a number of body systems. The body will strive to maintain pH balance as any changes in the acid base will affect the association of oxygen to haemoglobin and all body processes. An understanding of these processes can help to facilitate early interventions and treatments and serves to enhance the practice base of health care.

PATHOPHYSIOLOGICAL CHANGES TO THE ENVIRONMENT OF THE CELL

Fluid imbalance

Fluid and electrolyte management is a vital component of patient care. The main objective is to maintain tissue perfusion and safeguard against changes in plasma components.

Hypovolaemia

Hypovolaemia is defined as a diminished circulatory fluid volume (Edwards, 1998). Hypovolaemic shock is a further decrease in the circulating fluid volume so large that the body's metabolic needs cannot be met.

> **Case study 4.1**
>
> Dale was back home after spending the day at a picnic where he ate some 'spoiled' potato salad. He developed severe abdominal pain and cramps, vomiting and diarrhoea. After about 10 or 12 episodes of watery diarrhoea, Dale became so pale and weak he could hardly walk. His wife called for the ambulance. The paramedic team was concerned about his hydration and commenced an IV infusion as per ambulance protocol. Dale was thought to be suffering from shock.

Aetiology

- Haemorrhage – the loss of whole blood
  - Decreases the oxygen carrying capacity of the blood – hypoxia
  - Can develop into an acidosis (reduced pH)
- Plasma loss
  - Occurs in individuals with:
    - Large partial-thickness burns
    - Full thickness burns
    - Burns over more than 20% to 25% of the total body surface area

- Third space fluid shifts
  - Any type of trauma or cell damage will trigger an inflammatory response
  - The permeability causes movement of fluids, into the interstitial spaces
  - A patient can appear paradoxically 'dry' or hypovolaemic as fluid has moved into the intravascular spaces, yet can still have the same amount of body water
- Bleeding disorders
  - Platelet and coagulation disorders can cause or fail to prevent an internal or external haemorrhage
- Dehydration
  - Dehydration is more commonly seen in the elderly
  - If prolonged can induce hypovolaemic shock
  - It may be a consequence of a primary deficit of water, a primary deficit of salt or both e.g. vomiting and/or diarrhoea
- High temperature
  - The vasodilation observed during a high temperature can make a patient appear hypovolaemic
  - Fluid space has increased, yet there is still the same amount of circulating volume.

Pathology

- Results from a decrease in circulating blood volume and venous return produced by:
  - Continuous bleeding
  - Plasma loss
  - Water loss
  - Widespread vasodilation due to a high temperature (a relative rather than a true hypovolaemia).
- The loss is so great the body's metabolic needs cannot be met (Edwards and Coyne, 2013)
- The level of damage depends on:
  - The amount of blood lost
  - The rate at which the blood was lost
  - The age of the patient
  - The patient's ability to activate compensatory mechanisms.

(See Figure 4.5.)

Clinical features

- HCP should remain suspicious of hypovolaemia, even within the context of normal vital signs (Murch, 2005)

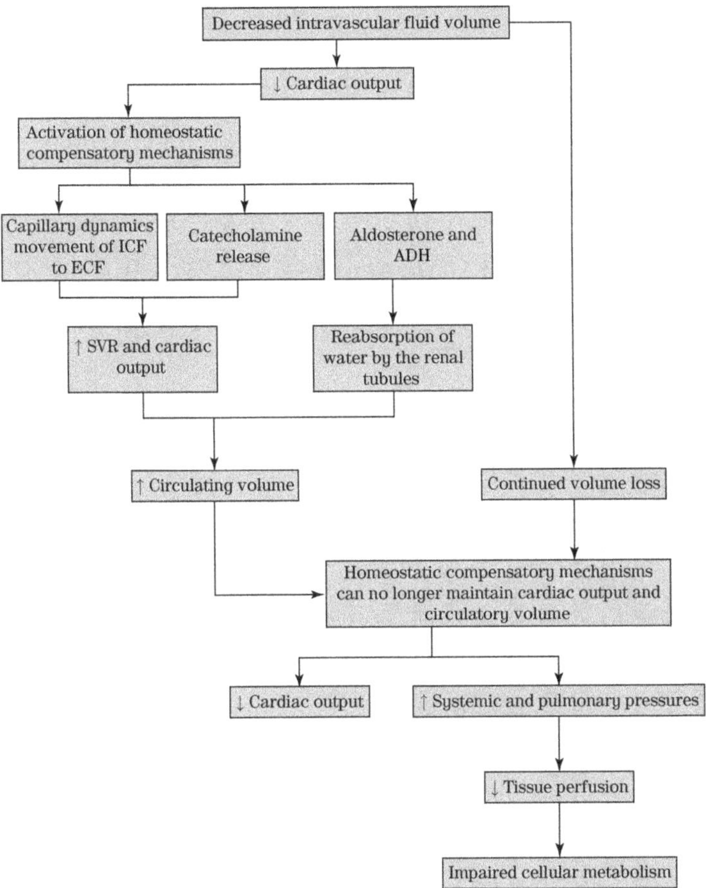

Figure 4.5 Hypovolaemic shock

- Signs of maintaining homeostasis (Table 4.1):
  - Normal or high blood pressure
  - Increased heart rate, respiratory rate
  - Reduced urine output
- Decreased cardiac output.

Increased systemic vascular resistance can be indicated by pale skin and cold to touch peripheries e.g. hands and feet.

Investigations

- Vital signs
- Urine output
- Central venous pressure (CVP)

Control mechanism	Stimulus	Result	Clinical implications
Release of catecholamines epinephrine and norepinephrine	Stimulate two classes of receptors: α-adrenergic receptors divided into 2 subclasses: α_1 and α_2 β-adrenergic receptors divided into 2 subclasses: β_1 and β_2 Epinephrine binds to and activates both α and β-adrenergic receptors Norepinephrine binds primarily to α-adrenergic receptors	Epinephrine enhances myocardial contractility, ↑ HR, venous return all improving CO and BP, ↑ blood flow to skeletal muscles, leads to a temporary hyperglycaemia, bronchodilatation and ↑ in RR, stimulates renin release from the kidney Norepinephrine ↑ BP by constricting peripheral and GIT blood vessels	A patient maintaining homeostasis will release epinephrine and norepinephrine within 3–5 seconds of the insult increasing HR, BP, and RR This can put an increase pressure on the heart and lungs All hospital patients have undergone some insult, anxiety and stress leading to the release of epinephrine and norephinephrine The receptors sites are the location of action for a variety of drugs e.g. beta blockers

Table 4.1 Homeostatic control mechanisms

Baroreceptors are stretch receptors located in the arch of the aorta and in the carotid sinus	↑ In firing when pressure on the receptors ↑ e.g. hypertension vasodilatation occurs to bring down BP ↓ In firing when the pressure on the receptors reduced e.g. hypotension vasoconstriction occurs to increase BP	The result is to: ↑ SNS discharge, which will cause vasodilatation to ↓ BP ↓ SNS discharge leads to vasoconstriction and an ↑ BP	When baroreceptor function is working normally homeostasis can be maintained in the event of a variety conditions e.g. and ↑ or ↓ in BP
Vascular compliance is the increase in volume a vessel is able to accommodate for a given increase in pressure	The ability of blood vessels to vasoconstrict or vasodilate in response to pressure changes	This allows a large volume of blood or fluid to be accommodated by the venous system A person with normal vascular compliance can be given a very large volume of fluid, and only gain a small ↑ in BP	Several conditions can lead to changes in vascular compliance Arteriosclerosis increases the rigidity or stiffness of arterial walls, which ↑ BP at a given volume of blood The volume of fluid in the circulation exerts a greater pressure on the vessels, which in a patient with arterial vessel stiffness, will result in a much higher BP with just a small volume of fluid and ↑ the risk of fluid overload

Table 4.1 Continued

Vascular resistance is the opposition to flow	Flow is determined by the diameter and length of blood vessels	The narrower the diameter of a blood vessel the greater the resistance The wider the diameter the less resistance	This can be effected in patients with changes in blood viscosity, baroreceptors, chemoreceptors, velocity and laminar flow
Renal autoregulation the kidneys play a complex role in restoring ECF volume or excreting excess fluid to maintain BP	Renin is released when there is a ↓ in BP, leads to stimulation of the RAA system ANF is released when fluid overload is threatened	RAA – there is reabsorption of sodium and water from the renal tubules and restores ECF volume to the circulation Angiotensin II effects norepinephrine and the release of ADH ANF – body's normal diuretic to an increase in circulating volume	When blood volume falls stimulation of RAA system is activated, ↑ circulating volume to maintain BP ANP prevents fluid overload
Central chemoreceptors are specialized areas in the brain stem sensitive to concentrations of carbon	Changes in acid base are sensed by nerves and in the CSF and transmitted to the brain stem	↓ In arterial pH can lead to vasoconstriction and an ↑ in BP ↑ In arterial pH can lead to vasodilation and an decrease in BP ↑ In CO_2 can cause vasodilatation and a decrease in BP	Patients with COPD suffering from a respiratory acidosis with an ↑ in CO_2 and a reduction in pH can have an ↑ in BP Patients suffering severe vomiting and a metabolic alkalosis can have an

Table 4.1 Continued

dioxide, hydrogen ions and pH		↓ In CO_2 can cause vasoconstriction and an increase in BP	increase in pH and a ↓ in CO_2 with a corresponding reduction in BP
Peripheral chemoreceptors are areas in the arch of the aorta and carotid arteries sensitive to reductions in oxygen	Transmit impulses to the medulla centres of the brain which regulates BP	↓ in arterial oxygen concentration will lead to vasoconstriction of blood vessels and a reflexive ↑ in BP	Patients with fluid overload, heart failure, pulmonary oedema, asthma can suffer varying degrees of hypoxia If they have additional problems such as varicose veins, this can further increase BP If fluid is administered there is an ↑ risk of fluid overload
Osmoreceptors are neurons located in the hypothalamus that are stimulated by an ↑ in plasma osmolality or a ↓ in circulating blood volume	Stimulated when there is a deficit of water or an excess of sodium in relation to water	Stimulates thirst and water drinking is increased ADH is released into the blood stream in response to activation of osmorecepters	ADH increases the permeability of renal tubules to water, and water is reabsorbed into the plasma Urine becomes more concentrated ↑ in urine SG, plasma osmolality is ↓, circulating volume is maintained, and BP is ↑

BP = blood pressure; CO_2 = carbon dioxide; RAA = renin-angiotensin-aldosterone; ↑ = increase; ↓ = decrease; ECF = extracellular fluid; COPD = chronic obstructive pulmonary disease; CSF = cerebral spinal fluid; ANF = atrial natriuretic factor; ADH = anti diuretic hormone; SG = specific gravity; SNS = sympathetic nervous system; HR = heart rate; RR = respiratory rate; CO = cardiac output

- Blood results e.g. haematocrit, urea and creatinine
- Check haemodynamic response to administration of a fluid challenge (Murch, 2005).

Practice point

When undertaking vital signs it is important to observe for patterns in the chart e.g. a gradual increase in heart rate, respiratory rate and blood pressure over a period of hours or days can be an indication of compensated hypovolaemia. Alongside, consider the urine output. A decrease over a 12–24-hour period e.g. a negative balance can indicate diminished circulatory fluid volume.

Treatment and drug therapy

- Administration of prompt oxygen therapy
- Correction of volume deficit
  - Early administration of fluids to maintain adequate blood pressure, tissue oxygenation and intravascular fluid volume
  - Colloid fluids give quick increases in plasma volume, but take a longer time to be excreted from the system
  - Crystalloid fluids, in comparison, are quickly lost from the circulation, but larger volumes are required to maintain the same increases in plasma volume to that given by colloid fluids (Table 4.2).

Practice point

A decrease in CVP does not necessarily indicate hypovolaemia, as CVP is unreliable in left ventricular failure (LVF), peripheral vascular disease (PVD), and valvular heart disease. The CVP can be difficult to determine and interpret, as peripheral vasoconstriction can maintain CVP despite hypovolaemia.

Fluid overload

An overload to the circulation may occur due to circulation problems, or due to fluid therapy, and can lead to cardiogenic shock (Edwards, 2000).

Aetiology

Circulation problems – certain conditions may hasten fluid overload:

- Hypertension – elevation of systemic arterial blood pressure and effects the circulation by damaging the wall of the systemic blood vessels

Fluid	pH/mOsm	Contents	Normal levels	Uses & why	Avoided in & why
0.9% Normal saline	Ph: 5 mOsm: 300	Na: 154 mmol/l Cl: 154 mmol/l	pH: 7.35-7.45 mOsm: 274-300 mmol/kg Na: 35-45 mmol/l K: 3.5-5.5 mmol/l Cl: 95-105 mmol/l Cal: 2.1-2.6 mmol/l Bic: 22-28 mmol/l Lactate: 0.3-1.4 mmol/l	Hypovolaemia Maintenance fluid (not recommended) Dilution of drugs	Dehydration Acidosis Oedema Hypernatraemia Neuro patients Diabetes insipidus Increased Chloride Heart failure
5% Glucose	pH: 4 mOsm: 300	Glucose: 25 gram/100 ml 420 kilo joules/L = 100 kcal (Yorkie bar 1500)		Cellular dehydration Insulin infusion Dilution of drugs	Hypovolaemia Feeding Neuro patients increased ICP
10% Glucose	pH: 4.15 mOsm: 604	Glucose: 50 gram/100 ml 836 kilo joules (200 kcal)			
Plasma Lyte (replaces Hartmann's solution)	pH: 6.5 – 8.00 mOsm: 295	Na: 140 mmol/l Cl: 98 mmol/l K: 5 mmol/l Sodium gluconate: 23 mmol/l Mg 1.5 mmol/l Acetate: 23 mmol/l		Hypovolaemia Maintenance during surgery	Hyperkalaemia Renal patients Acidosis

Table 4.2 Crystalloids and colloids: identifying the constituents of common fluids

Gelatins Isoplex 4% solution (replaces Gelofusine)	pH: 7.4 mOsm: 284	Gelotin 20 gram in 500 ml of water Na: 72.5 mmol/l Cl: 52.5 mmol/l K: 2 mmol/l Lactate: 12.5 mmol/l	Hypovolaemia	
Starches (Voluven, Volulyte)	pH: 4-5.5 mOsm:308	Voluven (starch in saline) Na: Volulyte (starch in water) Na: 137 K: 4 Cl: 110 Cal:	Hypovolaemia	Voluven Hypervolaemia Anaphylaxis Volulyte Clotting disorders

Table 4.2 Continued

- Heart failure (HF)
  - Left-ventricular failure (LVF) – a proportion of blood remains present in the left ventricle at the end of ventricular contraction, can continue to deteriorate the function of the heart and impairs the heart's ability to pump blood and trigger a series of events that result in heart failure
  - HF – four of the heart chambers overfill during subsequent cardiac cycles. The cardiac output drops considerably and blood velocity throughout the body slows down
- Peripheral vascular disease due to:
  - Arteriosclerosis a chronic disease of the arterial system characterised by abnormal thickening and hardening of the vessel walls, which diminishes the ability of the arteries to change lumen size
  - Atherosclerosis is a form of arteriosclerosis but the damage to the vessel walls is caused by soft deposits of intra-arterial fat and fibrin that harden over time
- Fluid overload due to fluid therapy given following surgery and/or following hypovolaemia:
  - Blood products and colloid solutions – blood velocity reduces and blood flow becomes slow
    - Blood pools in the peripheries, lungs, liver, kidneys and possibly the brain
    - Heart can no longer pump the increasing amount of volume around the circulation
    - The kidneys become swamped with fluid and start to receive a lower blood supply, renal failure ensues
    - Complications of pulmonary oedema, cardiac failure, renal failure, ascites, cerebral oedema and peripheral oedema can be very serious if not treated quickly
    - A diuretic is generally given either with each or every subsequent unit
  - Crystalloid and non-crystalloid solutions – fluid overload with crystalloid solutions (e.g. saline and polyionic solutions) and non-crystalloid solutions (e.g. dextrose solutions) cause similar problems but for different reasons
    - Under normal circumstances it is almost impossible to produce an excess of total body water, due to homeostatic mechanisms e.g. atrial natriuretic factor/peptide (ANF/P), osmoreceptors and anti-diuretic hormone (ADH)
    - When a patient's homeostatic responses are reduced, then fluid overload can occur during intravenous (IV) treatment given, with the different solutions (Table 4.2)

    - The effects can be an overload of both salt and water (isotonic volume excess) or just salt (hypertonic volume excess) or dilutional low sodium (hypotonic volume excesses) (Table 4.3)
- Cardiogenic shock – fluid overload from any of the previous aetiologies mentioned may precipitate cardiogenic shock:
    - A severe circulatory failure due to a primary defect of ventricular compliance and pumping activity of the heart
    - Ventricular preload, afterload, and contractility are all altered, compromising left ventricular function
    - Circulatory collapse leads to reduced myocardial contractility, an inability of the body to adequately compensate as cardiac output drops
    - An increased left ventricular filling pressure, decreased systolic blood pressure (BP), oliguria and impaired mental state (see chapter 8).

Pathology

There is an increase in volume in the circulation. This causes pressure on the baroreceptors – vasodilation takes place:

- The BP may be normal or slightly elevated
- As volume continues to increase the action of the baroreceptors is reduced
- Atrial natriuretic peptide or factor (ANP/F) is released from the atria of the heart in an attempt to off-load fluid
- Eventually as the signs of an overloaded circulation are evident, the heart may fail leading to heart failure (HF)
- If this becomes severe cardiogenic shock may ensue.

Clinical features

- Facial colour, pallor, flushed or cyanosed, cool or moist or dehydrated skin
- Respiratory difficulty e.g. rapid or shallow breathing
- Ischaemia of the eyelids, lips, gums and tongue
- Signs of left ventricular failure (LVF) and pulmonary oedema or heart failure (HF) with systemic oedema; increased or decreased body weight; pulsating neck veins
- Anxiety or distress; evidence of confusion, disorientation, apprehension, restlessness, agitation or calm.

Solutions	Type of overload	Fluid given	Causes/conditions leading to imbalance	Symptoms	Consequences
Isotonic has a sodium content approximately equivalent to that of the plasma	Isotonic volume excess (no swelling or shrinking of cells)	Excessive administration of a combination of IV fluid e.g. an overload of both salt and water	Gain or loss of extracellular fluid	Circulating volume increases: Weight gain and decrease in haematocrit and plasma proteins Neck veins distended Increased blood pressure leads to oedema formation	If circulating volume is great enough: Pulmonary oedema Heart failure may develop Leading to circulatory collapse Heart becomes dysfunctional and unable to pump blood from the heart
Hypertonic has a sodium content greater than that of the plasma	Hypertonic volume excess (cells shrink in a hypertonic fluid)	Inappropriate administration of hypertonic saline solution e.g. sodium bicarbonate and normal saline leading to a hypernatraemia	Hyperaldosteronism Cushing's syndrome Hyperglycaemia Diabetes insipidus Hypovolaemia (water loss) Hypervolaemia (salt gain) Pyrexia	Increase in extracellular sodium causes an osmotic attraction of water and intracellular dehydration Weight gain Breathlessness	Hypernatraemia Hypervolaemia If severe: Convulsions Pulmonary oedema being the most serious

Table 4.3 Causes and consequence of changes to tonicity in body water volume

Table 4.3 Continued

		or hyperchloraemia A water loss or solute gain		Thirst Decrease in urine output Confusion, coma	
Hypotonic has a sodium content usually half that of isotonic saline	Hypotonic volume excess (cells swell in a hypotonic fluid)	Replacement of fluid loss with intravenous 5% dextrose. This is a dilutional hyponatraemia (low sodium) A water gain or solute loss	Hyponatraemia Hypoaldosteronism Excessive diuretic therapy Nephrotic syndrome Cirrhosis Heart failure	Weight gain Intracellular oedema Ascites Jugular vein distension	Contents of the blood become low e.g. potassium, sodium, haemoglobin Cardiac, neurological and blood transport problems ensue Hypertonic hyponatraemia e.g. in hyperglycaemia

Investigations

- Urine output – in fluid overload with a reduced cardiac function blood flow to the kidneys becomes reduced with a decrease in urinary output; should also consider overall fluid balance and the quality of urine
- Weight – an important measurement in determining fluid overload and cardiac status, whether a patient is gaining weight the first indication of heart failure, and losing weight the first sign that diuretic therapy is working.

Treatment and drug therapy

- Clinical management of fluid therapy
- Monitoring and assessment to maintain adequate cardiac function
- The immediate restoration of an effective circulation is needed to minimise, prevent or reverse any overload, and/or cardiac failure or cardiogenic shock
- Prompt administration of diuretic therapy.

Oedema

This is an abnormal accumulation of fluid in tissues or cells (Edwards, 2003). Oedema is a problem of fluid distribution and does not necessarily indicate fluid excess.

Aetiology

There are two general forms of oedema: interstitial and intracellular. These 2 processes are not mutually exclusive, as one can lead to the other and vice versa:

- Interstitial oedema is caused by:
  - Changes in capillary dynamics due to increased hydrostatic pressure or decreased plasma oncotic pressure (Figure 4.6a, b):
    - Heart failure, hypertension (increase in hydrostatic pressure)
    - Malnutrition, renal disorders (the reduction in oncotic pressure)
  - Stimulation of the inflammatory immune response
    - Trauma, injury, infection (stimulation of the inflammatory immune response)
  - Lymphatic system obstruction
    - Cancer, surgical removal (blocked lymphatic system)
- Intracellular oedema: there is a lack of oxygen to the cells due to:

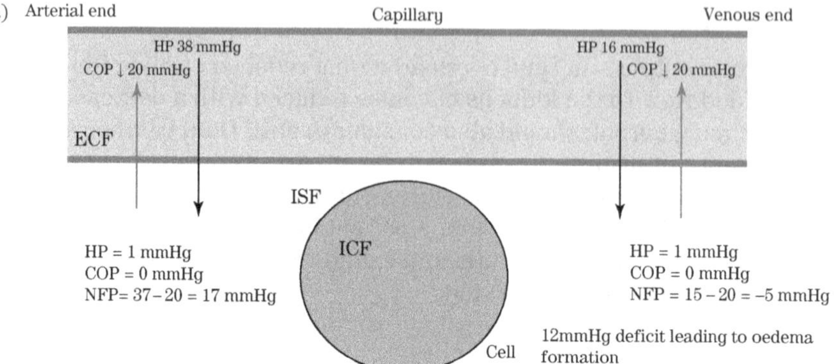

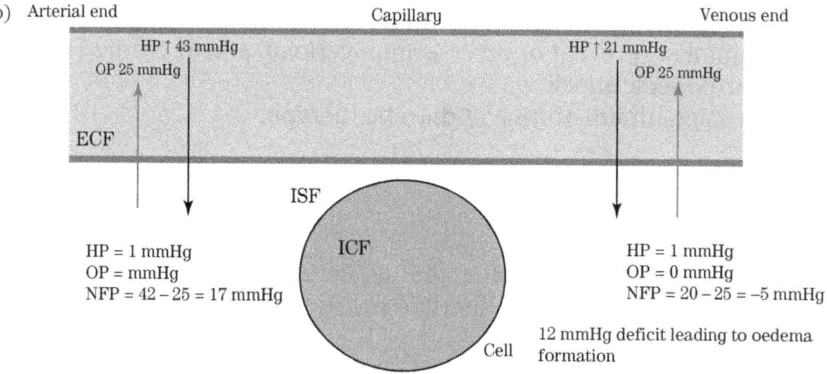

Figure 4.6 a) Oedema formation due to a reduced COP; b) Oedema formation due to an increase in HP

- Pressure ulcers
- Myocardial infarction
- Any of the above conditions from interstitial oedema.

Clinical features

The fluid is either in the interstitial (ISF) or intracellular (ICF) spaces. It is associated with:

- Generalised oedema
  - Weight gain
  - Diet high in sodium

    - Swelling and puffiness
    - Tight-fitting clothes and shoes
    - Limited movement of an affected area
    - Pain in the affected area
- Cerebral oedema signs of deteriorating mental state (see chapter 10)
- Pulmonary oedema increases breathlessness (see chapter 9)
- Systemic oedema is due to heart failure with swelling of legs, breathlessness, a common complication of a myocardial infarction (MI) (see chapter 8)
- Ascites signs of liver failure (see chapter 11)
- Skin lesions areas of redness due to pressure and immobility (see chapter 16)
- Swollen joints due to arthritis (see chapter 12)
- Signs of renal failure, oliguria, protein in urine, renal failure (see chapter 14).

Investigations

- Consider life style and personal habits, family and past medical history
- Blood tests e.g. albumin, sodium levels, liver function tests (LFT), urea and creatinine
- Physical examination of the cardiovascular system including blood pressure
- Respiratory assessment and examination
- Examination and assessment of abdomen e.g. auscultation, percussion and palpation (Quigley *et al*, 2012)
- Neurological assessment, mental status examination, behaviour, speech, cognitive functions
- Renal function tests, urine output studies, urinalysis.

Treatment

- As oedema is usually a symptom of an underlying condition, treatment involves treating the immediate cause
- If oedema is due to retention of sodium restricting intake is key
- Diuretics help to reduce swelling to increase sodium and water loss from the body
- Mannitol can be used in cerebral oedema when there is an emergency need to relieve pressure (Casey, 2004).

Electrolyte imbalance

Electrolytes are maintained within a very narrow range and concentration is balanced by an integration of renal, hormonal and neural functions (McCance and Huether, 2010). Any changes in electrolyte balance can affect many areas of the body e.g. pH balance, cardiac and muscle contraction, fluid shifts and can be life threatening. The treatment of electrolyte imbalance is not simply a matter of administering the electrolyte when there is a deficiency or increasing excretion when the concentration is too high, but may involve more complex interventions related to the treatment of the underlying cause.

Disorders of sodium balance

Hyponatraemia

Hyponatraemia is low sodium in the blood below 135 mmol/L.

- *Aetiology*:
  - Inadequate sodium intake or diuretic therapy
  - Excessive sweating stimulating thirst
  - Intake of large amounts of water which dilutes ECF sodium – compulsive water drinking
  - Vomiting, diarrhoea, gastrointestinal suctioning or burns
  - Heart failure
  - Hepatic cirrhosis
  - Diuretic phase of acute tubular necrosis
  - Adrenal insufficiency
  - Oversecretion of antidiuretic hormone (ADH)
- *Pathology*
  - Causes hypo-osmolality
  - Fluid moves into cells and cell swelling
  - Usually observed when there is:
    - Sodium loss
    - Inadequate sodium intake
    - Dilution of the body's sodium e.g. fluid regimes with excess intravenous 5% dextrose can lead to over-hydration and a dilutional hyponatraemia (Edwards, 2001)
- *Clinical features*
  - Behavioural and neurological changes e.g. headache, confusion, apprehension, seizures, coma
  - Lethargy
  - Isotonic hypovolaemia, simulation of compensatory mechanisms leading to increased blood pressure, tachycardia, decreased urine output
  - Dilutional hyponatraemia – interstitial oedema causing weight gain, ascites, jugular vein distension
- *Investigations*
  - Serum sodium is <135 mmol/L

    - Increase in plasma proteins and haematocrit
    - Urine specific gravity is <1.010 with a normal renal function
- *Treatment and drug therapy*
    - Related to the contributing disorder
    - Losses of sodium and water calculated and appropriate solutions are given for replacement.

Practice point

Severe hyponatraemia (serum sodium <120 mmol/L) is a common electrolyte abnormality observed in many hospitalised conditions or by administration of fluid regimes. Frequent checks on serum sodium levels and attention to subtle symptoms leading to early treatment and improved outcomes.

Hypernatraemia

Hypernatraemia is high serum sodium greater than 145 mmol/L.

- *Aetiology*
    - Inappropriate administration of saline solutions resulting in an increased load onto the circulation
    - Other causes of hypernatraemia are
        - Water depletion, excess sodium and loss of water
        - General fever or those caused by respiratory infections which increase the respiratory rate, enhance water loss from the lungs and sweating
        - Diabetes insipidus leads to increased loss of water and hypernatraemia
        - Diabetes mellitus
        - Severe vomiting and diarrhoea can cause water loss in relation to sodium
        - Insufficient water intake
        - Over secretion of aldosterone, as in primary hyper-aldosteronism, or Cushing's syndrome
- *Pathology*
    - An increase in dietary sodium is rarely the cause of hypernatraemia
    - Always associated with hyper-osmolality
- *Clinical features*
    - Intracellular dehydration leading to thirst and dry mucous membranes
    - Seizures, restlessness, coma

    - Pulmonary oedema
    - Pyrexia
    - Hypotension, tachycardia, low jugular venous pressure due to water loss
- *Investigations*
    - Serum sodium is >147 mmol/L
    - Urine specific gravity is >1.030
    - Haematocrit and plasma proteins are raised
- *Treatment and drug therapy*
    - Hypernatraemia
        - Administration of an isotonic salt-free solution e.g. 5% dextrose
        - Frequent measure of serum sodium to sodium level has returned to normal
    - Hypervolaemia
        - Treatment of the underlying condition.

Disorders of potassium balance

Hyperkalaemia

A high level of ECF potassium in the blood above 5.5 mmol/L is rare.

- *Aetiology*
    - The clinical features may be very few
    - If there are any symptoms changes in the ECG, this will show (Figure 4.3):
        - Peaking of the T waves
        - Followed by loss of P wave
        - Abnormal QRS complexes
    - Potassium levels are increased in:
        - Increased intake of potassium in diet
        - Renal failure
        - The use of potassium-sparing diuretics
        - Adrenal insufficiency
        - Acidosis (potassium increase tends to cause acidosis)
        - Potassium replacement due to loss
        - Cellular trauma or hypoxia
- *Pathology*
    - The severity of hyperkalaemia is related to:
        - The amount of potassium intake
        - The degree of acidosis, K^+ is exchanged for H^+ in cells
        - The rate of renal cell damage
- *Clinical features*
    - Muscle weakness or paralysis

    - Arrhythmias with changes in the ECG (Figure 4.3)
    - Mild hyperkalaemia
        - Neuromuscular irritability, restlessness
        - Tingling in the lips and fingers
        - Intestinal cramping
        - Diarrhoea
    - Severe hyperkalaemia
        - Loss of muscle tone
        - Depression of ST segment
        - Bradycardia, ventricular fibrillation
- *Treatment and drug therapy*
    - May be related to other underlying causes which need to be investigated and treatment instigated
    - Correcting potassium excess
    - Administration of calcium gluconate, glucose or glucose and insulin
    - Sodium bicarbonate corrects acidosis
    - Dialysis.

Hypokalaemia

A low level of serum potassium in the blood of less than 3.5 mmol/L.

- *Aetiology*
    - Severe hypokalaemia may be asymptomatic
    - Generally the clinical features of hypokalaemia are:
        - Constipation and paralytic ileus are the commonest problems
        - In addition there may be:
            - A decrease in excitability of the nervous system
            - Muscle weakness
            - Depression
            - Confusion
            - Arrhythmias, ECG changes (Figure 4.3)
    - Blood potassium levels are decreased in:
        - Diarrhoea and vomiting, excessive sweating
        - Use of diuretics (loop and thiazide-like diuretics)
        - Steroids
        - Salbutamol and other B_2 agonists
        - Nephrotic syndrome
        - Diabetes mellitus
        - Cushing's syndrome
        - Alkalosis (potassium depletion tends to cause alkalosis)
        - Over hydration
        - Laxative abuse

- *Pathology*
  - Potassium is distributed between ICF and ECF
  - This makes determining hypokalaemia difficult
  - Generally low serum potassium levels indicate a loss of body potassium, but this is not always accurate
  - Plasma potassium levels may be normal or high even when total body potassium is low
- *Clinical features*
  - Weight loss as carbohydrate metabolism is impaired leading to skeletal muscle weakness
  - Renal function can be impaired
  - Cardiac effects due to changes in membrane potential
  - Neuromuscular changes
- *Treatment and drug therapies*
  - Involves identification of the disorder related to the hypokalaemia
  - Correction of acid base balance
  - Eat food rich in potassium e.g. bananas and orange juice
  - Safe oral or IV replacement until normal levels are reached.

Disorders of calcium

Hypocalcaemia

- *Aetiology*
  - Is usually associated with inadequate dietary intake of calcium or vitamin D (Edwards, 2005)
  - Hypoalbuminaemia
  - Chronic renal failure
  - Acute haemorrhagic and oedematous pancreatitis
  - Diseases, which interfere with calcium absorption from the gut:
    - Respiratory alkalosis
    - Excessive use of loop diuretics because of excessive calcium loss
    - Patients suffering from burns – calcium can become trapped in burned tissue
    - Blood transfusion
    - Hyperparathyroidism – lack of parathyroid hormone leads to a drop in calcium levels
    - Low magnesium, which inhibits parathyroid function
    - A high level of phosphorus (hyperphosphataemia) is usually present

- *Clinical features*
  - Chvostek's sign is a positive twitch of the nose or lip caused by tapping the facial nerve just below the temple
  - Trousseau's sign is observed in severe hypocalcaemia, when arterial blood flow in the arm is occluded the muscles of the hand and fingers contract and spasm
  - Neuromuscular excitability
  - Tetany – severe muscle spasm which interferes with breathing
  - Paraesthesia
  - Muscle cramps
  - Spasms or seizures
  - Nausea
  - Weakness
  - Irritability
  - Confusion
- *Investigations*
  - Consideration of underlying pathological conditions that require further investigation
- *Treatment and drug therapies*
  - Depending on severity administration of IV or oral calcium gluconate
  - Serum levels of calcium monitored
  - Decrease in phosphate intake for long-term management
  - Prevention of complications:
    - Osteoporosis
    - Bone fractures
    - Convulsions
    - Muscle spasms
    - Heart failure
    - Bleeding.

Hypercalcaemia

A total serum calcium above 10 mmol/L or a free calcium level above 5.5 mmol/L.

- *Aetiology*
  - The condition is most often related to malignant tumours and prolonged immobility
  - Endocrine disorders that can increase bone calcium re-absorption include:
    - Acute adrenal insufficiency
    - Hyperparathyroidism

        - Level of PTH inappropriate to calcium level
        - Raised calcium with a raised or normal PTH
        - Primary usually due to parathyroid adenoma
        - Treatment – high fluid intake, surgery, watch and wait
        - Side effects – osteoporosis, renal failure, kidney/renal stones
    - Hypophosphataemia
    - Hyperproteinaemia
    - Hyperthyroidism
  - Familial hypocalciuric hypercalcaemia (FHH)
    - Leading to an asymptomatic hypercalcaemia
    - Normal/slightly elevated PTH
    - Differentiate from primary hyperparathyroidism
  - Renal dysfunction
  - Thiazide diuretics
  - Vitamin D intoxication
  - Granulomatous disorders e.g. tuberculosis and sarcoidosis
- *Pathology*
  - There is an increase in calcium inside cells and the membrane potential threshold becomes lengthened
  - Many of the clinical features are related to the inability of cell membranes to become excited
- *Clinical features*
  - Dependent on the rate of increase
  - Lethargy
  - Nausea and vomiting
  - Anorexia
  - Constipation
  - Polyuria
  - Kidney stones form as calcium salts are excreted in the kidney and solidify
  - Bradycardia and degrees of heart block
- *Treatment and drug therapies*
  - Treatment of underlying pathological condition
  - There may be a reciprocal decrease in serum phosphate
  - In the instance of normal renal function oral phosphate administration is recommended
  - Increased IV administration of normal saline to stimulate the excretion of excess calcium
  - Administration of calcitonin
  - Corticosteroids
  - Cytotoxic drug mithramycin (malignant disease).

Disorders of phosphate balance

Hyperphosphataemia

- *Aetiology*
  - Decreased renal excretion
    - Reduced glomerular filtration rate (GFR)
    - Increased reabsorption
      - Hyperparathyroidism
      - Acromegaly
  - Increased intake
    - Oral or intravenous
    - Phosphate containing laxatives/enemas
    - Vitamin D intoxication
  - Cell lysis
    - Rhabdomyolysis
    - Cytotoxic therapy leukaemia
    - Lymphoma
  - Lactic acidosis
  - Respiratory acidosis
  - Diabetic ketoacidosis
- *Clinical features*
  - Comparable to those observed in hypocalcaemia as high levels of phosphate can lower serum calcium levels
  - Muscle weakness
  - Calcification of soft tissue occurs in the:
    - Lungs leading to respiratory failure
    - Kidneys and renal failure
    - Joints causing swelling and pain
  - Decreased myocardial output
  - Rhabdomylolysis, a disease of skeletal muscles
  - Rickets/osteomalacia
- *Treatment and drug therapies*
  - Correction of the underlying condition
  - Aluminium hydroxide can be administered but can lead to neurological complications if not eliminated as deposited in the central nervous system
  - Dialysis if renal failure.

Hypophosphataemia

- *Aetiology*
  - Re-feeding syndrome (re-feeding of starved patients)
  - Respiratory alkalosis
  - Phosphate depletion is associated with a significant increase in urinary magnesium excretion and may cause hypomagnesaemia

  - Lowered renal phosphate threshold
    - Primary hyperparathyroidism
    - Renal tubular defects
    - Familial hypophosphataemia
  - Increased loss
    - Vomiting
    - Diarrhoea
    - Phosphate binding antacids
  - Decreased absorption
    - Malabsorption syndrome
    - Vitamin D deficiency
    - Poor diet
- *Clinical features*
  - Usually not identified until hypophosphataemia is severe
  - Reduced capacity for oxygen transport by red blood cells with diminish release of oxygen to the tissues
  - Hypoxia can occur
  - Muscle weakness may lead to respiratory failure
  - Bradycardia
  - Disturbed energy metabolism
  - Blood clotting impairment with potential for haemorrhage
  - Irritability, confusion, coma, numbness, convulsions
  - Signs of rickets or osteomalacia
- *Investigations*
  - Clotting factors
  - Patient history
  - Bone profile
  - Renal function tests
  - Magnesium and calcium levels
  - Vitamin D levels
  - PTH levels
- *Treatment and drug therapies*
  - Investigation of the underlying cause
  - Administration of phosphate salts is not recommended as it is dangerous
  - A low phosphate is not considered life threatening.

Disorders of magnesium balance

Hypermagnesaemia

- *Aetiology*
  - Rare and usually caused by renal failure

    - Excessive intake
    - Failure to excrete magnesium
    - Magnesium containing antacids
    - Enemas
    - Parenteral nutrition therapy
    - Magnesium therapy
- *Clinical features*
    - Depressed skeletal muscle contraction and nerve function
    - Depressed respiration
    - Cardiac arrest
    - Nausea and vomiting
    - Muscle weakness
    - Hypotension
    - Bradycardia
- *Treatment*
    - Avoidance of magnesium containing substances
    - Dialysis.

Hypomagnesaemia

- *Aetiology*
    - Diabetes mellitus both types 1 and 2 are the most commonest causes of magnesium deficiency
    - Associated with hypokalaemia and hypophosphataemia
        - Oral potassium is not retained if patient also has a magnesium deficiency
        - Associated with calcium deficiency with overlapping symptoms
        - Hypocalcaemia and hypokalaemia unresponsive to supplementation should prompt magnesium measurement
    - Poor nutritional status is often due to alcoholism
    - During treatment for metabolic acidosis
    - Re-feeding syndrome
    - Can lead to chronic diseases such as heart disease, high blood pressure, osteoporosis and type 2 diabetes
    - Renal losses
        - Chronic renal failure
        - Peritoneal dialysis
        - Inherited disorders
    - Observed in some patients with pancreatitis
    - Gastric intestinal disorders:
        - Prolonged nasogastric suctioning
        - Feeding is maintained on parenteral nutrition

    - Malabsorption
    - Bowel resection
    - Steatorrhoea, diarrhoea
    - Crohn's disease, ulcerative colitis, celiac disease
    - Fistulas
    - Acute pancreatitis
    - Decreased dietary intake
    - Chronic vomiting
  - Impairs PTH secretion
  - Drug therapies
    - Osmotic, thiazide and loop diuretics
    - Aminoglycosides including gentamycin, tobramycin and amikacin, viomycin and capreomycin
    - Cardiac glycosides
    - Cyclosporin an immunosuppressant agent
    - Theophylline
    - Amphotericin B e.g. pentamidine
- *Clinical features*
  - Early signs of magnesium deficiency include:
    - Loss of appetite
    - Nausea
    - Vomiting
    - Fatigue
    - Muscle weakness
  - Increased neuromuscular excitability, convulsions, irritability, increased reflexes, nystagmus
  - Results in a low calcium (see hypocalcaemia) and potassium (see hypokalaemia) levels
- *Treatment*
  - Administration of IV magnesium sulphate.

Acid base imbalance

Many respiratory conditions lead to changes in respiratory and metabolic acid base balance. In addition, systemic conditions lead to changes in metabolic and respiratory acid base balance. This is due to the ability of the body to maintain balance e.g. if there is a change in respiratory acid base balance for example respiratory acidosis, the body will maintain pH by altering metabolic acid base balance to a metabolic alkalosis. For the clinical features, investigations and treatment and drug therapies for conditions that lead to imbalances in acid base balance, please view the appropriate chapter.

A low pH corresponds to a high H^+ concentration – acidosis. A high pH corresponds to a low H^+ concentration – alkalosis (Edwards, 2008). The normal pH of arterial blood is 7.4

- If acid production is less than excretion, then HCO_3^- increases and H^+ reduces – an alkalosis results with a corresponding increase in pH
- If acid production is greater than excretion, then H^+ increases and HCO_3^- decreases – an acidosis ensues with a corresponding reduction in pH
- Acid base disorders are generally associated with:
  - Metabolic disorders where there are changes in HCO_3^-.
  - Respiratory disorders result from an accumulation or reduction of PCO_2 an acid increases H^+ concentration.

Measuring acid base balance

- By measuring the partial pressure and other values in arterial and venous blood can determine whether the patient is experiencing acidosis or alkalosis (Table 4.4)
- Arterial blood gases can determine the type of acid base disorder e.g. respiratory or metabolic and whether the kidneys are compensating the condition (Table 4.5)
- Many articles discuss their interpretation (Fletcher and Dhrampal 2003, Woodrow 2004). Once determined interventions can be instigated.

Respiratory acidosis

Respiratory acidosis occurs when the respiratory system is unable to eliminate CO_2. When there is an increase in CO_2 there is an increase in H^+ concentration and the body's pH starts falling below 7.35 (Figure 4.7). The increase in CO_2 stimulates central chemoreceptors to increase respiratory rate and changes in acid base balance occurs (see chapter 9).

Aetiology

- Determined by PCO_2 >5.7 kPa; pH <7.35, occurs in:
  - Any condition that impairs gas exchange or lung ventilation (chronic bronchitis, cystic fibrosis, emphysema, adult respiratory distress syndrome (ARDS), respiratory arrest)
  - Rapid, shallow breathing
  - Narcotic or barbiturate overdose or injury to brain stem
  - Under-ventilation via endotracheal tube (ETT)

Measure	Normal limits	Interpretation
pH	7.35 – 7.45	This indicates whether the person is in acidosis (pH < 7.35) or alkalosis (pH >7.45), but it does not indicate the cause
$PC0_2$	4.5 – 6.0 kPa (35 – 42 mmHg)	Check the PCO_2 to see if this is the cause of the acid-base balance. The respiratory system acts fast, and an excessively high or low PCO_2 may indicate either the condition is respiratory or if the patient is compensating for a metabolic disturbance ■ The PCO_2 is over 6.0 kPa (40 mmHg), the respiratory system cannot excrete $C0_2$ and a hypercapnia results ■ The PCO_2 is below normal limits 4.5 kPa (35 mmHg), the respiratory system is not the cause but is compensating
$P0_2$	12–14.6 kPa (90 – 110 mmHg)	This does not reveal how much oxygen is in the blood but only the partial pressure exerted by dissolved O_2 molecules against the measuring electrode
HCO_3^-	22–26 mmol/l	Abnormal values of the HCO_3^- are only due to the metabolic component of an acid base disturbance: ■ A raised HCO_3^- concentration indicates a metabolic alkalosis (values over 26 mmol/L) ■ A low value indicates a metabolic acidosis (values below 22 mmol/L)
BE	–2 – +2 mmol/l	Is the amount of acid required to restore 1 L of blood to its normal pH, at a PCO_2 of 5.3 kPa (40 mmHg)? The BE reflects only the metabolic component of any disturbance of acid base balance: ■ If there was a metabolic acidosis then acid would have to be added to return the blood pH to normal, the BE will be positive ■ If there is a metabolic acidosis, acid would need to be subtracted to return blood pH to normal, the BE is negative

Table 4.4 Measure of arterial blood gases

Acid base is separated into 4 categories:	The conditions/diseases that lead to acid base abnormalities
Respiratory acidosis – any disorder that interferes with ventilation (PCO_2 >6.0 kPa; pH <7.35)	■ Any condition that impairs gas exchange or lung ventilation (chronic bronchitis, cystic fibrosis, emphysema, pulmonary oedema) ■ Rapid, shallow breathing, hypoventilation ■ Narcotic or barbiturate overdose or injury to brain stem ■ Airway obstruction ■ Chest or head injury
Metabolic acidosis (HCO_3^- <22 mmol/L; pH <7.35)	■ Severe diarrhoea causing loss of bicarbonate from the intestine ■ Circulatory failure/hypovolaemia ■ Renal disease/failure ■ Untreated diabetes mellitus ■ Starvation ■ Excess alcohol ingestion ■ High ECF potassium concentrations ■ Lactic acid production
Respiratory alkalosis (PCO_2 <4.5 kPa; pH >7.45)	■ Direct cause is always hyperventilation (e.g. too much mechanical ventilation, pulmonary lesions) ■ Brain tumour or injury ■ Acute anxiety ■ Early stages of congestive obstruction airway disease ■ Asthma
Metabolic alkalosis (HCO_3^- >26 mmol/L; pH >7.40) is the result of excess base bicarbonate ion (HCO_3^-) or decreased hydrogen ion (H^+) concentration, caused by an excessive loss of non-volatile or fixed acids.	■ Vomiting or gastric suctioning of hydrogen chloride-containing gastric contents ■ Selected diuretics ■ Ingestion of excessive amount of sodium bicarbonate ■ Constipation ■ Excess aldosterone (e.g. tumours) ■ Loss of gastric-intestinal hydrochloric acid and potassium (e.g. severe vomiting or gastric suctioning) ■ Over-use of potassium wasting diuretics

Table 4.5 Acid base categories and related conditions

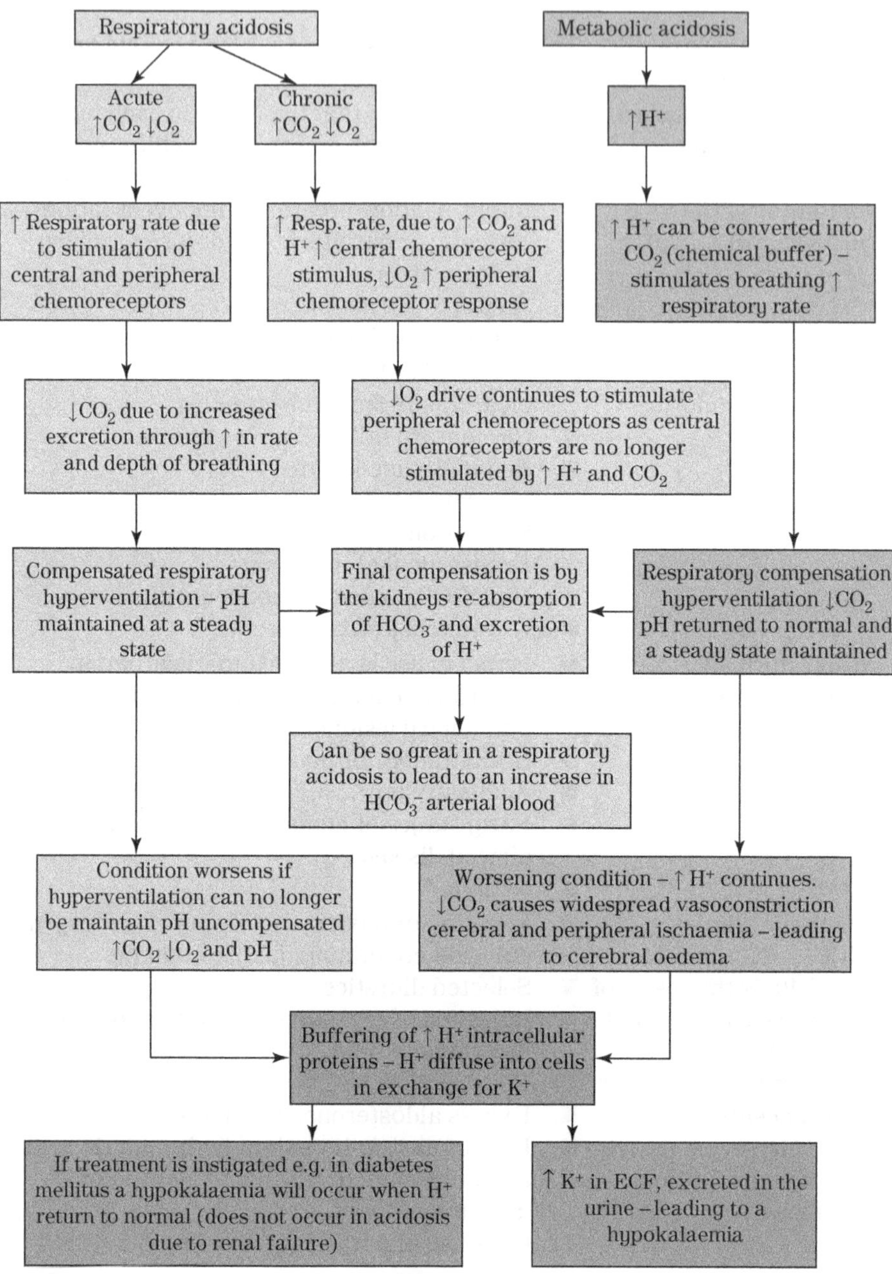

Figure 4.7 Processes involved in respiratory and metabolic acidosis

  - Airway obstruction
  - Chest or head injury
  - Severe and life threatening asthma.

Pathology

- The accumulation of CO_2
  - The Haldane effect is when CO_2 transported in blood is affected by the partial pressure of oxygen in the blood
  - A reduced partial pressure of oxygen cannot sufficiently facilitate the release of carbon dioxide from the Hb – eventually lowering pH
  - A reduction in PO_2 might not be picked up by oxygen saturation monitoring due to the oxygen disassociation curve
  - In some conditions the administration of oxygen will improve PO_2 and reduce the accumulated PCO_2
- Improved release of oxygen
  - In an acid environment less oxygen can be carried by haemoglobin
  - The acid environment in tissues causes the Hb to release O_2 more readily to cells – known as the Bohr effect
  - The increased hydrogen ions bind to the Hb in the RBC and alter the structure of the molecule temporarily causing it to release O_2.

Metabolic acidosis

Metabolic acidosis occurs when there is excess acid or reduced bicarbonate in the body.

Aetiology

- Determined by HCO_3^- <22 mmol/l; pH <7.35, occurs in conditions such as:
  - Severe diarrhoea causing loss of bicarbonate from the intestine
  - Circulatory failure/hypovolaemia
  - Renal disease/failure
  - Untreated diabetes mellitus
  - Starvation
  - Excess alcohol ingestion
  - High ECF potassium concentrations
  - Lactic acid production.

Pathology

- There is an over-production or excess of hydrogen ions, which will lead to decreased pH of less than 7.35 (Figure 4.7)

- This is followed by a reduction in HCO_3^- (used to buffer excess H^+) in an effort to return the pH to within the normal range (7.35–7.45)
- The slight change in H^+ concentration can cause alterations in body enzymes as these can only function in a pH range of between 6.80 and 7.80 and as such enzyme activity falls with a reducing pH with 50%
- There is reduced mortality rate with a blood pH ≤6.80
- Therefore, the body will work diligently to return pH to normal.

Compensation for an accumulation of acids

- In the lungs
  - An increase in $H^+ \uparrow CO_2$ production and stimulates the respiratory centre (CSF) via the equation:

$$CO_2 + H_2O \leftrightarrow H_2CO_3 \leftrightarrow H^+ + HCO_3$$

  - Oxygen saturation will decrease
  - There will be an increase in respiratory rate and depth of breathing – worsens as the acids continue to rise
- In the kidneys
  - Excess H^+ can be converted through the above equation
  - The H_2CO_3 dissociates to release free hydrogen (H^+) and bicarbonate ions (HCO_3^-), and stimulates the kidneys to retain (HCO_3^-) and sodium ions (Na^+), and excrete H^+
  - The bicarbonate is retained to circulate and buffer further carbon dioxide
  - The kidney can only retain so much bicarbonate
- Electrolyte exchange
  - If the concentration in H^+ rises to a level beyond the compensatory mechanism H^+ move into cells to be buffered by intracellular proteins
  - This is in exchange for potassium ions (K^+)
  - This leads to a hyperkalaemia and characteristic changes in the ECG can occur (peaked T waves and abnormal QRS complexes)
  - In normal renal functions the majority of the extracellular K^+ will be excreted in the urine.

Practice point

If normal ventilation is restored or the acidosis (e.g. diabetic ketoacidosis) is treated (with for example insulin and glucose) the potassium will return to the intracellular fluid in exchange for hydrogen ions and the patient can develop a hypokalaemia.

Respiratory alkalosis

Respiratory alkalosis occurs when the respiratory system eliminates too much CO_2. This reduction of PCO_2 below the range of 4.6 kPa (30 mmHg) causes hydrogen ions to be lost (Figure 4.8). The decreasing hydrogen ion concentration raises the blood pH above the normal range of 7.45.

Aetiology

- Any condition that causes hyperventilation, determined by a PCO_2 <5.6 kPa; pH >7.35, occurs in:
  - Direct cause is always hyperventilation e.g. too much mechanical ventilation, pulmonary lesions
  - Brain tumour or injury
  - Asthmatic attack (overcompensated)
  - Acute anxiety
  - Early stages of congestive obstructive airway/pulmonary disease.

Pathology

- When ventilation is increased above the normal rate e.g. in depth and rate large amounts of CO_2 is excreted in expired air:
  - A fall in PCO_2 (hypocapnia) causes a rise in pH and a reduction in carbonic acid (CSF)
  - When both CO_2 and H^+ are reduced they have a reduced effect on the respiratory centre and on the central chemoreceptors
  - Causing an ↑ in heart rate without a rise in blood pressure, this could lead to angina and ECG changes
  - Respiratory rate may be ↓ in both depth and rate
- The binding of Hb and O_2 in alkaline states:
  - A decrease in CO_2 and H^+ the pH will rise and more oxygen remains bound to Hb
  - The Hb molecule fails to release sufficient O_2 to the tissues under conditions of decreased hydrogen ion concentration
  - This will maintain O_2 saturation, but not cellular oxygen delivery.

Metabolic alkalosis

Metabolic alkalosis is the result of excess base bicarbonate ion (HCO_3^-) or decreased hydrogen ion (H^+) concentration (Figure 4.8).

Aetiology

- Determined by HCO_3^- >26 mmol/l; pH >7.45 occurs in:
  - Selected diuretics

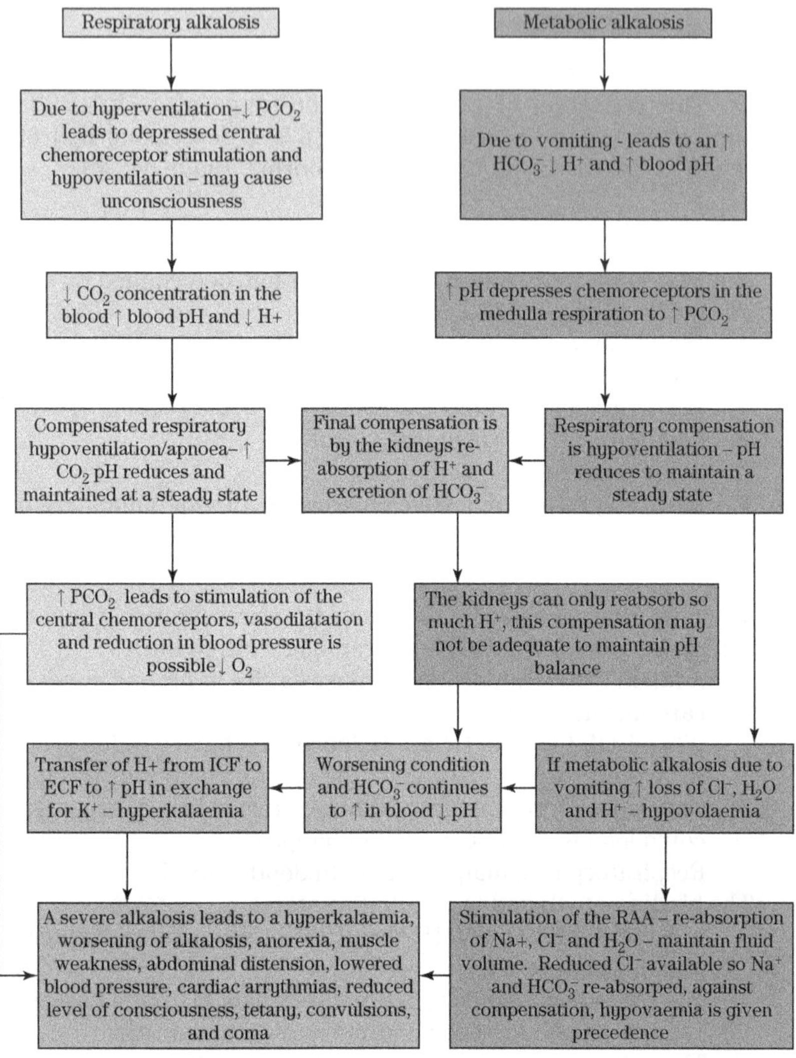

Figure 4.8 Processes involved in respiratory and metabolic alkalosis

- Ingestion of excessive amount of sodium bicarbonate
- Constipation
- Excess aldosterone release (e.g. tumours)
- loss of gastric-intestinal hydrochloric acid and potassium (e.g. severe vomiting or gastric suctioning)
- Over-use of potassium wasting diuretics.

Pathology

- Metabolic alkalosis overexcites the central and peripheral nervous systems
- The body finds it difficult to compensate in alkalosis as the body is programmed to maintain balance for acid environments
- An alkalosis can be seriously exacerbated if there is a severe drop in circulating volume e.g. in persistent vomiting
  - Electrolytes are no longer available to the body from the alimentary canal to replace those lost in the vomit and in urine (Na^+, Cl^-, HCO_3^-)
  - Hydrochloric acid is also lost as hydrogen and chloride ions
  - The loss of fluid and plasma volume can lead to hypovolaemia, which leads to activation of powerful compensatory mechanisms that are inappropriate in an existing alkalosis (Figure 4.8).

The retention of electrolytes and fluid during a hypovolaemia takes precedence over acid base homeostasis (Edwards, 2008).

> **Practice point**
>
> At this stage the patient could have bradypnoea, be hypoventilating or exhibit Cheyne Stokes respiration.

Compensation for alkaline environments:

- In the lungs
  - As base bicarbonate ions start to accumulate chemical buffers in ECF and cells bind to HCO_3^-
  - The unbound excess HCO_3^- elevates blood pH
  - To compensate the H^+ combine with HCO_3^- to form H_2CO_3
  - Blood and tissues give up more hydrogen ions as a compensatory response
  - An increase in blood pH depresses chemoreceptors in the medulla. This reduces respiration and increases blood PCO_2
  - The chemical reaction of $CO_2 + H_2O$ to form carbonic acid (H_2CO_3) is part of the respiratory compensation for a metabolic alkalosis
  - This is limited since it lowers O_2 levels
- In the kidneys
  - After approximately 6 hours the kidneys start to increase the excretion of HCO_3^- and reduce the excretion of H^+
  - This renal compensation returns the plasma hydrogen ion concentration towards normal and urine will be very alkaline

  - To maintain electrochemical balance, excess sodium ions (Na^+) and chloride ions (Cl^-) are excreted along with HCO_3^-. This can lead to a hyponatraemia
  - H^+ is returned to the blood to reduce the pH, chemoreceptors in the medulla increase respiratory rate and a compensatory hyperventilation may ensue
  - If the PCO_2 becomes too low due to the hyperventilation, metabolic compensation may not be adequate
  - A prolonged alkaline environment leads to vasoconstriction, which increases cerebral and peripheral hypoxia
  - If left untreated an alkalosis can overwhelm the heart and central nervous system
- Electrolyte exchange
  - Decreased H^+ levels in ECF cause them to diffuse passively out of the cells
  - To maintain balance of charge across the cell membrane, ECF K^+ move into the cells
  - When potassium cannot be replaced by absorption in the alimentary tract there is a severe depletion of the body's total potassium content (hypokalaemia), as a consequence of continued K^+ excretion, leading to confusion and arrhythmias
  - An alkalosis can be seriously exacerbated further if there is a severe drop in circulating volume e.g. vomiting.

CONCLUSION

The chapter has examined the chemical and physiological mechanisms that provide the optimal cell environment for survival. The kidney regulates water, electrolytes and acid base balance, made possible by a number of hormones, blood bound buffers and the respiratory system, which shoulders the main responsibility for acid base balance in the blood. Now that the topics discussed in chapters 2, 3 and 4 have been read, it is important to begin to make connections with other body systems and the changes that occur, which can lead to illness/disease or pathophysiology.

SELF-ASSESSMENT QUESTIONS

1. Outline the composition of and movement between fluid compartments of the body.
2. Briefly describe mechanisms involved in regulating electrolyte and water balance.

3. Define how the kidneys regulate hydrogen and bicarbonate ion concentrations in the blood.
4. Describe the importance of normal respiratory and renal compensation in acid base balance.
5. Explain the physiological processes involved in hypovolaemia, fluid overload, oedema formation and dehydration.
6. Outline the abnormalities of electrolyte imbalance.
7. Distinguish between acidosis and alkalosis resulting from respiratory and metabolic factors.

REFERENCES

Casey, G. (2004) Oedema: causes, physiology and nursing management, *Nursing Standard*, 18(51), 45–1.

Doherty, M. and Buggy, D.J. (2012) Intraoperative fluids: how much is too much? *British Journal of Anaesthesia*, 109(1), 69–79.

Edwards, S.L. (1998) Hypovolaemia: pathophysiology and management options, *Nursing in Critical Care*, 3(2), 73–82.

Edwards, S.L. (2000) Fluid overload and monitoring indices, *Professional Nurse*, 15(9), 568–572.

Edwards, S.L. (2001) Regulation of water, sodium and potassium: implications for practice, *Nursing Standard*, 15(22), 36–42.

Edwards, S.L. (2003) The formation of oedema, Part 1: pathophysiology, causes and types, *Professional Nurse*, 19(1), 29–31.

Edwards, S.L. (2005) Maintaining calcium balance: physiology and implications, *Nursing Times*, 101(19), 58–61.

Edwards, S.L. (2008) Pathophysiology of acid base balance: the theory practice relationship, *Intensive and Critical Care Nursing*, 24, 28–40.

Edwards, S. and Coyne, I. (2013) *A Survival Guide to Children's Nursing*, Edinburgh: Elsevier.

Fletcher, S. and Dhrampal, A. (2003) Acid base balance and arterial blood gas analysis, *Surgery*, 23(3), 61–65.

McCance, K.L. and Huether, S.E. (2010) *Pathophysiology: The Biologic Basis for Disease in Adults and Children*, 6th edn, Missouri: Mosby Elsevier.

Murch, P. (2005) Optimising the fluid management of ventilated patients with suspected hypovolaemia, *Nursing in Critical Care*, 19(6), 279–285.

Quigley, B., Palm, M.L. and Bickley, L. (2012) *Bates' Nursing Guide to Physical Examination and History Taking*, Philadelphia: Wolters Kluwer, Lippincott Williams & Wilkins.

Woodrow, P. (2004) Arterial blood gas analysis, *Nursing Standard*, 18(21), 45–52.

5 Body defence mechanisms

Sharon Edwards

The aim of the immune system is to provide protection through an intricate system of cells, enzymes and proteins. It provides resistance to infection by invading organisms such as bacteria, viruses and fungi, and parasites.

To survive infections the human body relies on 2 systems that respond immediately to protect it from foreign substances.

THE IMMUNE SYSTEM

The lymphatic system

This is a vascular system that detects excess tissue fluid and returns it to the blood stream (McCance and Huether, 2010).

The lymph system consists of the following:

- Lymph is mainly water with a few dissolved proteins
- Lymphatic vessels carry lymph away from tissues and return it to the circulation
- Lymphatic tissue contains a high concentration of lymphocytes and phagocytes
- Lymphatic nodes filter lymph
  - Lymphatic tissue consists mainly of lymphocytes
  - Lymphatic nodules consists of numerous loose connective tissue of digestive tract (Peyer's patches), respiratory, urinary and reproductive systems
- Tonsils
  - Large lymphatic nodules in nasopharynx and oral cavity
  - Provide protection against bacteria and other harmful substances, 3 groups:
    - Palatine
    - Pharyngeal
    - Sub-lingual

- Spleen
  - Located in left superior abdomen
  - Functions
    - Destroys and removes aged and defective red blood cells and platelets (RBCs) from the blood
    - Detects and responds to foreign substances
    - Limited reservoir for blood
- Thymus
  - Located in superior mediastinum, where it partially overlies the heart
  - The site of maturation of T lymphocyte cells.

Functions of the lymphatic system

- Fluid balance – any excess interstitial fluid enters lymphatic capillaries and becomes lymph
- Fat absorption – absorption of fat and other substances from the digestive tract
- Defence – micro-organisms and other foreign substances from digestive tract are filtered from lymph and lymph nodes and from blood by the spleen.

The immune system relies on 2 defence mechanisms; these are innate immunity and specific immunity that act both independently and cooperatively to provide resistance to disease (Figure 5.1).

Innate immunity

The innate immune system is the first response to any invasion by a foreign body. The response is the same for every micro-organism attacking the body. It responds immediately to protect the body from all foreign substances. The innate immune system provides 2 barriers that prevent entry to micro-organisms.

External body membranes

These include an intact skin and mucosa and are the first line of defence

- The skin:
  - Prevents entry of micro-organisms
  - Effective as long as the epidermis is unbroken
  - Provides a watertight barrier protecting internal organs
  - The acid of the skin secretions (pH of 3–5) inhibits bacterial growth

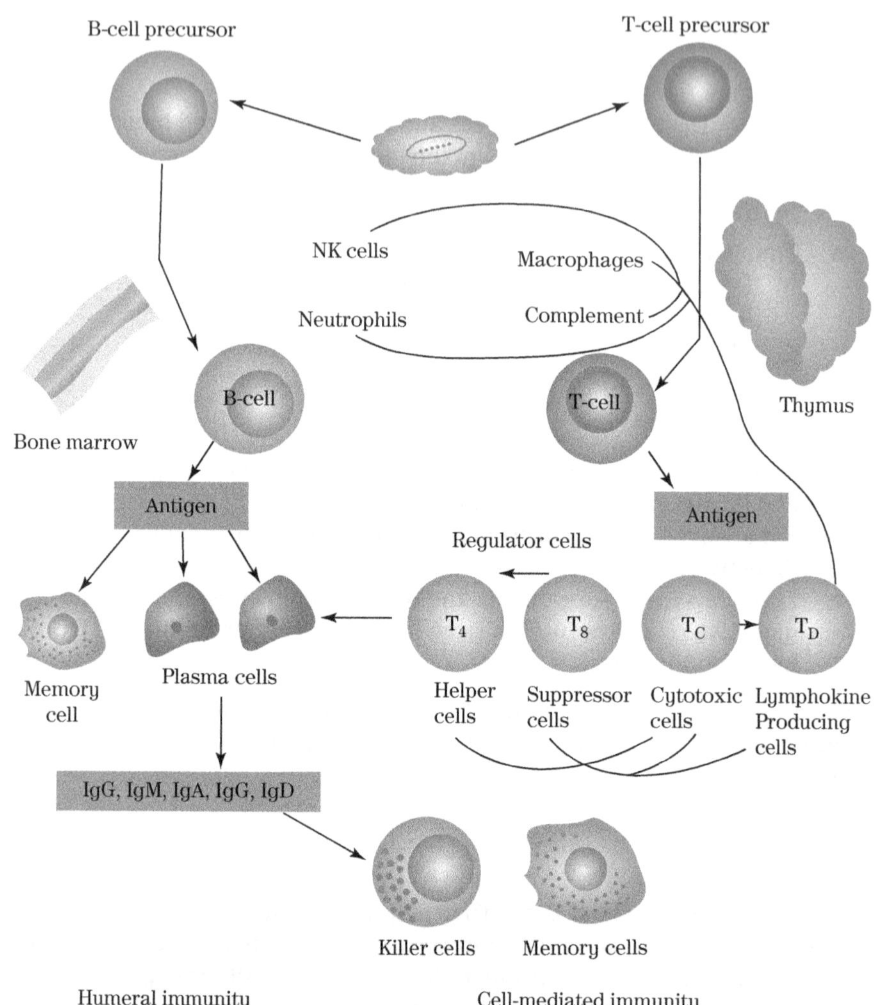

Figure 5.1 An overview of the immune system

- The sebum it secretes contains chemicals, which are toxic to bacteria
- Contains keratin, which presents a physical barrier to most micro-organisms

- Vaginal secretion
  - Acid medium of the vagina (pH 4.0–4.5) is maintained by the resident flora, notably *Lactobacillus*; acts upon the glycogen in the vagina to produce lactic acid, which forms a hostile environment for many fungi, bacteria and viruses

- Urine
  - A constant downward flow of urine through the ureter and bladder irrigates the urethra
  - The acid pH of urine tends to militate against ascending infections
  - The acidity of urine will kill most bacteria found in the urine
  - Effective response in the long male urethra, but less so in the female
- The stomach
  - Hydrochloric acid (pH 3) produced by the stomach and protein-digesting enzymes kill most organisms entering in food, drink or swallowed sputum
  - To a certain extent, the small and large intestines rely on the stomach's bactericidal activity
  - The resident flora of the large intestine such as *Escherichia coli*, non-haemolytic streptococci and anaerobic bacteroides ferment some of indigestible carbohydrates releasing acids and gases, and synthesise B complex vitamins and most of the vitamin K the liver requires to synthesise some clotting proteins
- Saliva
  - The buccal cavity is lined with a tough mucous membrane, which is irrigated by a constant backward flow of saliva (i.e. directed towards the throat)
  - The flow of saliva also prevents organisms from entering the salivary glands, and traps organisms, which can then be swallowed
- The nose and upper respiratory tract
  - Lined with small mucous-coated hairs, which trap small-inhaled particles
  - The mucosa of the upper respiratory tract is ciliated, sweep dust and bacteria laden mucus upward toward the mouth to be swallowed
  - Sneezing is a protective reflex, which expels irritants
  - Coughing is a defensive reflex, which removes particulate matter or excess mucus in the lower tract.

Internal body membranes

Even though the surface barriers are quite effective, they are breached occasionally by small cuts resulting from brushing your teeth or shaving. When this happens and micro-organisms manage to invade deeper tissues, the second innate defences come into play. This process uses chemical signals when the external defences are penetrated.

- Phagocytes engulf bacteria that get through the skin and mucosa into the underlying connective tissue 2 main types:

    - Neutrophils often called polymorphonuclear cells (PMNs) (see granulocytes)
        - Comprise the majority of blood leukocytes, making up 60% of all white blood cells
        - Release chemotaxic agents important for the killing of micro-organisms
        - Short lived, surviving for no more than a few days
        - Pivotal in stimulating the inflammatory response (Lydyard *et al*, 2000)
        - Monocytes develop in the bone marrow:
        - Circulate for 1 or 2 days in the blood, squeeze between cells of the blood-vessel wall and migrate into the tissues
        - Whereby they differentiate into macrophages, which make up only 6% of the white blood cells or leukocytes
        - Function is to dispose of micro-organisms and dead body cells through the process of phagocytosis. Can either be:
            - Free macrophages (monocytes) – which wander through the body's bloodstream in search of foreign invaders or cellular debris
            - Fixed macrophages such as the Kupffer cells in the liver and alveolar macrophages of the lungs are permanent residents of particular organs
- Natural killer cells (NKC):
    - Found throughout the tissues of the body, but mainly in the blood and lymph
    - Kill and lyse cancer cells and viruses before the immune system is activated
    - Will act against any target and can illuminate a variety of infected or cancerous cells by detecting the lack of 'self' cell surface membrane receptors
    - Not phagocytic, their mode of killing involves:
        - Attacking the target cell's membrane
        - Releasing several cytolytic chemicals to disintegrate the micro-organisms membrane and nucleus very rapidly
    - The potent chemicals enhance the inflammatory response
- Mast cells – found in connective tissues throughout the body, close to blood vessels and particularly in the areas of the respiratory, urogenital and gastrointestinal tracts
- Granulocytes
    - Neutrophils are the most numerous of the white blood cells (WBC), chemically attracted to sites of inflammation and are actively phagocytic and increase during acute bacterial infections

    - Oesinophils are in smaller amounts and attack parasites, which are too large for phagocytes to eat, and lessen severity of allergies by devouring the immune complexes
    - Basophils are the rarest WBC, present in very low numbers in the circulation
    - Granulated cells similar to basophils called mast cells, both bind to particular antibodies (immunoglobulin E), cause the release of histamine and prostaglandin, which attract other WBCs to the area
    - Both these cells are essential in the development of an acute inflammatory response
- Dendrite cells – present antigens to T and B cell lymphocytes (Lydyard *et al*, 2000).

Innate molecular defence against organisms

A variety of molecules mediate protection against pathogens during the period before specific immunity develops. Most of the molecules, which play a role in the innate immune system also, have functions associated with the specific immune system (Figure 5.1).

- Complement system provides a major mechanism for destroying foreign substances in the body:
    - Group of at least 20 plasma proteins
    - Normally circulate in the blood and body fluids in an inactive state
    - Activated directly by certain molecules associated with micro-organisms, or by antibodies bound to a pathogen or any other antigen, when activated:
        - Chemical mediators are released that amplify virtually all aspects of the (acute) inflammatory process
        - Attraction of neutrophils to the site of microbial attack (chemotaxis)
        - Enhancement of the attachment of the micro-organisms to the phagocyte (opsonisation) by coating the micro-organism and providing holders for the receptors of macrophages and neutrophils can adhere to, allowing them to engulf the particle more rapidly
        - Killing of the micro-organism activating the membrane attack complex (lysis)
    - A powerful mediator of inflammation and destruction can cause extensive damage to host cells if uncontrolled, luckily our cells are equipped with proteins that inactivate complement
    - Tightly regulated by inhibitory/regulatory proteins

  - Is part of innate immunity, but it complements and enhances both innate and specific immune defences
- Acute phase proteins are a group of plasma proteins that:
  - Work against bacteria and in limiting tissue damage caused by infection, trauma, malignancy and other diseases e.g. rheumatoid arthritis
  - Maximise activation of the complement system and opsonisation of invading pathogens. They include:
    - C-reactive protein (CRP)
    - Serum amyloid protein A (SAA)
    - Mannose binding protein (MBP)
- Interferon are proteins involved in protection against viral infections
  - Interferon is produced in response to particular viruses
- The inflammatory response is a localised response to invading micro-organism, triggered whenever body tissues are injured. Acute inflammation is caused by the release of inflammatory mediators from microbes, damaged tissue, mast cells and other leukocytes. The IR (see chapter 2):
  - Protects the body from invading micro-organisms and prevents the spread of damaging agents to nearby tissues
  - It limits the extent of blood loss and injury
  - Removes and disposes of dead cells, other debris and pathogens
  - Promotes rapid healing of involved tissues and as such is closely associated with wound healing
- High temperature or fever is a systemic response to invading microorganisms, this results in the hypothalamus thermostat is reset upward in response to chemicals called pyrogens which are secreted by leukocytes and macrophages exposed to bacteria and other foreign substances in the body (Marieb, 2012).

It is thought that specific immunity is not possible without the assistance of the mechanisms of innate immunity. This can occur in a number of ways (Figure 5.1).

Specific immunity

The specific immune response mounts an attack against particular foreign substances, and is different for each micro-organism. Specific immunity consists of lymphocytes, divided into 2 main classes:

- B-cells referred to as humoral immunity
- T-cells referred to as cell mediated immunity.

Specific immunity has the ability to target specific types of micro-organism and destroy them, and remember how this was achieved. The immune response is specific for individual stimulating antigens, which are substances that stimulate the immune system and cause an immune response. The features are:

- Specificity
- Diversity
- Memory.

It is an intricate system of cells, enzymes and proteins, which protects the body by making it resistant (immune) to infection.

Humoral immunity

The major cells involved in humoral immunity are the B-cell lymphocytes, which mature in the bone marrow.

The B-cell lymphocytes

- When exposed to an antigen B-lymphocytes become larger plasma cells:
  - Plasma cells are the result of B-cells preparing to destroy antigens
  - They grow larger (filled with plasma) and produce thousands of immunoglobulins (Ig antibodies) on their surfaces
  - Produce and secrete into the blood and lymph specific antibodies or immunoglobulins (Ig) in response to an antigen
  - Igs are Y-shaped groups of molecules which can alter their receptors at one end so that they can attach themselves to antigens so mediate phagocytosis
  - Some can stimulate the complement system of innate immunity, some die, some persist as memory cells that can be rapidly activated if exposed to same antigen
  - There are 5 classes of Ig:
    - IgG – makes up 70 + % of Ig, the smallest molecular weight, activates the classical pathway of the complement system
    - IgA – makes up 13% of Ig (90% in mucous membranes), very important as secreted in the body's secretions e.g. saliva, tears, colostrums, major Ig in mucosal secretions of nose, mouth, lungs, gut, etc.
    - IgM – makes up 6% of Ig, largest Ig and only found in large intravascular spaced, i.e. blood and lymph, a marker for acute infection
    - IgE – less than 1% of Igs are IgE, higher in atopic people, therefore associated with disease such as asthma and eczema, important in providing defence against parasites such as intestinal worms

        - IgD – makes up 18% of Ig, very small amounts only in the body, not much is known about IgD
    - Transported to the site of antigenic invasion leading to the destruction or neutralisation of the antigen
    - Two types = plasma cell and memory cell
    - B-memory cells are quickly stimulated if an individual is exposed to the same antigen, as the specific Ig for that particular antigen has been remembered and stored.

Cell mediated immunity

Does not make antibodies – is made up of T-cell lymphocytes.

- Some T lymphocytes need to pass through thymus to mature
- Re-enter circulation and settle in lymph and spleen
- Attach to antigens to destroy them
- Effective against fungi, intracellular viruses, parasites, foreign tissue transplants and cancer cells
- Reliant on cytotoxic T-cells, as these are the only T-cells that can directly attack and kill other cells, and other substances, such as:
    - Lysozymes
    - Macrophages
    - Interferon
- Secrete a variety of cytokines, which enhance the immune response, some of which regulate the function of other lymphocytes
- T-cells divide into four types:
    - T cytotoxic (killer) – Tc
        - Important in defence against viruses
        - They break up and hijack the cell DNA to produce hundreds and thousands of other viruses
        - Tc cells are capable of recognising infected cells and destroying them
        - Secrete cytotoxic substances (cytokines):
            - Lymphotoxins
            - Lymphokines
            - Interferon
            - Lysozymes
    - T helper – Th
        - Stimulate the immune system to proliferate and attack any antigens which enter the body
        - When the Th-cells come into contact, and interact, with an antigen, they release substances which help the Tc-cells and B-cells to react to that particular antigen
        - Assist plasma B-cells to secrete antibodies

    - Implicated in certain types of hypersensitivity reactions
    - Secrete interleukin-2 activated by interleukin 1 (IL-1) from macrophages
    - Interleukins also:
        - Amplify inflammatory responses
        - Elevate temperature
        - Aid scar tissue formation
        - Promote the release of cortisol
        - Stimulate mast cell production
- T suppressor – Ts
    - The purpose of these cells is to stop the immune system proliferation once an antigen has been destroyed
    - Failure to do so could cause the immune system to attack its own cells ('self' cells)
    - Limits the effect of cytotoxic secretions on self
    - Restrain killer and B-cell activities
    - Moderate responses
    - The regulation of the immune system depends upon the balance between Ts-cells and Th-cells
- The memory cells – Tm
    - These remember an encountered antigen and how it was destroyed
    - The memory cells are able to mobilise the immune system very quickly if re-infected with the same antigen
    - Known as secondary immunity and is very important
    - Retain the ability to recognise previously encountered antigens.

Primary response

- Occurs when first come into contact with specific antigen that has not been met before
- The response time is around 3–6 days after the antigen has entered the body
- Immune system remembers how to destroy this specific antigen.

Secondary response

- When the same antigen is encountered, memory cells come into play
- Immediately stimulate immune system, which can occur within hours after exposure and within 2–3 days the antibody blood levels are raised higher than that of the primary response
- IgG is released is important in this response
- This is the basis of immunisations and vaccinations.

Immunisation

Many deaths from infection could be prevented with immunisation. Because of immunisation, many serious diseases have almost disappeared from the UK but they are still around in other countries and they could return to the UK. Already some, such as TB, have returned to the UK. The childhood immunisation programme gives a child the best protection from many of these diseases.

Types of immunity:

- Natural immunity is obtained from parents
- Acquired immunity:
  - Active acquired immunity:
    - Natural exposure to an antigen (generally life long)
    - Immunisation either of the dead bacteria or its toxins
  - Passive acquired immunity:
    - Does not involve an immune response
    - P-antibodies or T-lymphocytes are given from a donor (human or animal) this is temporary.

Vaccination

A vaccine contains a small part of the bacterium or virus that causes a disease, or very small amounts of the chemicals produced by the bacterium. Vaccines are specially treated so that they do not cause the disease itself. Vaccines work by encouraging the body's immune system to make antibodies:

- If someone who has been vaccinated against a disease comes into contact with the disease, the antibodies will recognise it and be ready to protect the individual
- Immunisation does not just protect the individual – it can help to protect communities, especially those not vaccinated (herd immunity)
- This only occurs if there are sufficient people vaccinated against that disease to produce herd immunity
- Stimulates primary immune response, puts it into memory – when infected again it can be remembered – illness prevented
  - Poliomyelitis
    - Attenuated live oral vaccine (also known as the Sabin vaccination)
    - Excreted in the faeces for up to 6 weeks post-immunisation
    - An extremely small chance of developing polio from the vaccine – about 1 case in 1,500,000 doses used
    - There is a killed injected vaccine for those who may be immunosuppressed

- Diphtheria, tetanus, acellular pertussis (whooping cough) and poliomyelitis (DTP) and *Haemophilus influenza* (Hip)
  - Protects against diphtheria, tetanus and pertussis as well as *Haemophilus influenza* type B
  - DTP is a combination of diphtheria toxoid, tetanus toxoid and *Bordetella pertussis*
  - All 4 components are inactivated (killed) or toxoids – inactivated by treating with formaldehyde
  - Hib – cause of meningitis in very young
- Meningitis C
  - Inactivated vaccine which protects against infection by meningococcal group C bacterium which causes meningitis and meningococcal septicaemia
  - Babies and people aged 15–27 most at risk
  - The Men C vaccine was introduced in 1999
  - In 1998, there were 1530 cases of Men C meningitis and septicaemia and 150 people died and has now been a 90% drop in the number of under 1-year-olds who get meningitis C meningitis or septicaemia
- Measles, mumps and rubella (MMR)
  - Protects against measles, mumps and rubella
  - Live vaccine which contains egg protein
  - The 3 separate vaccines may have different side effects at different times
    - Fever and measles-type rash (6–20 days after)
    - Small bruise-like spots (very rarely) – within 6 weeks
    - Mild form of mumps (very rarely) after 3 weeks
    - Febrile convulsion (1:1000)
  - Should be at least 3 months between live vaccines
- Bacillus calmette-guerin vaccine (BCG)
  - Protects against TB (*Mycobacterium tuberculosis* or *Mycobacterium bovis*)
  - Live, attenuated strain derived from *Mycobacterium bovis*
  - Given intradermally
  - Promotes cell-mediated immunity
  - Blister or sore will appear where the injection occurs – may leave a small scar
- Hepatitis B
  - Inactivated viral surface antigen (HBsAg)
  - Made biosynthetically using recombinant DNA technology
  - Given to babies whose mothers or close family have been infected with hepatitis B
  - First dose is given within 2 days of birth

- Second dose at 1 month
- Third dose at 2 months
- Booster dose and blood test at 12 months.

PATHOPHYSIOLOGY OF BODY DEFENCE MECHANISMS

Factors that suppress the immune response

The innate immune response and specific immunity can be suppressed, and certain factors are known to reduce immunity. This might be due to:

- The individual patient's general condition
  - There are many body processes that deteriorate due to age; older adults are at greater risk from developing complications due to this
- The inability of the patient to take nutrition or fasting practices in hospital
  - Nutrition is required to produce the cells and molecules of innate immunity, as most phagocytes, complement, acute phase proteins, clotting factors, mediators are made from proteins, vitamins, minerals, carbohydrates and fats
  - Fasting practices observed on the wards, the mechanisms of inflammation cannot be switched off, and due to reduction in anti-inflammatory molecules, in this event can lead to serious complications, such as adult respiratory distress syndrome (ARDS), systemic inflammatory response syndrome (SIRS) and multisystem organ failure (MSOF)
  - Wound healing requires an adequate protein intake:
    - Proteins supply the amino acids necessary for repair and regeneration of tissues, and produce many of the proteins involved in the innate immune response
    - Fibrous tissue is protein based and hence scar tissue will have poorer tensile strength in those who are protein depleted
    - Vitamin A is necessary for re-epithelialisation and vitamin C is required for collagen synthesis and capillary integrity
    - Zinc deficiency is thought to be associated with delayed wound healing
    - Zinc supplements can help to promote venous ulcer healing in those with zinc depletion
    - A reduced nutrition affects the body's ability to fight infection
    - A patient admitted to hospital may have suppressed nutrition due to a medical condition
- Intravenous (IV) lines that pierce the skin

- It might be due to prescribed treatments or drug therapies:
    - Non-steroidal anti-inflammatory drugs (NSAIDs) – prescribed to relieve pain, work by reducing the release of prostaglandin during the inflammatory response and as such healing mechanism may also be delayed
    - Prostaglandin has a number of roles in the body:
        - Sends messages to the brain and pain may be felt
        - Simulates the inflammatory response and leads to swelling and pressure on localised nerve endings resulting in pain
        - Stimulates the clotting cascade, so any interference with its release can induce bleeding of the nose, vagina, from wounds etc.
        - It controls renal blood flow and if prostaglandin is reduced then glomerular filtration rate (GFR) will be reduced leading to sodium and water retention
    - Broad spectrum antibiotics – destroy invading bacteria but also devastate the normal flora present in the mucous membranes, destroying resident flora living in the mouth and vagina, allowing pathogens (commonly *Candida albicans*, which causes thrush) to colonise leading to fungal infections
    - Antacids neutralise the acidity of the gastric juice and can give rise to an increase in production of bacteria living in the stomach, small and large intestine, which can lead to diarrhoea
    - Chemotherapy and radiotherapy depress the bone marrow, which produces neutrophils and monocytes, which mature to become macrophages – increased risk of patients becoming neutropenic
    - Steroids such as corticosteroids are anti-inflammatory and suppress the immune response, which aids healing.

Stress and immunity

One of the earliest responses to injury is neuroendocrine activation, which is intimately linked to the stress response and the control of tissue function. The increased sympathetic activity affects almost all elements of the cardiovascular system, and stimulates a highly complex series of events that leads to stimulation of the peripheral sympathetic system and adrenal medulla resulting in the release of numerous substances into the circulation:

- Catecholamines – released via the adrenal medulla in response to IL-1 from damaged endothelium. The sympathetic nervous system is mobilised and the neurones secrete the catecholamines:
    - Adrenaline:

    - A potent stimulator of the heart and metabolic activities and as a result increases heart rate, cardiac output, metabolic rate and causes dilatation of bronchioles
    - Stimulates the conversion of glycogen from the liver and skeletal muscles to be converted into glucose raising blood glucose levels
  - Noradrenaline:
    - Causes peripheral vasoconstriction (together with an increase in heart rate raises blood pressure)
    - Blood is diverted from temporarily nonessential organs to the brain, heart and skeletal muscles (Marieb, 2012)
- Glucocorticoids (cortisol)
  - Regulated by a negative feedback system which is interrupted by acute stress and IL-1 release and via the sympathetic nervous system:
    - The hypothalamus releases corticotrophin releasing hormone (CRH)
    - The anterior pituitary gland in turn secretes adrenocorticotrophic hormone (ACTH)
  - Stimulates the release of cortisol from the adrenal cortex of the adrenal gland and leads to gluconeogenesis, glycogenolysis, proteolysis and lipolysis, anti-inflammatory and cell-protective events to prevent damage from excessive activation of the metabolic response
  - This process mobilises body proteins to be used as a source of energy:
    - To produce adenosine triphosphate (ATP) for the use by cells for body organ function (the heart, lungs, brain)
    - Causing a reduction in protein and other nutrients available for the production of innate immune system molecules and cells such as phagocytes, interferon, complement and reduces the body's own innate defence mechanisms
    - Leading to a reduction in phagocytes, interferon, complement and reduces the body's own innate defence mechanisms.

Hypersensitivities

Hypersensitivity reactions arise from the usual adaptive immune responses.

- The ways in which they work depends on immunological memory for a particular antigen or allergen
- The intensity increases with repeated exposure
- These reactions are exaggerated or inappropriate forms of adaptive responses

- The response damages one's own tissue in the process of producing the immune reaction directed at destruction of the foreign antigens.

Allergy

- In modern usage, allergy is synonymous with hypersensitivity
- The antigen capable of eliciting an allergic or hypersensitive state is known as an allergen
- Anergic means the opposite of allergic – i.e. the individual shows no immune response to an antigen that he/she has met previously
- There are 4 different types of allergic reactions, types I – IV:
  - Immunoglobulin IgE-mediated reaction – involving mast cells e.g. asthma or anaphylaxis
  - Tissue-specific reaction – IgG and IgM immunoglobulin involving macrophages in tissues e.g. some autoimmune diseases such as Graves disease
  - Immune complex-mediated reaction – IgG and IgM involving neutrophils e.g. systemic lupus erythematosus (SLE)
  - Cell-mediated reaction – no immunoglobulins involved involves lymphocytes and macrophages e.g. contact dermatitis or graft rejection.

Atopy and anaphylaxis

Atopic disorders

- Some individuals appear to be 'prone' to IgE mediated allergies – atopic
- Atopic individuals produce higher concentrations of IgE and have more Fc receptors on their mast cells
- There is a family history
  - In families in which one parent has an allergy – allergies develop in about 40% of the offspring
  - If both parents have atopic disease – the incidence in offspring is approximately 80%
- Atopic disorders include conditions such as:
  - Asthma – see chapter 9
  - Eczema
  - Hay fever.

Anaphylaxis

This is mediated through IgE-dependent mechanisms stimulated by food and drug allergies, bee and wasp stings (Figure 5.2).

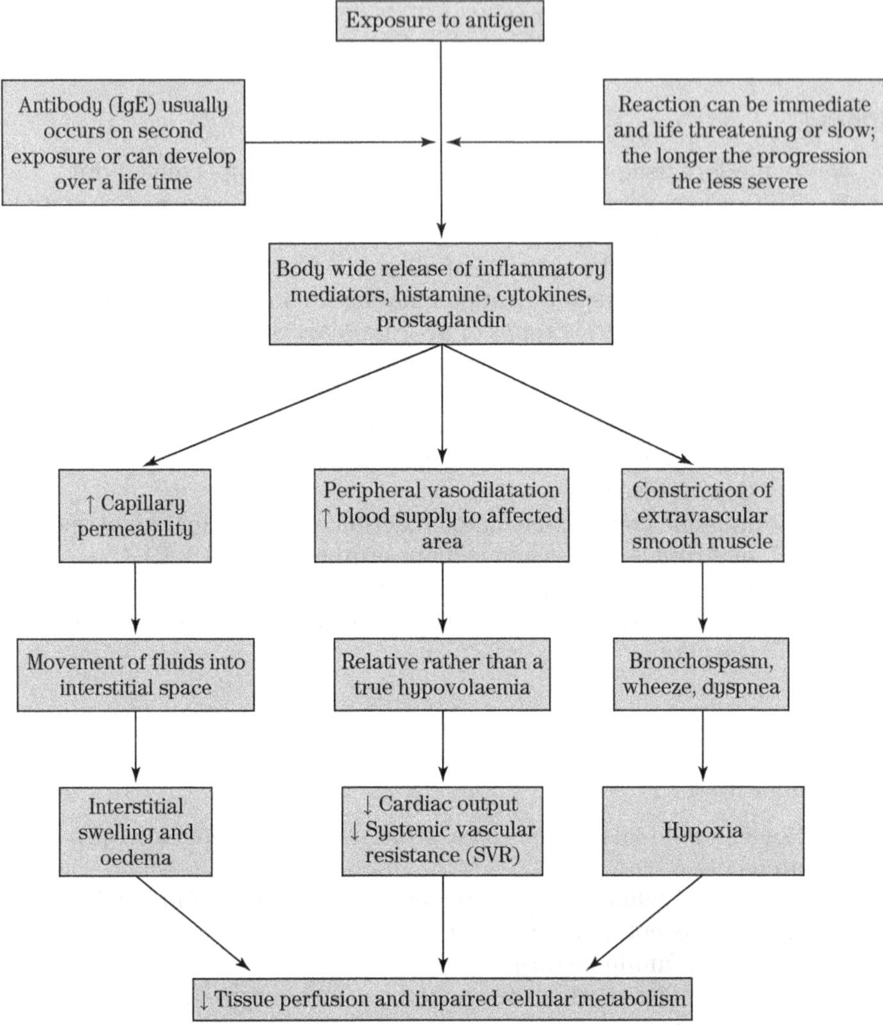

Figure 5.2 The progression of anaphylactic shock

Case study 5.1

David and his daughter Jane were walking and playing in the park. Jane had been eating peanuts; when she had finished the peanuts she ran and placed the empty packet in the nearest bin. Jane ran from the bin smiling to where her father was standing and clasped his hand. The traces of peanut oil on Jane's hand set off a potentially fatal allergic reaction in her father.

First, David began to itch, his hand began to swell and the skin blistered, then the arm and the rest of his body were affected. His face and mouth became so swollen that his breathing was restricted. A passer-by called the paramedics.

You arrive at the scene to find David's breathing is worse with inspiratory stridor, wheezing, a high respiratory rate and dizziness. David had since vomited.

Considerations in anaphylaxis are the variables that affect the course of the condition:

- Age:
  - The elderly are more at risk of developing late stage organ problems following anaphylaxis than a younger person due to:
    - Slowed blood circulation
    - Structural and functional changes in the skin
    - Decrease in heat-producing conservation activities
    - Slowed metabolic rate
    - Sedate lifestyle
    - Decreased vasoconstrictor response
- General state of health.

Aetiology

Anaphylaxis is a severe systemic allergic reaction, in which a person is hypersensitive to an antigen (Edwards, 2001):

- It can have a rapid and severe onset or it can be of slow and of less severe onset
- Anaphylaxis causes the cardiovascular system to fail to perfuse body tissues adequately bringing about a widespread disruption of cellular metabolism, which results in functional disturbances at organ/tissue level which affects:
  - Blood volume
  - Blood pressure
  - Cardiac function.

Pathology

- Atopy and anaphylaxis occur when a sensitised person is exposed to an antigen (a substance they are allergic to) – an allergic reaction
- The antigen enters the body and combines with immunoglobulin E (IgE) antibodies (antigen-antibody reaction) on the surface of mast cells and basophils found in:

  - The lungs
  - Small intestines
  - Skin
  - Connective tissue
- An antigen-antibody reaction occurs which induces abnormal over-stimulation of the inflammatory immune response bodywide (Edwards, 2001)
- The consequences are the release of mediators from mast cells and basophils into the blood:
  - Histamine and prostaglandins cause:
    - Extreme vasodilatation, this results in:
      - Reduced cardiac output
      - Low arterial pressure
      - Cellular perfusion fails to meet the metabolic demands
    - Selective vasoconstriction in the:
      - Pulmonary bed
      - Hepatic circulation
      - Other large veins
  - Cytokine activation
- This causes the movement of circulating fluids into the interstitial space causing a relative hypovolaemia and shock (Figs 2.2 Cellular death and 2.3 The inflammatory immune response).
- This leads to:
  - Reduced systemic vascular resistance (SVR) and cardiac output (CO)
  - Reduced cellular perfusion inadequate flow of nutrients and oxygen to the cell
  - Disruption to the cellular membrane
  - Changes in cardiac function
  - Reduced contractility and dysrhythmias may occur.

Clinical features

- Urticaria
  - itching
  - raised wheals diffusely distributed and evanescent
- Angio-oedema
  - Tingling
  - Swelling of lips, eyes, hands
  - No heat or erythema
- Laryngeal oedema
  - Hoarseness
    - Dysphagia

        - Lump in throat
        - Airway obstruction
        - Sudden death
    - Inspiratory stridor leading to cyanosis
- Bronchospasm
    - Cough, dyspnoea, chest tightness
    - Wheezing, high respiratory rate
- Severe bronchospasm
    - Chronic inflammatory changes
    - Pulmonary oedema
    - Mucous plugging/reduced tidal volume/atelectasis
    - Airway obstruction/difficulty in breathing
    - Tachypnoea, hypoxia, cyanosis
- Hypotension
    - Dizziness
        - Syncope
        - Confusion
    - Hypotension (mild to severe), tachycardia, oliguria
- Rhinitis
    - Nasal congestion
        - Itching and fluid accumulation in the upper airways
        - Mucosal oedema
- Conjunctivitis
    - Tears and itching
    - Lid oedema
- Gastroenteritis
    - Cramping
        - Diarrhoea
        - Vomiting
    - Normal on examination.

Investigations

- This is an emergency and therefore two potentially life-threatening features should be present for diagnosis:
    - Respiratory difficulty due to laryngeal oedema
    - Hypotension.

Treatment and drug therapy

Emergency management (Resuscitation Council, 2005):

- Reassure patient
- Immediately assess responsiveness and severity of condition
- Immediately stop possible cause of anaphylaxis

- Immediately assess:
  - Airway
  - Breathing
  - Circulation
- If unconscious instigate full cardio-pulmonary resuscitation (CPR) procedures
- Call for additional nursing support from within the clinical area
- Call cardiac arrest team if available/call for an ambulance
- Need to have access to adrenaline immediately
  - IM injection related adult/child dose
  - Epipen fixed delivery doses 2 strengths:
    - 0.3 ml 1:1000
    - 0.3 ml 1:2000
- If in doubt, it is safer to give adrenaline than withhold it if anaphylaxis is developing
- If the patient remains conscious:
  - If feeling faint lie flat and elevate legs to help hypotension
  - If respiratory difficulty sit up and administer 100% oxygen (if available)
- Monitor (if available):
  - Blood pressure
  - Attach ECG monitor
- Reassess patient – 1st line drug treatment may need to be repeated in 5 minutes if no clinical improvement (Johnson and Peebles, 2004)
- If available/possible ensure patient has a patent cannula – IV fluids may be required later
- Obtain other drugs that may be prescribed:
  - Chlorphenamine
  - Hydrocortisone
  - Salbutamol
- Take notes and document/record in relevant notes, and give to the ambulance when it arrives:
  - The time the injection was given
  - Used syringe
  - Any personal details
- If patient recovered may need to get a detailed history, if cause not immediately obvious
- Ensure adequate follow up/admission to ward.

Prevention of complications and organ dysfunction

- Some organs bear the brunt of a decrease in systemic pressure e.g.:
  - Kidneys – the renal tubules can undergo necrosis and acute kidney injury

    - Lungs – respiratory failure can occur if treatment is not instigated immediately
    - Heart failure of the circulatory pump and insufficient oxygen delivery
    - Brain is the most susceptible to hypoxic injury and irreversible brain injury can occur
    - Gastro-intestinal tract (GIT) suffers early when there is a reduction in oxygen delivery and produces large amounts of lactic acid.

Continuous care

- Allergy clinics
    - Serology allergy testing
    - Total and specific IgE antibodies to allergen
- Desensitisation:
    - Immunotherapy
        - Weekly injections for 3 months
        - Reduced dose of venom/stings
        - Maintenance dose monthly or increase in intervals of 3 years
    - Expensive, generally unnecessary and can be dangerous
- The role of the dietician:
    - Exclusion in diet
    - Adequacy of diet
- Alternative therapies
    - Homeopathy
    - Acupuncture
    - Hypnosis.

Autoimmune disease

The response of the immune system against self, protected by self-tolerance, affects about 5–7% of the population. May be:

- Organ specific
- Systemic.

Organ specific

- *Aetiology*
    - Organ specific diseases include:
        - Addison's disease – adrenal glands
        - Haemolytic anaemia – RBC membrane protein and destruction of erythrocytes

    - Graves' disease – thyroid stimulating hormone (TSH) over-stimulation of the thyroid gland
    - Hasimoto's thyroiditis – thyroid proteins uptake of iodine is reduced leading to a reduced production of thyroid hormones
    - Type 1 diabetes mellitus – destruction of the pancreatic beta cells
    - Myasthenia gravis – antibodies to acetylcholine receptors on muscle cells are gradually destroyed leading to progressive muscle weakness
    - Pernicious anaemia is a failure to absorb vitamin B_{12} in the stomach, as antibodies destroy the intrinsic factor released by gastric parietal cells.
- *Pathology*
  - Immune response is directed to a target antigen unique to a single organ or gland
  - Manifestations limited to that organ
  - Organ may be subjected to direct cellular damage or may be stimulated or blocked by antibodies
  - Lymphocytes or antibodies bind to cell membrane antigen causing lysis and/or an IR
  - The cellular structure of the organ is replaced by connective tissue and the organ function declines.

Systemic autoimmune disease

- *Aetiology*
  - Systemic auto-immune diseases include:
    - Ankylosing spondylitis – vertebrae
    - Multiple sclerosis – white matter in CNS is destroyed leading to inflammation affecting the nervous system (see chapter 10)
    - Rheumatoid arthritis – connective tissue IgG (see chapter 12)
    - Systemic lupus erythematosus (SLE) – Inflammatory disorder involving a number of body systems, antibodies to DNA, nuclear protein, RBC and platelet membranes
- *Pathology*
  - The response is directed towards a large number of target antigens and involves a number of organs and tissues
  - A defect in immune regulation which results in hyperactive T and B cells
  - Tissue damage is widespread both from cell mediated immune responses and from direct cellular damage caused by auto-antibodies

- *Treatment and drug therapies*
  - Aimed at reducing the autoimmune response but leaving the rest of the immune system intact
  - Current therapies available are palliative
  - Reduce symptoms to ensure a reasonable quality of life
  - Immuno-suppressive drugs to slow down proliferation of lymphocytes
  - Increased risk of infection and cancer
  - Removal of thymus gland for myasthenia gravis
  - Plasmapheresis may help some patients.

Immune deficiencies

Immune deficiency disorders result from impaired function of one or more of the components of the immune system, resulting in a susceptibility to infection (McCance and Huether, 2010).

Primary immune deficiencies

- *Aetiology*
  - Primary deficiencies are caused by a genetic anomaly:
    - SCIDS (severe combined immune deficiencies)
    - X-linked agammaglobulinaemia
    - Wiskot Aldrich syndrome
    - Complement deficiency
    - Neutropenia
    - Chronic granulomatous disease (CGD)
    - Common variable immunodeficiency (CVID)
- *Pathology*
  - In the primary immune deficiency conditions there is a single gene defect:
    - A family history is rare, but the condition usually occurs in utero and before birth
    - Sometimes the signs and symptoms of one of the conditions does not appear until after the first 2 years of life
- *Clinical features*
  - Susceptibility to infection
  - Severe documented pneumonia
  - Recurrent otitis media
  - Sinusitis
  - Bronchitis
  - Septicaemia or meningitis
  - Opportunistic infections microorganisms that are usually not pathogenic lead to infection in unusual sites

- *Treatment*
  - Antibiotics
  - Antiviral drugs
  - Antifungal drugs
  - Monoclonal antibodies
  - Immunoglobulin replacement
  - Cyclosporin A
  - Cytotoxic chemotherapy
  - Radiation therapy
  - Gene therapy
  - Bone marrow transplants
  - Peripheral blood stem cell transplants
  - Cord blood transplants
  - Nutrition
  - Isolation (temporary)

Secondary immune deficiencies

- These are far more common, and are complications of other conditions, such as:
  - Medical interventions e.g. chemotherapy, radiation/radiation therapy, steroids
  - Trauma
  - Metabolic diseases e.g. diabetes, cystic fibrosis, alcoholic liver disease, sickle cell disease, SLE
  - Malignancies
  - Dietary insufficiencies e.g. malnutrition
  - Physiological stress
  - Infections e.g. rubella, hepatitis B, HIV and AIDS – HIV mainly replicates and destroys T_4 helper cells and eventually reduces the effectiveness of the whole immune system, as T_4 cells play a major role in establishing an immune response (Figure 5.1).

SEPTIC SHOCK

Septic shock is the end product of a progressive dysfunction beginning with systemic inflammatory response syndrome (SIRS), then sepsis, then severe sepsis and finally septic shock (McCance and Huether, 2010).

Aetiology

- Suspected or known infection
- SIRS

  - Any major insult to the body:
    - Burns
    - Acute pancreatitis
    - Myocardial infarction
    - Trauma
- 6 most common infection sites
  - Pneumonia
  - Bloodstream
  - Intravascular catheter
  - Intra-abdominal
  - Urine/kidney
  - Surgical wound infection.

Pathology

- The significant change in severe sepsis or septic shock are an exaggeration of the normal immune response to infection or an insult (Robson *et al*, 2005)
- Inflammation should normally be restricted to the site of infection or insult
- In septic shock the inflammatory response is over stimulated or can not be switched off by suppressor cells of specific immunity and inflammatory mediators enter the bloodstream:
  - Histamine
  - Prostaglandins
  - Cytokines:
    - Tumour necrosis factor
    - Interleukins
- Blood vessels dilate causing blood pressure to drop
- Capillaries become permeable to water leading to widespread oedema
- This produces a hypovolaemia leading to hypotension
- Coagulation becomes activated and small blood clots form, which can interfere with blood flow to major organs
- The combined hypotension, hypovolaemia and micro-emboli can lead to poor perfusion and organ failure.

(See Figure 5.3).

Clinical features

- SIRS
  - High or low temperature more than 38°C or less than 36°C
  - Heart rate more than 90 bpm
  - Respiratory rate more than 20 bpm or arterial carbon dioxide partial pressure (PCO_2) of less than 4.2 kpa

  - High or low white blood cell (WBC) count more than 12,000 per millilitre or less than 4000 per millilitre
- Severe sepsis
  - Hypotension a systolic >90 mmHg, MAP >60 mmHg or 40 mmHg from patients normal without other cause of hypotension
  - Poor perfusion capillary refill <2 seconds
  - Altered mental state confused, disorientated

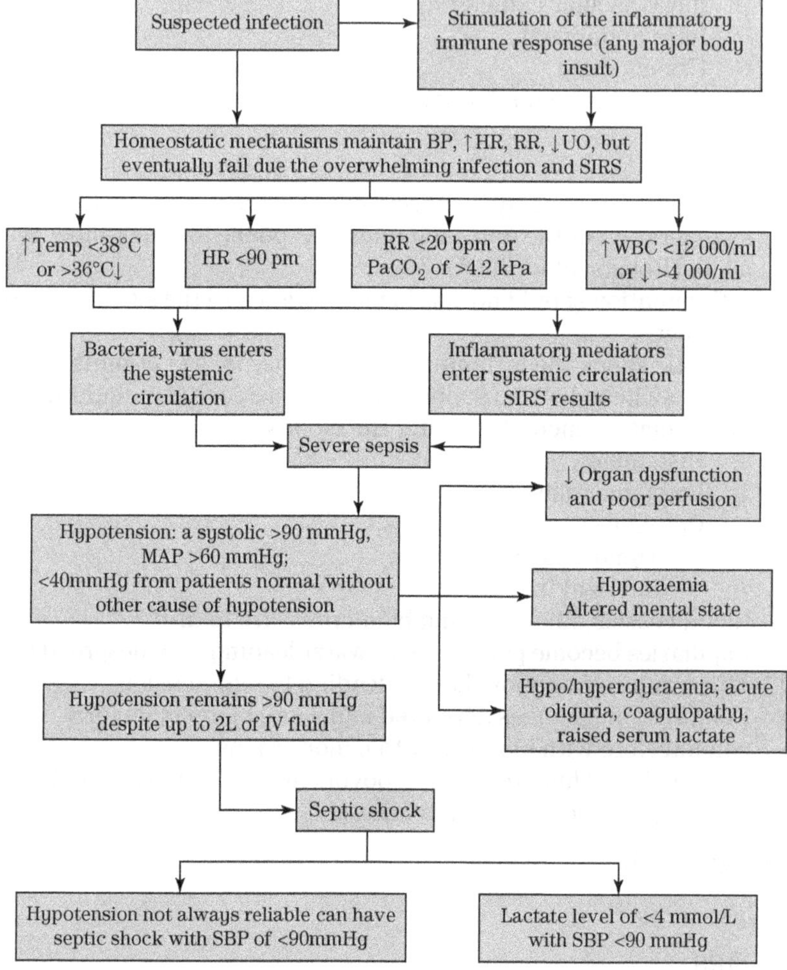

RR = respiratory rate; HR = heart rate; bpm = breaths per minute; bpm = beats per min; SBP = systolic BP; SIRS = systemic inflammatory response syndrome; MAP = mean arterial pressure

Figure 5.3 The progression of septic shock

  - Hyperglycaemia/hypoglycaemia measure blood glucose level (BGL)
  - Hypoxaemia measure oxygen saturation level or ABGs
  - Acute oliguria check urine output should not be <0.5 ml/kg/hr
  - Bloods to check coagulopathy and for raised serum lactate
  - Raised serum lactate
  - All organs can be affected the cardiovascular, lungs, liver, kidneys and brain
- Septic shock
  - Hypotension that does not respond to adequate fluid resuscitation
  - Systolic blood pressure remains at 90 mmHg despite receiving 2 litres of IV fluid
  - Septic shock can be observed in patients with a blood pressure of above 90 mmHg, and hypotension alone is not always a reliable indicator of septic shock
  - Lactate level of more than 4 mmol/L and a blood pressure less than 90 mmHg – patient considered to have septic shock.

Investigations

- Baseline observations and vital signs:
  - Heart rate
  - Blood pressure
  - Temperature
  - Respirations
  - Oxygen saturation
  - Level of consciousness
- Venous blood specimens for:
  - Full blood count (FBC)
  - Urea and creatinine to check renal function
  - Electrolytes as a low bicarbonate level (less than 20 mmol/L) can be an indicator that lactate is high
  - Glucose screen shows a high or low glucose level in the absence of diabetes
  - Clotting screen such as the international normalised ratio (INR) normal value should be >1.5
  - Blood cultures (taken before antibiotics are commenced)
  - Haematocrit levels
  - Liver function tests (LFT)
- Arterial blood specimen for:
  - Arterial blood gases (ABGs)
  - Arterial lactate is an indicator of tissue perfusion and >4 mmol/L
- Urine catheter to measure urine output oliguria is a sign of renal impairment.

Practice point

It is important to remember that due to homeostatic mechanisms BP will be maintained at all cost and as such BP is not a good indicator of shock. Therefore, all other observations and investigations given above should be interpreted together, and patterns of deterioration or improvement should be noted.

Treatment

- Treatment generally follows the surviving sepsis campaign guidelines for managing severe sepsis outlined by Dellinger *et al* (2004) and Rivers *et al* (2001):
  - Oxygen therapy
  - IV broad-spectrum antibiotics administered promptly
  - IV fluid challenges of approximately 500 ml up to total of 2 L
  - If no improvement then commence inotropic support
  - Add noradrenaline if patient does not respond
  - Blood transfusion if haematocrit is low
  - Insertion of central venous pressure (CVP) line and maintain between 8–12 mmHg
  - Mechanical ventilation may be required (Peel, 2008).

CONCLUSION

The immune system provides defence against disease. It includes a diverse set of cellular interactions and chemicals. Innate immunity includes a variety processes and responses that prevent invasion by microorganisms. Specific immunity provides B-cells, which produce antibodies against bacteria, and T-cells, which destroy foreign antigens such as viruses and cancer cells. These systems are closely interlinked, each amplifying the response to improve defences or blocking the response to reduce defences when the crisis is over.

SELF-ASSESSMENT QUESTIONS

1. Provide an outline of the structure and distribution of lymphatic vessels, lymph transport and lymph organs and note their important functions.

2. Explain innate immunity, its protective functions and the specific function of the inflammatory immune response.
3. What is the humoral immune response and its relationship to B lymphocyte immunity?
4. What is cell-mediated immune response and its relationship to T lymphocyte immunity?
5. Explain the mechanisms of immune system dysfunctions.

REFERENCES

Dellinger, R.P., Carlet, J.M. and Masur, H. (2004) Surviving sepsis campaign guidelines for management of severe sepsis and septic shock, *Critical Care Medicine*, 32(3), 858–873.

Edwards, S.L. (2001) Shock: types classifications and explorations of the physiological effects, *Emergency Nurse*, 9(2), 29–38.

Johnson, R.F. and Peebles, R.S. (2004) Anaphylactic shock: pathophysiology, recognition and treatment, *Seminars in Respiratory Critical Care Medicine*, 25(6), 695–703.

Lydyard, P.M., Whelen, A. and Fanger, M.W. (2000) *Instant Notes on Immunology*, Oxford: BIOS Scientific.

Marieb, E. (2012) *Essentials of Human Anatomy and Physiology*, 9th edn, San Francisco, CA: Benjamin Cummings.

McCance, K.L. and Huether, S.E. (2010) *Pathophysiology: The Biologic Basis for Disease in Adults and Children*, 6th edn, Missouri: Mosby Elsevier.

Peel, M. (2008) Care bundles: resuscitation of patients with severe sepsis, *Nursing Standard*, 23(11), 41–46.

Resuscitation Council UK (2005) *The emergency Medical Treatment of Anaphylactic Reactions for First Medical Responders and for Community Nurses*, London: Resuscitation Council UK.

Rivers, E., Nguyen, B. and Havstad, S. (2001) Early goal directed therapy in the treatment of severe sepsis and septic shock, *New England Journal of Medicine*, 345(19), 1368–1377.

Robson, W., Newell, J. and Beavis, S. (2005) Severe sepsis in A&E, *Emergency Nurse*, 13(5), 24–3.

6 Cellular proliferation and cancer

Ann Richards

A tumour or neoplasm is a mass of cells produced by abnormal cell proliferation. Some neoplasms are benign and do not spread to other areas of the body. An example is a lipoma which is a fatty growth that commonly occurs on the back. It is unsightly but harmless and can be easily removed as it is enclosed in a capsule. Other tumours spread and are malignant. These are called cancers (from the Latin for 'crab') and occur when a cell multiplies without control. The tumour has no capsule and may spread locally invading and destroying adjacent tissues, or spread to distant areas of the body via the lymphatic system or the bloodstream.

Cancer is the second commonest cause of death in the UK after cardiovascular disease. There are over 200 different types of cancer and this abnormal cell growth can occur in almost any tissue in the body. The study of tumours is oncology.

NAMING TUMOURS

Tumours are named according to the body tissue they originate within.

- Benign tumours usually end in *–oma* which is added to the tissue of origin e.g. lipoma, adenoma (glandular tissue)
- Carcinoma is a general term that refers to all cancers of epithelial tissue. These are the commonest cancers as epithelial tissue is constantly being replaced as it covers and lines the body. It is because of the constant cell growth needed that there is more chance of mutations occurring and a cell becoming cancerous
- An adenocarcinoma is a cancer of glandular tissue
- Sarcoma is a general name for cancers originating in connective tissue such as bone e.g. osteosarcoma (arising in bone)
- Cancers of the blood are leukaemias.

CAUSES OF CANCER

There is no one cause of cancer and carcinogenesis is a multistage process. Cancer is a multifactorial disease and although we know the risk factors for some types of cancer there are others that we do not understand. We are going to look at some of the known causes or risk factors for certain cancers here.

Most cancers occur because of a mutation within the genetic material (DNA) in the cell nucleus. Most cells are dividing at different rates throughout their lives and at any of these cell divisions mistakes could occur that cause a cell to start reproducing in an uncontrolled manner. Usually there are DNA repair proteins that will put right any mistakes that occur but if there is a lack of repair protein, the mistake cannot be corrected. Cells also communicate with each other and if cells start to multiply and contact other cells, growth is stopped. If this growth signalling goes wrong, contact inhibition fails to occur.

- The risk of some cancers is genetically transmitted. An example is familial breast cancer caused by mutations in the BRCA1 and BRCA2 genes. The protein in these cells cannot bind a DNA repair enzyme, Rad51, so that it can repair DNA breaks. This makes breast cancer much more likely in the woman's lifetime and some of those carrying these genes have had a bilateral mastectomy as a preventative measure. Other common cancers where there is a genetic predisposition include cancer of the colon
- Lifestyle and the environment e.g. some chemicals are carcinogens and have a direct link to cancer. One example here is cigarette smoke that is linked to lung cancer. Other carcinogens include radiation. Melanoma is linked to exposure to the ultraviolet rays of strong sunshine
- Dietary factors are important but still not fully understood. Eating too much red and processed meat appears to be linked to gastric and bowel cancer and eating more than 5 portions of fruit and vegetables daily appears to be protective. Heavy consumption of alcohol is linked to a higher incidence of mouth and throat cancer
- Age is an important risk factor and most cancers occur more frequently in the elderly. This is partly because cell mutations may accumulate over time and exposure to carcinogens within the environment has been occurring for a longer period. There have to be a number of changes to the DNA within a cell before it becomes cancerous and the immune system is less efficient at preventing the growth of abnormal cells as we age
- Viruses – some cancers such as cervical cancer (human papilloma virus – HPV) and certain lymphomas (Epstein-Barr virus) are linked to viruses. Hepatitis B and C viruses are linked to primary liver cancer.

This may be an increasing list as we discover more about the long-term effect of viruses on the cell. Not everyone who has been infected with these viruses develops cancer and other factors are involved
- Bacteria were not thought to be involved in cancer but it has now been found that stomach cancer may be linked to infection with *Helicobacter pylori*, a bacterium that causes inflammation of the stomach lining and can be treated by a combination of antibiotics (chapter 11)
- If the immune system is compromised cancer is more likely. Examples include people who have had organ transplants and are taking drugs to decrease the activity of the immune system in order to lessen the risk of organ rejection. People with AIDS are also more at risk of certain cancers
- Some cancers are hormone dependent, for example oestrogen dependent breast cancers.

OCCURRENCE RATES

- Breast cancer is the commonest cancer in women, worldwide
- Prostate cancer is the commonest cancer in men in the developed world
- Colorectal cancer is the third most common cancer in men and the second in women, worldwide. The regional incidence rates vary up to 10-fold, though being highest in Eastern Europe
- In men, in 2011, lung cancer caused most deaths (22% of all cancer deaths), followed by prostate cancer (13%) then bowel cancer (10%). In women lung cancer caused 21% of all cancer deaths, breast cancer 15% and bowel cancer 9%. These figures are from Cancer Research UK.

SPREAD

A malignant primary tumour (cancer) is capable of spreading both locally into surrounding tissues and to distant areas of the body where secondary tumours (metastases) may develop.

- Cancer cells are fragile and can break off from the tumour. They may be carried in the lymphatic drainage of that area to the nearest lymph gland. Here, they are trapped, rather like a sieve. The cancer cell is capable of multiplying in its new site though and a swollen lymph gland may occur. The cancer may spread to other lymph glands via the lymphatic system. Breast cancer spreads to the axillary lymph nodes and these are biopsied when breast cancer is present

- Some cancer cells may penetrate the walls of blood vessels and be carried within the circulation to distant organs of the body where a secondary tumour is produced. Veins are thinner than arteries and so cancer tends to follow the venous system. Different cancers tend to spread to different areas of the body. An example is breast cancer which commonly spreads to the brain, bronchus or bone. The cells that produce the tumour in these distant organs are still breast cells however and the tumour is not bronchial cancer but metastatic breast cancer. Cancers of the gut commonly produce liver metastases (as venous blood from the gut goes to the liver via the hepatic portal vein, this is not surprising)
- Cancer cells may also spread across membranes and into body cavities. An example here is the spread of ovarian cancer into the peritoneal cavity producing ascites and the spread of lung cancer into the pleural space
- Sometimes metastases (secondary tumours) are found without a primary tumour being detected and the primary tumour may never be found.

DETECTION AND DIAGNOSIS

- Screening can be done to detect the presence of cancer in an asymptomatic person. Breast, cervical and bowel cancer screening are examples but screening is not possible for all cancers
- Sometimes screening is targeted at high risk individuals such as those with a strong family history. Colonoscopy rather than the testing for occult blood in the faeces is used in those with a strong family history of colon cancer
- Once a patient is symptomatic then investigations will be done. The symptoms may be due to the primary tumour or the metastases or even be paraneoplastic where they are not directly due to the local presence of the cancer but perhaps because of hormones or cytokines released by the tumour
- There may be other non-specific symptoms such as lethargy, weight loss and tiredness.

STAGING OF CANCERS

- Staging is done to guide treatment and prognosis for the patient. Staging systems vary according to the type of tumour but the TNM (tumour, node, metastases) system is the commonest one for solid tumours

- The tumour is staged according to the size of the primary tumour, the presence of lymph nodes and the detection of metastases
- An example of TNM classification for breast cancer is shown in Figure 6.1. The cancer research website at www.cancerresearchuk.org/cancer-help/type/breat-cancer/treat,ment/tnm-breast-cancer-

T is for tumour and the T stages assess the size of the tumour		
TX	The size cannot be assessed	
Tis	Ductal cancer in situ	
T1	2 cm across or less	Can be further divided (T1a, T1b etc.)
T2	More than 2cm, less than 5 cm across	
T3	More than 5 cm across	
T4	The tumour has spread locally	Can be further divided depending on whether the spread is into the chest wall, the overlying skin or both
N is nor nodes and the N stage assesses the spread into the lymph nodes		
NX	Lymph nodes cannot be assessed	(lymph nodes may have been removed)
N0	No cancer found in nearby nodes	
N1	Cancer cells in the upper levels of lymph nodes in the axilla	Not fixed to underlying tissue
N2a	Cancer cells in axilla	Fixed to underlying tissue
N2b	Cancer cells in internal mammary lymph nodes	No evidence of cancer cells in axilla
N3a	Cancer cells in lymph nodes below collar bone	
N3b	Cancer cells in axilla and internal mammary nodes	
N3c	Cancer cells in lymph nodes above the collar bone	
M is for metastases		
M0	No sign the cancer has spread to other parts of the body	
M1	The cancer has spread to other parts of the body	Commonest are the brain, bone and lung
(Adapted from information at Cancer Research UK, 2014)		

Figure 6.1 The TNM Classification System for Breast Cancer

staging has some excellent diagrams that will help you to understand the staging method.

TREATMENT

- The patient with cancer needs to be managed by a multidisciplinary team (MDT). The team depends on the type of cancer but may include a surgeon, an oncologist, a radiologist, a physician, a specialised nurse and a dietician
- The treatment plan should be discussed with the patient at each stage so that they can make informed choices about their own care and management
- If a tumour is surgically removed there may be adjuvant therapy after the removal such as radiotherapy, hormone treatment or chemotherapy
- This may be given even if there are no metastases detectable as there may be micrometastases that have not been detected.
- Sometimes treatment may be given before surgery in an attempt to shrink the tumour
- Individual cancers are described in the relevant chapters of the book.

Chemotherapy

- The aim here is to prevent the cancer cell dividing and there are many different chemotherapy drugs in use
- They do not just affect the division of the cancer cell but also the division of normal body cells that are rapidly dividing in the bone marrow and the gut
- This leads to side effects such as a low white cell count and susceptibility to infection, low platelets and a tendency to bleed, anaemia, a sore mouth (due to failure to replace the epithelial cells) and sterility which may not be reversible
- Chemotherapy is given in cycles to reduce these side effects. Normal cells recover faster than cancer cells and some normal functioning can occur between treatments
- Some chemotherapy agents have a direct effect on the vomiting centre and cause severe nausea and vomiting. An example is cisplatin
- Antiemetics such as ondansetron must be given alongside the therapy.

Radiotherapy

- Radiation is used to cause dividing cells to die by breaking strands of DNA in the nucleus
- It is commonly used as a treatment in lung cancer but does have complications such as redness of the skin (erythema), nausea, vomiting, diarrhoea and mouth ulcers as well as general side effects such as loss of energy and lethargy.

Endocrine therapy

- Some breast cancers are oestrogen dependent and some prostate cancers are androgen dependent
- It is possible to block the effects of these hormones and so prevent them acting as growth factors
- Tamoxifen is an example of such a drug used in some breast cancers. Flutamide is an androgen blocker used to treat prostate cancer.

Other therapies

- Most of these involve the administration of protein molecules that are made by genetic engineering
- The group includes interferons which are antiproliferative, interleukin 2 used in renal cell carcinoma and melanoma and anti-growth factors such as cetuximab which is added to chemotherapy to enhance the response and erythropoietin used to stimulate red cells in anaemia.

CONCLUSION

This chapter has introduced the subject of abnormal cellular proliferation and cancer. It has looked at the naming of tumours, their spread around the body and the means of staging the disease. It can be seen that cancer is a very wide and complex subject area where our knowledge is incomplete. Treatments vary according to whether the tumour is operable or responds well to chemotherapy or radiotherapy. Cancers affecting various parts of the body are looked at in the relevant chapters of the book.

SELF-ASSESSMENT QUESTIONS

1. Describe what is meant by the term 'cancer'.
2. List six possible risk factors for cancer.

3. Describe how cancer may spread from its primary site and around the body.
4. Explain what is meant by the 'staging' of a cancer.
5. Describe what is meant by 'screening' for cancer.
6. List three possible treatments for cancer.

FURTHER READING

Cancer Research UK at www.cancerresearchuk.org/cancer-help/type/breat-cancer/treat,ment/tnm-breast-cancer-staging (accessed 2nd March 2014).

Herrington C.S. (ed.) (2014) *Muir's Textbook of Pathology,* 15th edn, London: CRC Press.

Richards A. and Edwards S. (2012) *A Nurse's Survival Guide to the Ward,* Edinburgh: Elsevier.

7 Diseases of the blood (haematological disorders)

Ann Richards

Blood is examined in the diagnosis of disease more than any other tissue, not only due to its accessibility but also because most disease processes will be reflected by changes in composition of the blood.

FUNCTIONS OF THE BLOOD

Blood and the cardiovascular system link the body's internal and external environments.

Blood is not only important in transporting oxygen and nutrients throughout the body but is also involved in regulation and protection against disease. These functions can be divided into the three areas of transport, regulation and protection.

Transport

- Delivery of oxygen from the lungs to the tissues
- Delivery of nutrients from the digestive tract to the body cells
- Transport of metabolic waste products from the cells to the kidneys for elimination
- Transport of carbon dioxide from the cells to the lungs for excretion
- Transport of hormones from their endocrine glands to their target cells
- Transport of inorganic ions such as sodium, potassium and chloride (electrolytes)
- Many insoluble substances are carried in the blood bound to plasma proteins.

Regulation

- Maintenance of body temperature – distribution of heat
- Maintenance of body pH – acid base balance
- Maintenance of adequate fluid volume in the circulatory system

Protection

- Prevention of blood loss – haemostasis. Clotting and clot breakdown (fibrinolysis) are functions of plasma
- Defence against microbial invaders and trauma. The white blood cells and the inflammatory response are part of the immune system
- B-lymphocytes produce antibodies.

PHYSICAL CHARACTERISTICS OF BLOOD

Blood is a sticky, opaque fluid that has a salty taste and is about five times thicker (more viscous) than water.

The colour of blood varies according to the amount of oxygen it is carrying. When fully oxygenated it is bright red (scarlet) and when it is carrying little oxygen it is dark red. This means that arterial and venous blood can be recognised by their colour.

Blood is slightly alkaline, having a pH that is maintained between 7.35 and 7.45 in health.

Components

Blood makes up 6–8% of body weight.

- This is equivalent to 70 ml/kg body weight and a healthy 70 kg male would have approximately 5 L of blood
- The average female weighs approximately 51 kg and will have about 3.5 L of blood.

Blood is a complex connective tissue with living blood cells suspended in a fluid matrix called plasma.

The cells present are:

- red blood cells (erythrocytes)
- white blood cells (leucocytes)
- platelets (thrombocytes).

The solid components of the blood are about 45% of its volume. Most of this is made up of red blood cells and is known as the red cell volume or haematocrit. White blood cells and platelets make up only 1% with the plasma making up the remaining 55% of the volume.

The sum of the red cell volume and the plasma volume gives the total blood volume.

Plasma is a straw coloured fluid that is 90% water and contains over 100 different solutes. It also contains clotting factors such as fibrinogen. Plasma without the clotting factors is called serum. Plasma also contains other proteins such as albumin and globulin that are manufactured in the liver and have an osmotic effect, important in the maintenance of blood volume and the formation and reabsorption of tissue fluid. If osmotic pressure becomes abnormally low oedema may result.

OVERVIEW OF THE CIRCULATION

- Oxygenated blood leaves the heart in the arteries – these branch again and again until they become tiny capillaries which are only one cell thick
- Oxygen and nutrients diffuse from the capillaries to the tissues and carbon dioxide and waste products diffuse from the tissues into the capillaries
- The capillaries flow into the veins which return the deoxygenated blood to the right side of the heart
- The right ventricle of the heart pumps the blood to the lungs where oxygen is picked up
- The blood is returned to the left side of the heart to again be pumped around the body.

Organic substances transported in the blood include:

- Nutrients. Glucose is the most abundant. Amino acids, fatty acids, cholesterol and vitamins are also present in varying amounts
- Waste products of metabolism include urea, uric acid and creatinine as well as bilirubin
- Hormones e.g. cortisol, thyroxine – attached to plasma proteins
- Enzymes. The levels of certain enzymes in the serum can help in the diagnosis of disease. Examples include serum amylase that is raised in pancreatitis and creatine kinase that is raised in myocardial infarction.

BLOOD IN HEALTH CARE

Obtaining venous blood is a relatively simple procedure and yet the blood can give vital information as to what is happening within the body. Changes in the composition of blood are usually secondary to disease elsewhere in the body, however, primary disorders of the blood are also important and have widespread effects on bodily functions.

Practice point

Handling blood and blood products

- Precautions need to be taken such as wearing protective gloves and safely disposing of sharps.
- Disease can be transmitted by blood borne organisms.
- Two important examples are HIV and hepatitis B.

Any fluid replacement into the bloodstream must be isotonic with the plasma or cell damage may occur. An example of an isotonic fluid is normal saline (0.9%).

BLOOD CELLS

Erythrocytes

These are red blood cells whose main function is to carry oxygen to the tissues. They are full of a special protein called haemoglobin (Hb) that combines reversibly with oxygen to form oxyhaemoglobin. This enables uptake of oxygen in the lungs and delivery to the tissues. In the tissues, where the partial pressure of oxygen is lower, the oxygen dissociates from the Hb and is given up to the cells – deoxyhaemoglobin results. 20–30% of the carbon dioxide in the blood is carried on the Hb as carbaminohaemoglobin.

The main function of haemoglobin is:

- Oxygen uptake in the lungs
- Carriage of oxygen in the blood
- Oxygen release in the tissues.

Erythrocytes are biconcave, non-nucleated discs that look like miniature doughnuts under the microscope. Their peculiar shape gives them a large surface area to volume ratio ideally suited for gaseous exchange. Red blood cells can change shape and need to do so as they pass through some of the smaller capillaries. Their life span in the circulation is approximately 120 days. They lack a nucleus so are unable to divide or to make new proteins.

Production of red blood cells (haemopoiesis)

Haemopoiesis in the adult occurs in the red bone marrow where all blood cells (RBCs) are made. The red cell goes through several stages in development and is released into the circulation as an immature red cell called a reticulocyte. The reticulocyte forms less than 2% of the red cells and matures in the circulation within 2–4 days. A reticulocyte count can be used as a measure of the rate of red cell formation.

There is maintenance of a balance between production and destruction of red blood cells and numbers remain remarkably constant.

- Having too few would lead to lack of oxygen in the tissues (hypoxia) and having too many makes the blood too viscous (polycythaemia)
- New cells are made at the rate of about 2 million per second and this is controlled by a hormone in the kidney – erythropoietin. Production is increased in hypoxia and is dependent upon sufficient supplies of protein, iron and certain vitamins
- Erythropoietin is inactivated by the liver and excreted in the urine.

Practice point

Oestrogens depress the erythropoietic response and androgens stimulate it which, along with blood loss in menstruation, accounts for the lower red cell count in women.

Dietary requirements

- Proteins are needed for the synthesis of the globin part of the Hb molecule
- Iron – available in the diet and absorption is controlled by intestinal cells according to the need
- B-complex vitamins – folic acid and vitamin B_{12} are needed
- Vitamin C is needed for normal folate metabolism and aids the absorption of iron
- Lack of any of these constituents may lead to anaemia.

Destruction of red cells

- Red blood cells gradually become more rigid as the plasma membrane is damaged in travel and after about 100–120 days become trapped in the capillaries of the spleen – known as the 'graveyard of the red cell'
- They are engulfed and destroyed by large white blood cells – macrophages
- Other organs that can destroy the red cell are the liver, the bone marrow and the lymph nodes
- Defective red cells such as those in sickle cell disease may haemolyse in the circulation
- Iron is removed from the haem and reutilised or stored in the liver to be used again

- The remainder of the haem molecule is degraded to bilirubin – a yellow pigment which travels in the blood attached to plasma albumin and is conjugated in the liver to become water soluble and is secreted into bile
- The protein component of haemoglobin is broken down to amino acids.

Leucocytes

Although there are many less of these, they are crucial to the body's defence against disease. White blood cells are able to slip out of the bloodstream and into the tissues to help in the defence of the body.

- There are 4000–11,000 white blood cells per cubic millimetre of blood
- During infection the body speeds up its production of white blood cells (WBC). There are two major categories of WBC – those with granules called granulocytes and those without granules called agranulocytes.

Granulocytes

All larger than the RBC and have lobed nuclei. They are able to phagocytose (engulf particles).

- Neutrophils – there are more of these than any other type of WBC, around 3000–7000 /mm^3 blood normally. They can move and are attracted to sites of inflammation where they engulf bacteria and dead tissue. They kill the bacteria by chemical means and live from 6 hours to a few days depending on their tasks

Practice point

Numbers of neutrophils **increase** drastically in **acute bacterial infections** such as meningitis or acute appendicitis.

- Eosinophils – 1% to 4% of all WBCs – 100–400 per cubic millilitre. Attack small parasitic worms – too large to be phagocytosed. They gather around the worm and release their enzymes onto the parasites surface thus digesting it away
- Basophils – only 0.5% of leucocytes – about 20–50 per mm^3 blood. Cytoplasm contains large, coarse histamine containing granules. Histamine is an inflammatory chemical that vasodilates and attracts other WBCs to the site. Cells similar to these are found in the tissues and are called mast cells. They are involved in an allergic response and are responsible for the symptoms of hay fever, for example.

Agranulocytes

- Lymphocytes – large numbers exist in the body but only a small proportion are found in the blood stream (1500–3000/mm^3). The rest are firmly enmeshed in lymphoid tissue. They have a very important role in immunity. B lymphocytes make antibodies and T lymphocytes help protect us against viral illnesses and act against tumour cells. T lymphocytes also help the B lymphocyte to produce antibodies by releasing certain chemicals
- Monocytes – the largest WBCs that move into the tissues and become mobile macrophages which are very important phagocytes especially in chronic infections e.g. tuberculosis.

Platelets (thrombocytes)

- Platelets are essential for the clotting process. They first of all form a platelet plug which becomes a clot when fibrin threads are enmeshed around it
- 250,000–500,000 platelets per cubic millilitre of blood
- Age quickly as they have no nucleus and only live 7–10 days.

PATHOPHYSIOLOGY OF THE BLOOD

Haematology is the study of the blood.

Disorders may affect the red cells, the white cells or the platelets.

> Any word that ends in ***-aemia*** relates to the blood. Examples include anaemia, polycythaemia and leukaemia.

Anaemias

Anaemia is a decrease in the level of haemoglobin which could be due to a decrease in the number of red cells or the amount of haemoglobin within them. The decrease in haemoglobin means that the transport of oxygen in the blood is less efficient. In severe cases this will lead to hypoxia.

Normal values for haemoglobin(Hb) in grams per dL (100 ml) of blood are:

- 12.5–18 g/dL in adult males
- 11.5–16 g/dL in adult females.

Aetiology

There are various causes of anaemia and these are shown in Table 7.1.

Problem	Cause
Increased loss of red cells	Blood loss ■ Acute ■ Chronic
Increased breakdown of red cells – haemolysis	Abnormality of the red cell ■ Genetic – thalassaemia and sickle cell ■ Acquired e.g. paroxysmal nocturnal haemaglobinuria Antibody mediated destruction e.g. autoimmune haemolytic anaemia Direct action e.g. malaria
Reduced red cell production due to deficiency	Iron deficiency anaemia Lack of Vitamin B12 – pernicious anaemia Lack of folate
Failure of bone marrow to produce cells	Aplastic anaemia
Chronic disease	e.g. chronic renal failure liver disease chronic alcoholism hypothyroidism
Invasion of bone marrow by malignant cells	Leukaemias Other malignancies

Table 7.1 Causes of anaemia

Clinical features

- May be pallor of the hands or conjunctiva
- Spoon shaped nails (koilonychia) that split easily may occur in chronic iron deficiency
- If mild or of insidious onset, there may be no symptoms.

If severe or more rapid onset then:

- Fatigue
- Swollen feet (peripheral oedema)
- Breathlessness – this is worse if there is already any heart or lung disease
- Heart failure may be accentuated.

Case study 7.1

Adele is a 43-year-old lady who has been feeling increasingly tired over the past 6 months. She has noticed that in the evenings her feet are slightly swollen and that if she walks briskly up the 2 flights of stairs to her flat, she becomes breathless.

On visiting the GP, Adele is asked about her diet and says she is vegetarian. The doctor sends her to have bloods taken and her haemoglobin level comes back as 9 g/dL. The GP makes a diagnosis of anaemia, probably due to iron deficiency, and Adele starts a course of ferrous gluconate tablets as iron therapy.

In anaemia there is a problem with oxygen transport to the tissues. This arises because of a lack of haemoglobin. The symptoms produced will depend on the body's demand for oxygen. This means that if the person is sedentary and sits at a desk they may be asymptomatic. Were the same person to try training for a marathon they would have severe problems.

Sickle cell trait and anaemia

Aetiology

This is a hereditary condition where the sickle cell gene results in one of the amino acids in haemoglobin being abnormal. This abnormal haemoglobin tends to polymerise leading to a change in shape. The red cell becomes deformed and elongates into a sickle shape – thus the haemoglobin is called HbS. When in the deoxygenated state, HbS causes a change in shape of the red cell known as sickling. This is reversible at first when the Hb becomes oxygenated but eventually the cell membrane of the haemoglobin becomes damaged and the cell is then irreversibly sickled.

In sickle cell trait there is one normal gene and one abnormal gene. Fifty per cent of the Hb is HbA (normal). Sickling only occurs when anoxia is present such as in poor anaesthesia or severe infections.

In sickle cell disease the abnormal cells are present all the time and are destroyed more rapidly, leading to anaemia.

- Sickle cells can also block small blood vessels and this is extremely painful. It is known as a sickle cell crisis and requires strong analgesia (e.g. opioids). Minor dehydration or infections can bring on a crisis
- Pain may occur in the limbs, abdomen or back
- Poor vision may result from occlusion and vascular proliferation in retinal vessels.

Thrombocytopenia

This is an abnormally low number of platelets in the circulating blood. The other name for a platelet is a thrombocyte.

The normal platelet count is 200,000/mm^3 to 400,000/mm^3.

Clinical features

- Platelets are involved in haemostasis (stopping bleeding) and prevent loss of blood from small blood vessels as part of the normal wear and tear process. A low platelet count is thus associated with petechial haemorrhage
- If a patient has less than 5000 platelets per mm^3 they are at high risk of spontaneous bleeding. This may be in the form of an epistaxis or, more dangerously, into the central nervous system
- Thrombocytopenia is treated by platelet transfusion but because platelets only live for about 2 days, it is difficult to treat effectively
- Idiopathic thrombocytopenic purpura – this is immune mediated and the cause is not known. It is treated with corticosteroids to induce remission and rarely a splenectomy is needed to reduce the destruction of platelets
- Cancer chemotherapy can also cause a low platelet count.

Disorders of white blood cells

- Neutropenia is a decreased number of neutrophils and agranulocytosis is a complete lack of neutrophils. The cause may be drug related e.g. a side effect of cytotoxic drugs, autoimmune or malignancy. The main danger is infection
- Leucocytosis is an increased number of white cells. This may be neutrophils only, and if so is commonly due to infection. It is a normal response.

Leukaemias

Leukaemia is a malignant condition with an increased number of white cells in the blood. There are many types of leukaemia which may be classified according to whether they are acute or chronic and the white cell type they affect.

Acute leukaemias (AL)

The effects of all ALs are due to bone marrow failure where the malignant immature white cells crowd out the normal haemopoietic (blood cell manufacturing) cells. This leads to a shortage of all types of blood cell resulting in anaemia, bleeding and a high risk of infection.

The onset is often acute with malaise, pyrexia and sometimes bone pain.

Acute myeloid leukaemia (AML)

- An expansion of myeloid blasts in the bone marrow
- Average age of onset is 60 years and the prognosis is poorer than for acute lymphatic leukaemias
- Risk factors include radiation, previous chemotherapy, chemicals such as benzene and viruses
- Classified by the World Health Organization (WHO) into many different types.
- May start with myelodysplastic syndrome which is a precancerous state.

Acute lymphoblastic leukaemia (ALL)

- A proliferation of either B lymphocytes (85% of cases) or T lymphocytes (see chapter 5)
- Mainly affects children but can affect adults. It is the commonest form of malignancy in children
- Symptoms include anaemia, bleeding, infection, lymphadenopathy (swollen lymph glands) and splenomegaly (an enlarged spleen). There may be CNS involvement especially if there is a relapse
- Cure can now be achieved in over 80% of children using chemotherapy.

Chronic leukaemias

Chronic lymphocytic leukaemia (CLL)

- May be discovered on routine blood count or may present with lymphadenopathy
- Insidious development of anaemia and perhaps infections
- Often there is enlargement of the spleen, liver and some lymph nodes

- Treatment is with chemotherapy and the disease is usually controlled although it cannot be cured.

Multiple myeloma

This is a malignant condition of the bone marrow that occurs more in the elderly. The plasma cells proliferate in the bone marrow and this leads to destruction of bone and osteoporosis. The disease affects places in the body where there is bone marrow such as the spine, the skull, the pelvis and the legs and arms. Bone pain, fractures and collapsed vertebrae may occur.

Clinical features

- Anaemia may be accompanied by low platelets and neutrophils
- Immune complexes may block the renal tubules leading to renal dysfunction
- Bone pain
- Treatment: bone pain may be relieved by local radiotherapy
- Chemotherapy is with melphalan or other regimens. This may produce a remission. Steroids are also given
- About 35% of those diagnosed live for 5 years or more.

Diseases of the lymph nodes

Lymph nodes are small bean-like structures which occur along the lymphatic system and filter the lymph. They can trap foreign particles, including cancer cells. They can also mount an immune response and so become enlarged when infection is present e.g. the cervical glands become swollen (lymphadenopathy) in pharyngitis.

The lymph nodes can also be affected by malignancies.

Malignant lymphomas

Usually arise in the lymph nodes and are classified as Hodgkin lymphoma or non-Hodgkin lymphomas.

Hodgkin lymphoma

- About a quarter of malignant lymphomas are of this type and causation in some types has been linked to Epstein–Barr virus (EBV) (glandular fever)
- Peak incidence is in early adult life
- The patient develops painless, swollen lymph glands and diagnosis is by lymph node biopsy. Lymph nodes may or may not be tender and may fluctuate in size

- There may be a low grade fever, weight loss and sweating at presentation
- There are several types of Hodgkin's lymphoma but with chemotherapy and radiotherapy there is a good cure rate.

Non-Hodgkin lymphoma

- There are many types of lymphoma with a complex classification
- Low-grade tumours cannot be cured but grow slowly and may be spread widely before they cause symptoms
- High-grade tumours are more localised but grow rapidly. Fever, anorexia and weight loss may be present. The disease may be cured by chemotherapy.

Metastatic tumours of the lymph nodes

- By far the greatest number of tumours in the lymph nodes are secondary to a primary cancer elsewhere
- Almost all carcinomas spread first through lymphatic drainage to the local lymph glands e.g. enlarged axillary nodes in breast cancer
- Enlarged lymph glands may be the first indication of a tumour
- If the nearest lymph node (the Sentinel node) to a cancer is clear of any tumour at biopsy, this is a good prognostic sign.

Coagulation disorders

These may be hereditary or acquired.

Hereditary disorders

Haemophilia A

This is also known as classic haemophilia. It is a hereditary defect of the X-chromosome that is recessive. This means it is carried by females but affects males. The male has only one X-chromosome and so if this is defective he will have the disease. The female has two X-chromosomes and as the gene is recessive it will not produce the disorder as long as there is one normal gene. This inheritance pattern is shown in Figure 7.1.

- There is a very low amount of one of the clotting factors (Factor VIII) in the blood
- The disease usually presents when a baby starts to crawl or walk and he/she will bruise easily
- There is often bleeding into joints (haemarthrosis) which occurs spontaneously. This may lead to restriction of movement when it occurs repeatedly

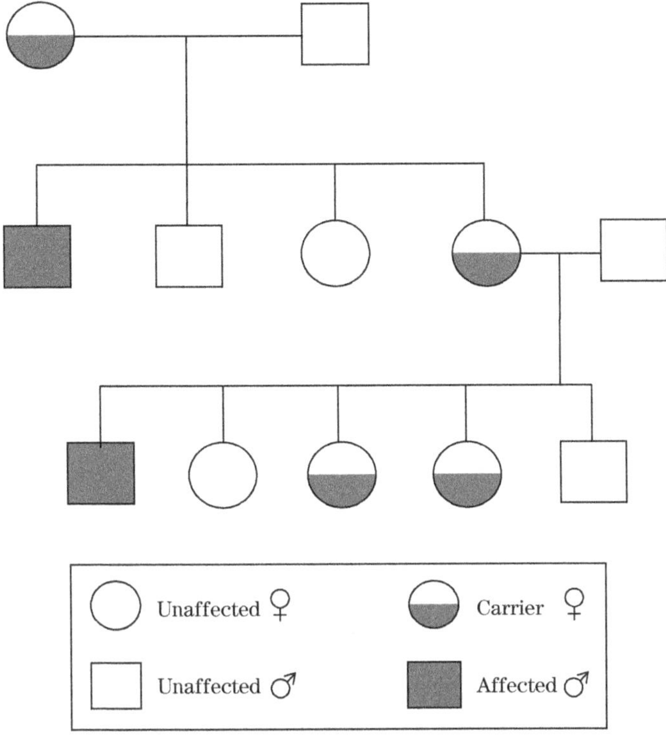

Figure 7.1 A family tree showing the inheritance pattern of haemophilia

- Bleeding into joints is very painful and good analgesia is needed
- Injected Factor VIII is the treatment and patients may keep a stock of factor VIII at home. In severe cases regular injections are given.

Von Willebrand's disease

- This is transmitted on a dominant gene and if the abnormal gene is present the person will develop the syndrome.
- There are different types with a deficiency in different clotting factors
- Bleeding results but it is less severe than in haemophilia and may only become apparent when a tooth is removed.

Acquired coagulation disorders

These may be due to:

- Vitamin K deficiency (vitamin K is needed for the formation of some clotting factors)

- Liver disease (the liver manufactures clotting factors)
- Disseminated vascular coagulation (DIC)
- Drugs such as heparin
- Immune mediated disease.

CONCLUSION

This chapter has given an overview of the blood in health and has looked at some of the commoner haematological disorders. As can be seen, these may affect the red cells, the white cells or the platelets. Other disorders affect coagulation and the clotting cascade. Some of these, such as haemophilia, may be genetically transmitted.

SELF-ASSESSMENT QUESTIONS

1. List the functions of the blood.
2. Describe the different types of blood cell in a normal blood sample.
3. Explain what is meant by 'anaemia'.
4. Describe the disorder 'sickle cell anaemia'.
5. Explain what is meant by 'thrombocytopenia'.
6. Describe the three main types of leukaemia.
7. Explain the abnormality found in haemophilia and its impact on coagulation.
8. Describe what is meant by a 'lymphoma'.

FURTHER READING

Herrington C.S. (ed.) (2014) *Muir's Textbook of Pathology,* 15th edn, London: CRC Press.

Hoffbrand V. and Moss P. (2011) *Essential Haematology,* 6th edn, Oxford: Wiley-Blackwell.

8 The cardiovascular system

Sharon Edwards

CARDIAC ANATOMY

Circulation can be considered as the circuit of blood around the body. It involves the heart and blood vessels. On average there are about 5 litres of blood travelling through the circulation and this passes through the heart every minute. There are two separate but interconnected systems, which are separated by intact septal membranes:

- The right side of the heart pumps blood to the lungs
- The left side of the heart pumps blood through the systemic circulation using arteries, arterioles, capillaries and veins which form the vascular system and are discussed later
- The veins and lymphatic system remove waste products of metabolism from tissue cells.

Structure of the heart

The heart walls consist of distinct layers of tissue in both the atria and ventricles (Figure 8.1):

- The pericardium is a sac that surrounds the heart (McCance *et al*, 2010):
  - Prevents displacement during movement
  - Protects the heart from infection
  - Contains pain receptors and mechanoreceptors that can initiate reflex changes to maintain blood pressure and heart rate
- The epicardium is the innermost layer of pericardium
- The myocardium is the thick contractile muscular middle layer:
  - Is composed of specialised cardiac muscle cells
  - The thickness varies between the different ventricular chambers, dependent on the amount of pressure required to eject blood
  - The muscle fibres of the myocardium contract together

- The endocardium is the interior layer of the myocardial wall (Carlene, 2010):
  - Is made of delicate endothelial tissue
  - Contains small blood vessels.

Chambers of the heart

The heart consists of 4 chambers. The circulation through the chambers, and consequently the body, is determined by pressures within each chamber (Figure 8.1):

- The 2 atria are the upper chambers and receive blood returning to the heart, and are separated by the inter-atrial septum:
  - Right atria – a thin-walled, low-pressure chamber, it receives deoxygenated blood from the systemic circulation via the superior and inferior vena cava, and immediately flows into the right ventricle, which gives little resistance
  - Left atria – also a thin-walled, low-pressure chamber, which is smaller but has thicker walls than the right ventricle. It receives oxygenated blood from the lungs via the 4 pulmonary veins, 2

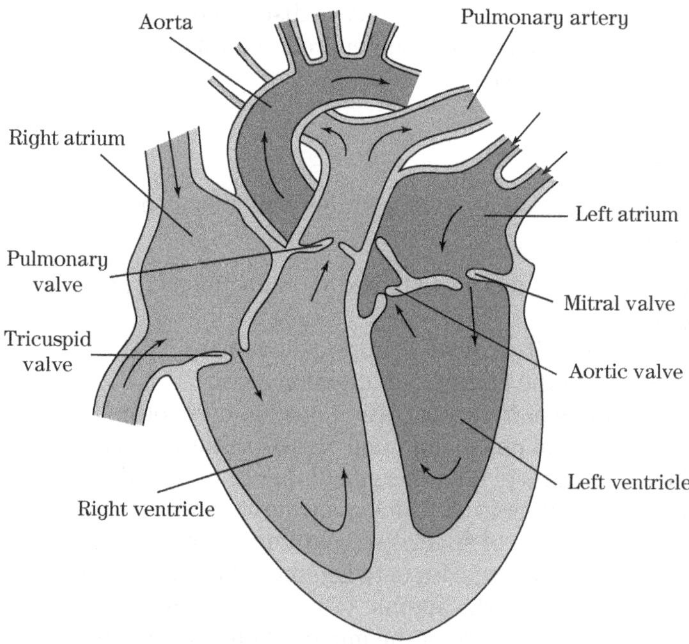

Figure 8.1 Structure of and circulation through the heart

    from each lung and flows into the left ventricle, which gives little resistance
- The 2 ventricles are the inferior chambers; they are larger and have thicker walls than the atria. They receive blood from the atria, and are separated by the inter-ventricular septum:
    - Right ventricle – a thicker walled chamber, with a higher pressure (up to 28 mmHg), as it is required to pump blood into the pulmonary artery, which gives a greater resistance
    - Left ventricle – the main pumping chamber, with thicker walls than the right ventricle and has the greatest pressure (up to 140 mmHg), it has to pump blood through the aorta to the rest of the body, which gives the greatest resistance. The blood is pumped into the aorta for distribution around the body.

Valves of the heart

- Between each of the 4 chambers is a valve, which facilitates the flow of blood in a one-way direction, preventing backflow through the heart. There are 2 atrio-ventricular (AV) valves and 2 semilunar valves (Figure 8.1):
    - The AV valves separate the atria from the ventricles, the cusps are attached to chordae tendineae, which prevent the valve being forced open when the ventricles contract:
        - Right atrio-ventricular (AV) valve (between the right atria and ventricle) is the tricuspid valve, as it has 3 cusps, and prevents backflow from the right ventricle into the right atrium
        - Left atrio-ventricular (AV) valve (between the left atria and ventricle) is a bicuspid (2 cusp) valve also referred to as the mitral valve, and prevents backflow from the left ventricle into the left atrium
    - The semilunar valves:
        - Right semilunar valve (between the right ventricle and the pulmonary artery) is the pulmonary valve, which prevents backflow from the pulmonary artery into the right ventricle
        - Left semilunar valve (between the left ventricle and the aorta) is the aortic valve, which prevents backflow from the aorta into the left ventricle.

The cardiac cycle

The action of the heart is determined by relaxation termed diastole, and contraction, termed systole (Figure 8.2):

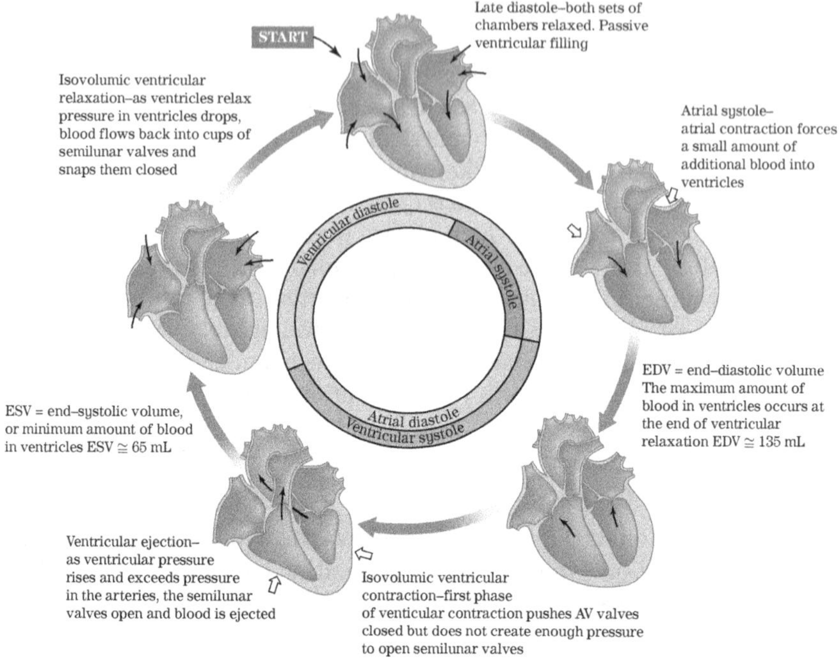

Figure 8.2 The cardiac cycle

- Diastole is the time when the atria and ventricles are relaxing
  - The two atria are filling, the right atria with blood from the systemic circulation, and the left with blood from the lungs
  - The pressures in the atria increase, and the 2 AV valves are pushed open
  - Blood flows from the higher-pressure atria into the relaxed ventricles
- Systole is the time when the atria and ventricles contract
  - The atria contract and push the remaining blood into the ventricles through the open AV valves
  - The increase in ventricular pressure causes the 2 AV valves to close preventing backflow into the atria
  - The ventricular pressures increase further, and the 2 semilunar valves open
  - The ventricles contract and blood is pushed out of the ventricles and into the pulmonary veins and aorta
  - After ventricular contraction and ejection, intra ventricular pressures falls and the pulmonary and aortic semilunar valves close preventing backflow into the right and left ventricles.

Coronary arteries

The coronary arteries receive blood from the opening behind the left cusp of the aortic semilunar valve in the aorta called the coronary ostia (Figure 8.3):

- The right coronary artery travels to supply the right ventricle and posterior sections of the atrium and ventricle. There are 3 branches:
  - Conus supplies blood to the upper right ventricle
  - The right marginal branch, which traverses the right ventricles to the apex
  - The posterior descending branch supplies smaller branches to both ventricles
- The left coronary artery divides into two branches:
  - The left anterior descending (LAD) artery supplies blood to portions of the left and right ventricles, much of the intra-ventricular septum and the apex
  - The circumflex artery supplies blood to the left atrium and the lateral wall of the left ventricle and branches to the posterior section of the left atrium and ventricle
- Collateral arteries are connections between two branches of the same coronary artery (McCance *et al*, 2010):
  - The development of a collateral circulation is important as it protects the heart from ischaemia

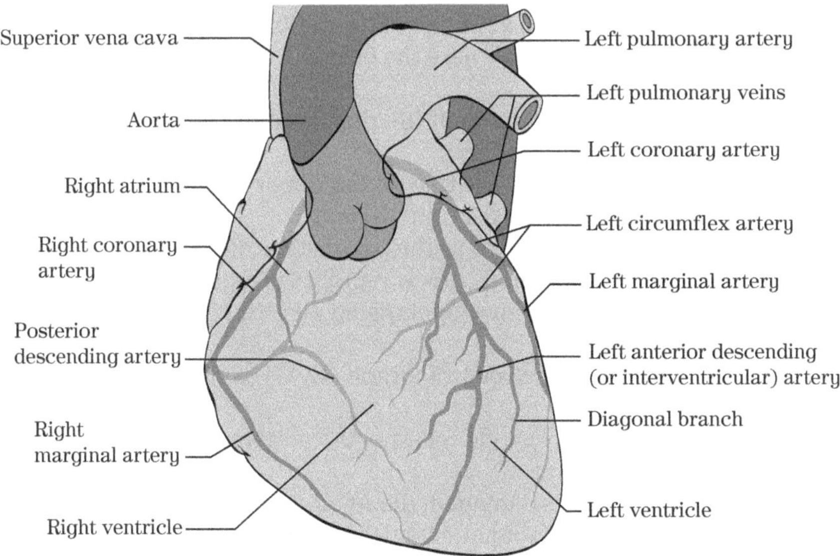

Figure 8.3 Coronary arteries

  - Growth is stimulated by gradual coronary occlusion
- Regulation of coronary blood flow
  - Often referred to as coronary perfusion pressure (CPP)
  - CPP is the difference between the pressure in the aorta and pressure in the coronary vessels (McCance *et al*, 2010)
  - The aortic pressure determines adequate blood supply to the myocardium despite resistance from the pumping action of the heart and shifts in CPP
  - Most coronary artery perfusion occurs during diastole.

CARDIAC PHYSIOLOGY

The contraction of the atria and ventricles of the heart, during systole depends on the transmission of electrical impulses. The impulses travel through the atria and ventricles to the myocardium and are termed cardiac action potentials (McCance *et al*, 2010).

Electrical conduction through the heart

- Electrical conduction consists of pacemaker cells, which all have 3 unique characteristics (Carlene, 2010) (Figure 8.4):
  - Automaticity – the ability to generate an electrical impulse
  - Conductivity – the ability to transfer the impulse to the next cell
  - Contractility – the ability to shorten fibres to eject blood
- Sino-atrial (SA) node is where the electrical impulse arises, and sets the pace for the heart:
  - Located in the junction of the right atrium and superior vena cava
  - Generates around 75 action potential per minute or beats at around 6–100 beats per minute (bpm)
  - Sometimes referred to as the pacemaker of the heart
  - Each action potential travels rapidly through specialised conduction pathways depolarising all atrial cells causing both atria to contract
  - Shows on the electrocardiograph (ECG) as the P wave (see Figure 8.5)
- Atrioventricular (AV) node receives the action potential from the atria:
  - If the SA node is damaged, the AV node can become the pacemaker initiating about 40–60 bpm

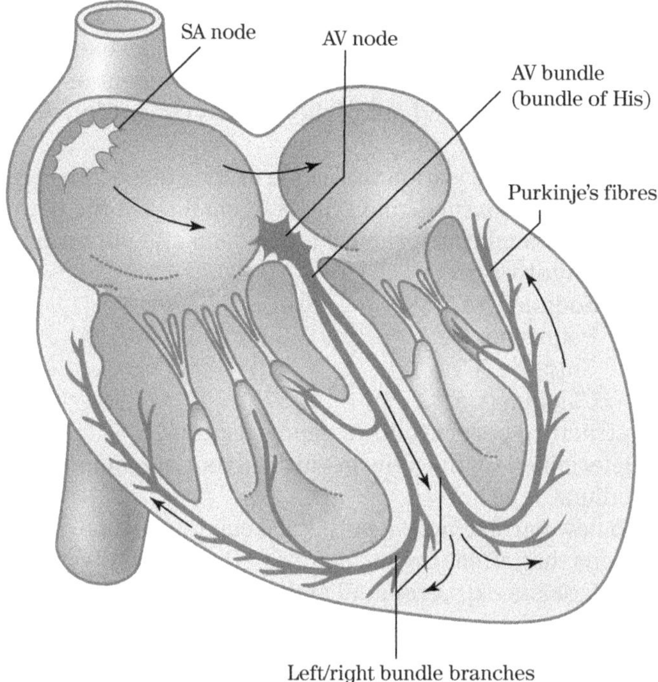

Figure 8.4 Electrical conduction of the heart

  - The fibres join in the superior part of the inter-ventricular septum to form the bundle of His
- Bundle of His gives rise to the right and left bundle branches:
  - The right bundle branch (RBB)
  - The left bundle branch (LBB) divides into 2 branches or fascicle
    - The left anterior bundle branch (LABB)
    - The left posterior bundle branch (LPBB)
- The Purkinje fibres are the terminal branches and extend into the ventricles:
  - Following the P wave on the ECG is a straight isometric line
  - This is the time it takes the action potential to travel from the AV node to the Purkinje fibres to reach the myocardium for ventricular depolarisation, the QRS on the ECG (see Figure 8.5).

These fibres are capable of independent depolarisation but only at a rate of around 30–40 bpm.

Depolarisation and repolarisation of cardiac cells

- Depolarisation is the electrical activation of muscle cells:
  - Depolarisation is determined by the movement of electrically charged ions in and out of the cells and the difference between them
  - During depolarisation the inside of the cell becomes less negatively charged, and relates to changes in the permeability of the cell membrane primarily to sodium and potassium. The major ions involved are:
    - Sodium (Na^+)
    - Potassium (K^+)
    - Chloride (Cl^-)
    - Calcium (Ca^{++})
- The refractory period follows depolarisation:
  - Determined by the slow inward current of calcium and sodium
  - No new cardiac action potentials can be stimulated
  - Drugs that effect the refractory period are known as calcium antagonists e.g. verapamil and can be used to:
    - Slow down or alter heart rate
    - Treat some cardiovascular disorders
- Repolarisation is deactivation of cardiac muscle cells:
  - Repolarisation is the return of the electrically charged ions to their normal resting membrane potential.

The normal electrocardiogram

- Depolarisation
  - The P wave
    - Is the first positive deflection, upwards from the isometric base line, that is seen
    - It should be no longer than 0.11 sec, or three small squares on the ECG trace, amplitude is normally 0.5 to 2.5 mm
    - A QRS complex should always follow the P wave, unless conduction disturbances are present
  - The PR interval
    - Measured from the beginning of the P wave to the beginning of the QRS complex irrespective of whether the QRS complex begins with a Q or an R wave
    - It varies between 0.12–0.20 sec, or 3–5 small squares
    - Dependent on the heart rate and conduction of AV node
    - Normal tracing indicates electrical impulses have been conducted through the correct conduction pathways

- The QRS complex
    - Consists of three waves, Q, R and S, which results from ventricular depolarisation
    - Should be narrow and sharply pointed
    - Represents ventricular contraction (depolarisation), marking the beginning of ventricular systole, and can be:
        - Predominately positive (upright)
        - Predominately negative (inverted)
        - Biphasic (partly positive, partly negative)
    - Varies between 0.04–0.11 sec, or 2–3 small squares, amplitude varies from less than 5 mm to more than 15 mm
- The ST segment
    - Is the resting period between ventricular contraction and the returning of the cardiac muscle to its resting stage
    - Early repolarisation, should always return to the baseline, depressed or elevated in abnormalities

- The refractory period
    - The QT interval is the period from the beginning of ventricular depolarisation (onset of the QRS complex) until the end of ventricular repolarisation, or the end of T wave
    - During this period the heart is fully refractory (the absolute refractory period)
    - During the latter period of the interval (from the peak of the T wave onward), the conduction system is relatively refractory
    - Drugs may prolong the QT period
- Repolarisation
    - The T wave represents repolarisation of the ventricular myocardial cells
    - The wave is usually slightly rounded
    - Deep and symmetrical inverted T waves suggest cardiac ischaemia
    - T waves elevated more than half of the height of the QRS complex (peaked T waves) can indicate hyperkalaemia.

(See Figure 8.5.)

Nervous control of the heart

The heart is able to transmit its own action potentials without stimulation from the nervous system. The heart will continue to beat in the absence of any central nervous system input.

- Reflexes that indirectly effect the heart:
    - Baroreceptor reflex mediated by pressure receptors in the aortic arch and carotid arteries:

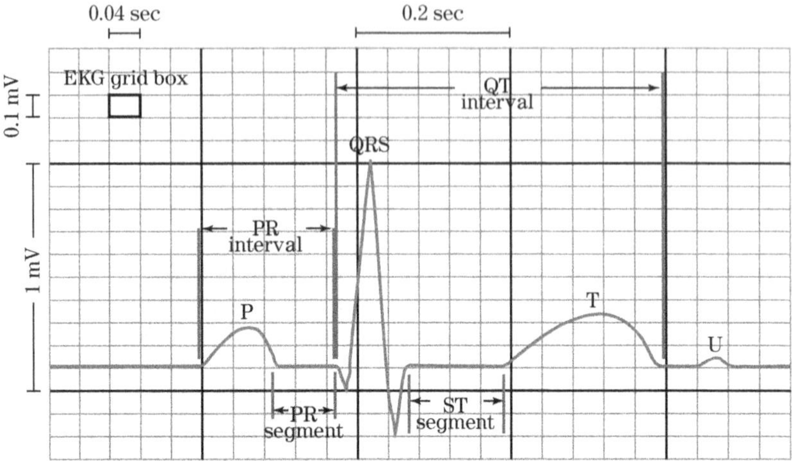

Figure 8.5 The normal electrocardiogram (ECG) rhythm strip

- If blood pressure is decreased, the baroreceptors reduce their firing rate of action potentials to the medulla, accelerating heart rate and causing vasoconstriction of blood vessels, raising blood pressure back toward normal limits
- If blood pressure is increased, the baroreceptors become stretched and increase their firing rate to the medulla in the brain, causing vasodilation lowering blood pressure and allowing heart rate to decrease

- Atrial receptors are stimulated when there is an increase in blood volume, the result is an increase in urine volume because they:
  - Reduce the release of antidiuretic hormone (ADH)
  - Mediate the release of atrial natriuretic peptide (ANP) a powerful diuretic, decreasing blood volume and pressure

- The heart is under sympathetic and parasympathetic nervous system control (see chapter 10), as these are needed to increase or decrease the cardiac cycle e.g. increase or decrease heart rate
- Sympathetic nerves effect heart rate and myocardial performance, it does this by using:
  - Catecholamines:
    - Adrenaline (epinephrine) (which strongly stimulates all 4 adrenergic receptors, but more β than α receptors)
    - Noradrenaline (norepinephrine) (stimulates the 2 α adrenergic receptors)
  - Adrenergic receptors which bind specifically with neurotransmitters of the sympathetic nervous system:

  - Beta 1 (β_1) – found mostly in the heart, adrenaline binding with β_1 receptors, increase heart rate and strength of myocardial contraction
  - Beta 2 (β_2) – found mostly in the coronary arterioles and cause vasodilation when stimulated by adrenaline, therefore increasing overall cardiac blood flow
  - Alpha 1 (α_1) – noradrenaline binding with α_1 receptors found in the systemic and coronary arteries causes vasoconstriction
  - Alpha 2 (α_2) – noradrenaline binding with α_2 receptors found in the GI tract leads to vasoconstriction, thus increasing systemic vascular resistance (SVR), providing another safety mechanism to maintain cardiac stability
- Parasympathetic nervous system uses acetylcholine to slow heart rate, and block action potentials transmitted from the atria at the AV node and bundle of His.

Cardiac output

This is the volume of blood pumped out of the heart per minute (Carlene, 2010), and is usually around 5 litres per minute (L/min).

- The cardiac output (CO) is determined by multiplying the heart rate (HR) (bpm) and the stroke volume (SV) (ml per minute), the amount ejected from the heart with each heart beat:

$$CO = SV \times HR$$

- If heart rate is around 70 bpm and stroke volume is approximately 70 ml: $4900 = 70 \times 70$
- Cardiac output is affected by 4 factors:
  - Preload is the pressure generated in the left ventricle at the end of diastole or left ventricular end-diastolic pressure (LVEDP)
  - Afterload relates to the pressure the ventricular muscles need to generate to overcome the higher pressure in the aorta, so blood can be pumped out of the heart
  - Myocardial contractility determines the amount of blood ejected from the blood during systole and depends on:
    - The ability of the myocardial fibres to stretch
    - Sympathetic activation on the ventricles
    - Adequate supply of oxygen to the myocardium
  - Heart rate is affected by, hormones such as thyroxin and other chemical factors such as adrenaline.

THE VASCULAR CIRCULATION

The vascular circulation includes the blood vessels, which pulsate, constrict, dilate and proliferate and form the delivery system of nutrients and gases from the heart to cells.

The structure of blood vessels

Blood vessels vary in thickness depending on their function, and are made up of three layers:

- The tunica intima is the inner layer
- The tunica media is the middle layer
- The tunica adventitia is the outer layer.

(See Figure 8.6.)

Arteries

- Arteries carry oxygenated blood away from the heart (Figure 8.6) (with the exception of the pulmonary artery which carries deoxygenated blood). They have thick muscular elastic fibre walls

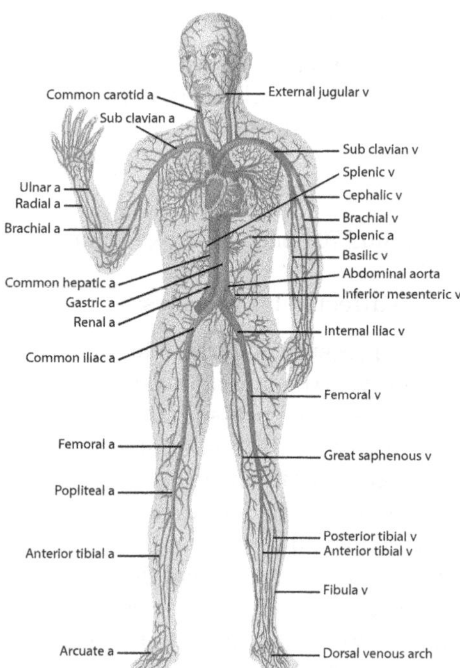

Figure 8.6 The vascular system showing both arteries and veins

- There are two types:
  - Elastic arteries:
    - Allows the artery to stretch during systole
    - Have a thick lining
    - Include the aorta and its major branches, the pulmonary trunk
  - Muscular arteries:
    - Are found further away from the heart and have less need to stretch
    - Major function is to distribute blood around the body
    - Control blood flow as they can constrict (vasoconstriction) and dilate (vasodilatation)
    - Arteries branch into smaller arterioles and then the fine network of capillaries.

Arterioles

- Arterioles contain little elastic muscle tissue, do not vasodilate or constrict to changes in blood pressure
- Main role is to control blood in to the capillaries by vasoconstriction and vasodilation.

Capillaries

- Capillaries carry blood from arteries to veins
- They have very thin and leaky walls to allow exchange of gases (oxygen and carbon dioxide) and nutrients between the blood and tissues
- They branch into venules, which join to form larger veins.

Endothelium

- All cells require a blood supply, and this relies on the endothelial cells that line blood vessels
- Endothelial cells form tissues, which release mediators and chemicals to:
  - Remodel and repair of blood vessels
  - Promote contraction or relaxation
  - Activate anti-thrombogenesis and fibrinolysis
- Injury to and dysfunction of the endothelium is significant in many cardiovascular disorders e.g. hypertension and atherosclerosis (McCance *et al*, 2010).

Veins

- Veins have thin walls and are more numerous than arteries
- They carry deoxygenated blood towards the heart (Figure 8.6) (with the exception of the pulmonary veins which carry oxygenated blood)

from the capillaries in all parts of the body, and deliver it back to the heart
- The veins in the lower limbs contain valves that maintain a one-way flow of blood back to the heart, facilitated by the contraction and relaxation of skeletal muscles in the leg
- This function is referred to as venous return
- The veins and the lymphatic system drain the heart and systemic circulation eventually emptying into the superior vena cava and back to the heart.

Factors that affect blood flow

Flow of blood through the systemic circulation is regulated by a number of processes.

Pressure

- Pressure in the arteries and veins determines blood flow through the pulmonary and systemic circulation:
  - Usually higher in the arteries (left side of the heart) and lower in the veins (right side of the heart)
  - Blood will flow from a high pressure to a low e.g. from the left side of the heart to the right.

Resistance

- Resistance is the opposition to the force given by the pressure:
  - In the cardiovascular system resistance is given by:
    - The pulmonary and systemic circulation or the blood vessels themselves determined by vessel diameter
    - An increase in resistance leads to a decrease in blood flow
  - Resistance to flow is:
    - Greater in longer vessels as resistance increases with length
    - Greater in the major arteries, approximately 60 mmHg, and less in the capillaries, approximately 15 mmHg
  - Viscosity of blood:
    - Thick blood moves slowly and causes a greater resistance, for example, the greater the amount of red blood cells, the more viscous blood becomes (expressed as haematocrit)
    - Thin blood causes a lesser resistance and moves quickly.

Velocity

Velocity is the distance the blood has to travel in a unit of time and is directly related to blood flow:

- In wide vessels the blood will flow slowly
- In narrow vessels the blood will flow quickly.

Laminar and turbulent flow

- In a laminar flow blood moves in a straight line
- In a turbulent flow blood is obstructed, the vessel turns or blood flows over rough surfaces; with this resistance increases.

Vascular compliance

Vascular compliance is the ability of the blood vessels to constrict or dilate in response to an increase or decrease in pressure.

The opposite of compliance is stiffness e.g. in arteriosclerosis when there is an increased rigidity of arterial walls (McCance *et al*, 2010).

Blood pressure (BP)

BP is the force exerted on the wall of blood vessels by its contained blood and when measured in clinical practice usually refers to BP in the arteries near the heart. BP varies with age, gender, weight, stress levels, mood, posture and physical activity. BP is dependent on compliance (the heart's ability to stretch) and stroke volume (the volume of blood pushed out of the heart per beat).

BP is constantly regulated (see below) to maintain circulation of blood, which is crucial for tissue and cellular perfusion. This is despite changes to the physiological conditions:

- Body position
- Muscular activity
- Circulating blood volume.

Pressure gradients

A pressure gradient through the circulation keeps the blood flowing:

- Varies through the vascular system
- BP is highest and most variable in the aorta and other elastic arteries, decreases through the arterioles and capillaries:
    - Aorta 80–120 mmHg
    - Major arteries 60 mmHg
    - Arteries 45 mmHg
    - Arterioles 35 mmHg
    - Veins 15 mmHg and less.

Systolic and diastolic pressure

BP rises during ventricular systole and decreases during diastole, giving two distinct readings systolic and diastolic pressure:

- Systolic pressure is the pressure in the arteries during ventricular systole (cardiac contraction)
- Diastolic pressure is the pressure in arteries during ventricular diastole (resting/filling period)
- 2 other pressures can then be determined:
  - The pulse pressure is the difference between systolic and diastolic pressure
  - Mean arterial pressure (MAP) is the average pressure in the main arteries:
    - Useful because aortic pressure fluctuates up and down with each heart beat, and MAP is the actual pressure that propels the blood to tissues
    - Is not as simple as adding the diastolic and systolic together and dividing them by 2, as diastolic time is longer, therefore MAP = diastolic pressure plus pulse pressure divided by 3.

Regulation of blood pressure

- Neural control:
  - Baroreceptors are stimulated when there is an increase or decrease in BP
  - Arterial chemoreceptors located in the same position as baroreceptors e.g. in the arch of the aorta and carotid arteries and respond to changes in oxygen only if very low, blood pH (hydrogen ions) and carbon dioxide levels
- Chemical control
  - Catecholamines are chemicals that act on vessels, heart or blood volume e.g. norepinephrine causes vasoconstriction and epinephrine leads to vasoconstriction in some organs and vasodilation in others
  - Antidiuretic hormone (ADH) which stimulates water reabsorption
  - Atrial natriuretic peptide (ANP) antagonises aldosterone and causes general vasodilation and increase in diuresis
  - Inflammatory mediators leads to vasodilation, nitric oxide is a powerful vasodilator
  - Angiotensin II is:
    - Created when renin splits off a polypeptide from angiotensinogen to generate angiotensin I

    - Converted to angiotensin II by the angiotensin-converting enzyme (ACE)
    - Angiotensin II is a powerful vasoconstrictor and stimulates the secretion of ADH from the pituitary gland and aldosterone from the adrenal gland, and the thirst mechanism
  - Alcohol inhibits ADH secretion and depresses the vasomotor centre
- Renal control
  - Renin is released by the juxta-glomerulus apparatus in the kidney, and stimulates the conversion of angiotensin I to angiotensin II by the ACE stimulating the release of aldosterone
  - The net effect of circulating aldosterone in the renal tubules of the kidney is the re-absorption of sodium and water
  - Renin is released in response to:
    - A drop in BP
    - Reduced plasma sodium
    - Increase in plasma potassium
    - Stress
- Capillary dynamics is the movement across a capillary gradient, which can be a:
  - Solute gradient (diffusion)
  - Water gradient (osmosis)
  - Pressure gradient (hydrostatic pressure)
  - Oncotic gradient (albumin).

Practical significance of BP

If systolic BP drops to below 100 mmHg, all body processes are in danger and if further reduced to 80 mmHg or below all body processes may cease and all organs of the body can die or become seriously damaged.

- The body will maintain BP at all costs, as our survival depends on it, by:
  - Changing blood vessel diameter
  - Releasing chemicals
  - Reabsorbing fluid back into the circulation.

Knowledge of this is essential for effective interpretation of a patient's condition.

> **Practice point**
>
> BP can be an unreliable measure with regards to determining shock as it will initially be maintained during injury or disease.

DISORDERS OF THE HEART

More than 40% of patients admitted to medical wards in the UK have some form of heart disease (Richards and Edwards, 2012). These are degenerative disorders which occur over time and can be insidious, symptoms only emerging when the disease has progressed.

Acute coronary syndromes

Acute coronary syndromes (ACS) occur when there is some degree of coronary artery occlusion. The plaque is fatty atheromatous deposits that build up over time and cause narrowing and partially occlude blood flow. It is difficult to differentiate between unstable angina and a myocardial infarction (MI), therefore, ACS is now used to describe both. An MI is usually termed as a heart attack or coronary thrombosis. About 105,000 people die in Britain each year from acute coronary syndromes; half of these die in the first hour usually due to cardiac arrhythmias (Richards and Edwards, 2012). The level of occlusion is represented as:

- Unstable angina
- ST-segment elevation myocardial infarction (STEMI)
- Non-ST-segment elevation myocardial infarction (NSTEMI).

Aetiology

- The focus is on primary prevention, but some risk factors cannot be changed:
  - Age, gender, family history
- Other risk factors can be changed or modified:
  - High-fat, high-carbohydrate diet leading to a raised cholesterol and lipids
  - Hypertension
  - Diabetes mellitus
  - Lack of exercise
  - Smoking
  - Obesity
  - Diet high in saturated (animal) fats leading to hyper-lipoproteinaemia
  - Menopause
  - Stress.

Pathology

ACS begin with an increase in plasma lipoprotein concentrations, these include:

    - Low-density lipoproteins (LDLs), an increase in serum concentration of LDLs is an indicator of coronary risk; lowering of LDLs with diet and cholesterol-lowering drugs decreases the risk of ACS
    - High-density lipoproteins (HDLs), a low level serum concentration of HDLs is a strong indicator of coronary risk of ACS; high levels may be more protective, as HDLs return excess cholesterol from the tissues to the liver and are eliminated as bile; some drugs work to increase HDL.

If an increase in plasma lipoproteins occurs, they are deposited as fatty streaks within the endothelium of the lumen of an artery, which progresses to narrowing of the vessel:

- Eventually may leak and/or rupture
- Attracts platelets and forms a thrombus
- Resulting in acute coronary syndrome.

Clinical features

Angina is pain in the chest, felt as a result of lack of blood supply (*ischaemia*) to the heart. There is a narrowing of the coronary vessels, due to deposits of atheroma.

- Stable angina:
    - Pain is usually in the chest but may extend down the left arm or both arms or into the neck; some experience pain just in the arm, the neck or the back
    - Described as a tightness or squeezing pain or discomfort
    - Brought on by exertion, fades fairly rapidly on rest
    - A glyceryl trinitrate (GTN) tablet sublingually or spray relieves the pain
    - Distribution of the pain will be the same each time but in more severe attacks it may extend further
    - Sometimes the pain of angina is mild and confused with heartburn and the patient ignores it
- Unstable angina:
    - May be a sign of an impending heart attack
    - Episodes of pain are more frequent
    - Occur without obvious cause and at rest
    - Can present with pleuritic pain, indigestion or dyspnoea
    - Usually requires admission to hospital
    - Urgent angiography is required for diagnosis and treatment
- Myocardial infarction:
    - Chest pain, which is tight or crushing in nature; 80% of patients
    - Pain:

  - Similar to unstable angina but more severe
  - Lasts longer than 20 minutes, and may radiate to the arms, throat and jaw
  - Not relieved by sublingual GTN
- Nausea and vomiting may occur
- Sweating, pallor
- Hypotension, tachycardia
- Anxiety
- The older adult, diabetic patient or some female patients may sometimes have a 'silent' MI where no chest pain is experienced.

Investigations

- Observations of BP, HR monitored half hourly at first
- 12-lead ECG daily until discharge, contributes to determining worsening or improving condition:
  - May be normal or inconclusive in the first few hours, abnormalities may include:
    - ST-segment depression in a NSTEMI
    - ST-segment elevation and Q waves in a STEMI, representing necrosis
- Coronary angiography may reveal:
  - Coronary artery stenosis or occlusion
  - Development of a collateral circulation
  - The state of the arteries past the narrowing
  - Blood will be sent to the laboratory for cardiac markers, FBC, biochemistry, lipids and glucose
- Cardiac markers:
  - Released into the blood stream by the damaged myocardium:
    - *Cardiac troponins I and T* highly specific to damaged cardiac muscle, may be undetected within the first 12 hours
    - *Creatine kinase* (CK) peaks within 24 hours of MI and falls back to baseline by 48 hours
    - *Aspartate aminotransferase* peaks at 24 hours and falls to baseline by 48 hours
    - *Lactate dehydrogenase* peaks at 3–4 days and remains raised for 10–14 days. It is useful when the patient has not been diagnosed immediately as having had an MI.

Treatment/drug therapy

Stable angina can be managed by the GP:

- Medical therapy:
  - Nitrates e.g. GTN, isosorbide mononitrate and isosorbide dinitrate

    - Beta-blockers e.g. atenolol to reduce the workload and oxygen demands of the heart
    - Calcium antagonists if angina is caused by coronary artery spasm
    - Aspirin
    - Lipid-lowering drugs such as statins e.g. atorvastatin.

Unstable angina: usually the patient is admitted to hospital:

- The immediate administration of oxygen to improve oxygenation, reduce ischaemia and pain (Lemone and Burke, 2004)
- Insertion of IV cannula in the incidence of deterioration
- May include some of the treatments for stable angina with the addition of other drugs:
    - Anti-platelet drugs are vital, aspirin 75–150 mg / day has been shown to reduce mortality or others such as clopidogrel
    - Low-molecular weight heparins (LMWH) given once daily by subcutaneous injection e.g. dalteparin and tinzaparin
    - Statins and ACE inhibitors to stabilise the plaque and to reduce cardiac work
    - Pain assessment and management is vital (Alexander *et al*, 2006)
    - Drugs given early in patients with an evolving MI:
        - Beta-blockers IV and continued orally
        - Angiotensin-converting enzyme (ACE) inhibitors for MIs with ST-segment elevation to reduce afterload and preload
- Coronary angioplasty and stenting – percutaneous transluminal coronary angioplasty (PTCA)
- Surgical treatment of angina – coronary artery bypass grafts (CABG).

Myocardial infarction

- The treatment and drug therapy options given above
- Offer reassurance, using a calm and confident manner
- Continued serial 12 lead ECGs to determine worsening or improving condition
- IV cannula will be inserted to allow drugs to be given easily and immediately analgesia – IV diamorphine 2.5–5 mg and an antiemetic e.g. metoclopramide 10 mg
- Fibrinolytic drugs (clot busters)
    - Streptokinase derived from bacteria:
        - Contraindicated if a patient has been administered streptokinase therapy 5 days to 12 months previously
        - This means the drug cannot be used and an alternative may be sought. This is due to the presence of antibodies in the circulation, from a recent streptococcal infection
- Genetically engineered alternative is alteplase, which is more frequently used

- Others include tenecteplase, which is administered by pre-hospital practitioners, only one bolus dose is necessary
- Any delay will lessen the effectiveness of the treatment
- Contraindications for this therapy include:
  - Recent haemorrhage, trauma or surgery
  - History of cerebrovascular disease
  - Severe hypertension
  - History of peptic ulceration and pregnancy
- Cardiac monitoring to determine complications such as cardiac arrhythmias, the commonest and most lethal complication of an MI:
  - The most dangerous irregularity is ventricular fibrillation (VF), which immediately precedes a cardiac arrest
  - Immediate treatment of VF using defibrillation (DC shock) may be lifesaving
- Different arrhythmias that can be observed following an MI are given in more detail in the section below.

Heart failure

Heart failure – the heart is no longer acting as an efficient pump and cannot respond to the demands made upon it (Nicholas, 2004). The heart is really two pumps – the right side of the heart and the left side – and either side may fail independently; however as all chambers are linked together as one structure, if one side fails then it will effect the other (Waugh and Grant, 2010). There may be a failure of both sides or left heart failure may lead to right.

Left ventricular failure (LVF)

In most cases the left ventricle fails first. LVF is damage to, or overload of, the left ventricle (Figure 8.7a), which leads to pulmonary oedema (Figure 8.7b).

Aetiology

- Cardiovascular disorders that lead to heart failure:
  - Hypertension
  - Mitral and aortic valve disease
  - Cardiac arrhythmias
  - Over transfusion e.g. fluid overload
  - Myocardial infarction
  - Congenital heart disease
  - Cardiomyopathy
- Non-cardiovascular causes of heart failure
  - Pregnancy and childbirth
  - Thyrotoxicosis

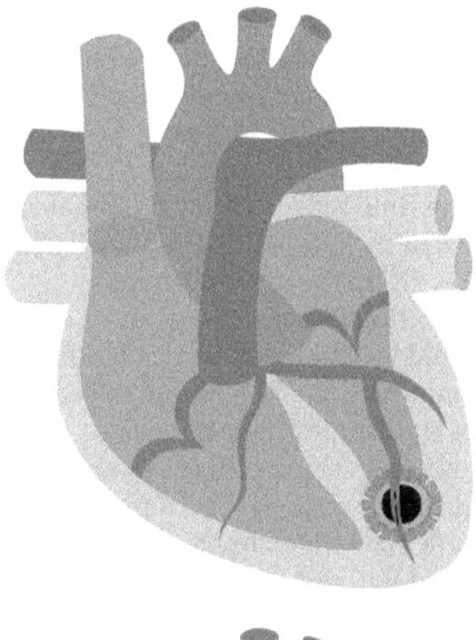

a)
- zone of death
- zone of ischaemia
- zone of inflammation

b) If treatment is instigated and oxygen therapy administered, blood can be restored to the area of ischaemia and repaired. This can potentially prevent an extension of the MI

c) The area of inflammation will gradually subside and repair

d) The zone of death is irreversible

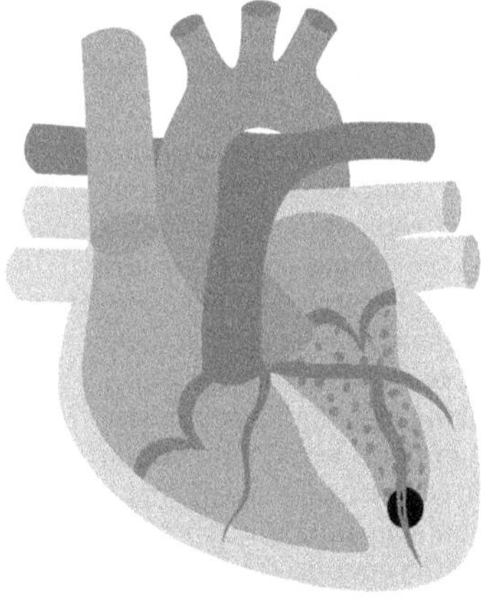

a) Over time (this can be a number of days, weeks, months or even years) the area of dead cardiac muscle leaves the left ventricle weakened and unable to pump effectively

b) This can lead to a small amount of blood collecting in the LV after each beat

c) There is an increase in pre load and after load

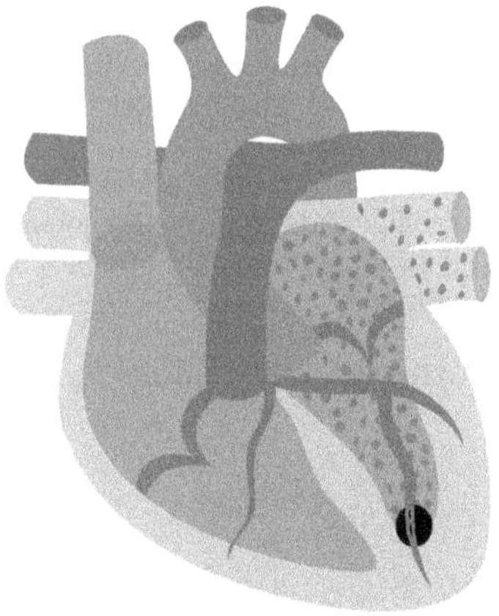

a) If the accumulation of blood in the LV is allowed to continue, blood will back track into the LA

b) Consequently blood will move through the LA into the pulmonary veins increasing HP in the pulmonary circulation

c) This can lead to pulmonary oedema (see Fig. 8.7b)

Figure 8.7a The pathophysiological processes of left ventricular failure (LVF)

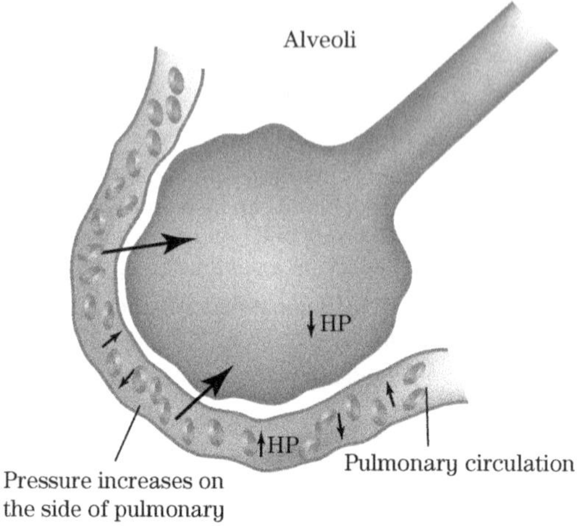

a) The increased collection of blood in the pulmonary circulation increases HP and changes capillary dynamics
b) When HP exceeds oncotic pressure fluid moves
c) The fluid moves from an increased HP in the pulmonary capillaries to a low HP in the alveoli due to filtration pressure
d) Fluid is usually picked up by the lymphatic system, but when the flow of fluid out of the capillaries exceeds the lymphatic system's ability to remove it then pulmonary oedema will occur
e) Fluid will accumulate in the alveoli spaces
f) Rapid filling of alveoli spaces with fluid leads to pulmonary oedema

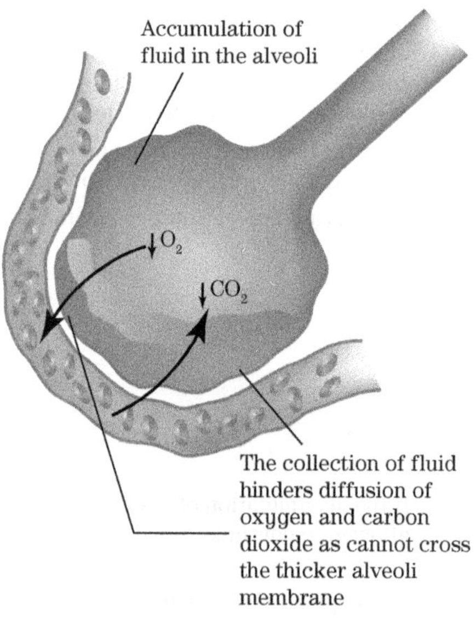

a) The fluid in the alveoli spaces will prevent efficient movement/ diffusion of oxygen from the alveoli to the haemaglobin and carbon dioxide carried by haemaglobin and plasma back into the alveoli
b) This will lead to dyspnea, orthopnea, hypoxaemia and increased work of breathing
c) In severe cases the patient can cough up pink and frothy sputum or frothy sputum
d) The administration of oxygen will ↑ the PP of oxygen in the alveoli making it greater than capillary HP, forcing more oxygen across the fluid membrane
e) This will facilitate the release of carbon dioxide from haemoglobin and rapidly improve the patient's condition

Figure 8.7b The physiological processes of the formation of pulmonary oedema

- Hypovolaemia/hypervolaemia (fluid overload)
- Pulmonary embolism
- Sepsis
- Anaemia
- Chronic obstructive pulmonary disease (COPD).

Pathology

- The myocardium becomes weak; this impairs the ability of the heart to pump efficiently
- With each beat blood (the amount depending on the severity of the weakness) remains in the left ventricle, decreasing the amount of blood pumped out from both ventricles
- Nervous stimulation will increase heart rate to maintain cardiac output for a while, but the blood continues to build up in the left ventricle leading to a back flow from the left ventricle into the lungs
- This will raise the hydrostatic pressure (HP) in the blood vessels into the lungs leading to pulmonary oedema.

Investigations

- Physical examination is required following airway, breathing, circulation, disability and exposure (ABCDE)
- Blood tests:
  - Full blood count (FBC)
  - Urea and creatinine to determine kidney function
  - Transaminase and bilirubin to determine liver function
- ECG may show atrial and/or ventricular enlargement
- Chest X-ray to determine size of the heart e.g. enlarged
- Echocardiography – repeated scans can show response to treatment
- Trans-oesophageal echocardiography can show hypertrophy, valve disorders
- Cardiac catheterisation can show coronary artery occlusion, any disorders of the valves e.g. stenosis, insufficiency.

Clinical features

- Severe breathlessness
- Moist, wheezy breathing
- Anxiety – feeling of suffocation
- Tachycardia
- Cold, clammy skin
- White, frothy sputum – may be pink in terminal stages.

Treatment and drug therapy

- Sit up in bed allowing maximum lung expansion
- Administer oxygen as prescribed – high concentration

- A portable chest X-ray may be performed
- Urgent diuretics are needed to relieve the pulmonary oedema
- A small dose of diamorphine (2.5 mg) – relieves the panic and anxiety but also helps to reduce the strain on the heart.

Heart failure (HF)

This is when the increased pressure pushes backwards into the pulmonary artery and into the right side of the heart leading to failure of the right side (Nicholas, 2004) (Figure 8.7c). Heart failure is commonly associated as a complication of MI, as in the case of George (Case study 8.1).

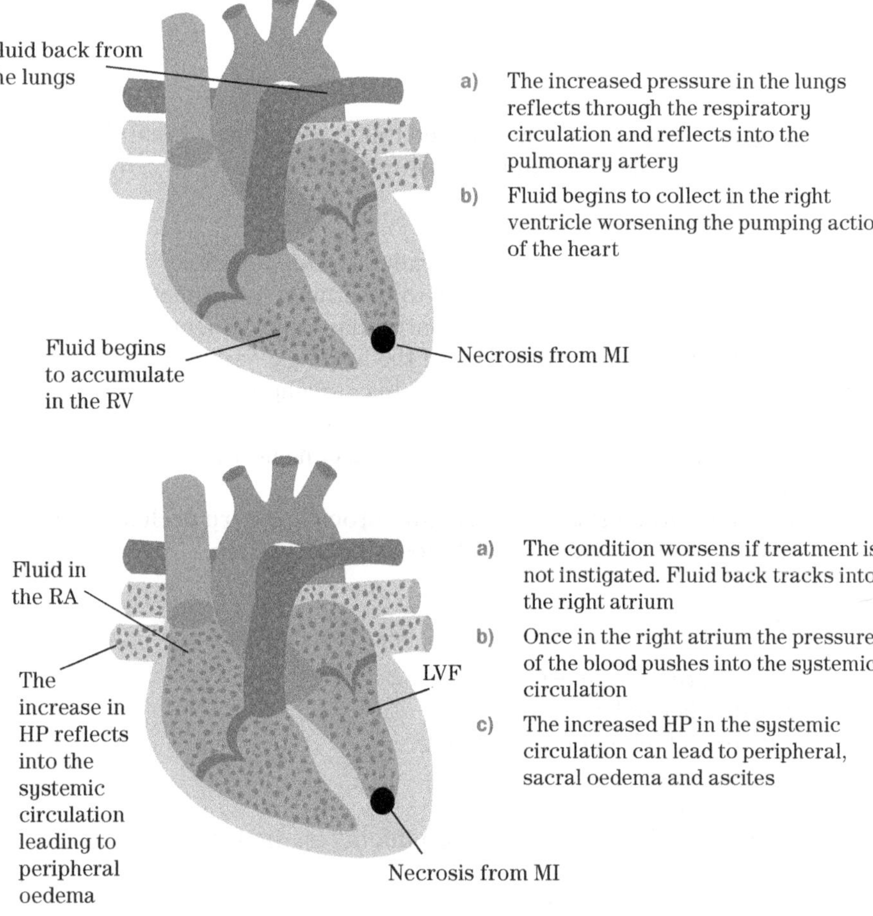

Figure 8.7c The pathophysiological processes leading to heart failure (HF)

Case study 8.1

George is a 65-year-old man who had a myocardial infarction (MI) 3 months ago. He was found wandering in the local shopping centre in a confused state. George was carrying his current medication, which consisted of a cardiac glycoside and a thiazide diuretic. He had distended neck veins, oedema of the ankles, rapid respiratory rate, a raised pulse and a high blood pressure. He had a diagnosis of heart failure following his recent MI. George was given an IV bolus of furosemide.

- *Pathology*
  - The stress on the heart from the necrotic muscle reaches a critical level
  - There is impaired contractility of the cardiac muscle and cardiac output declines
  - There is an increase in volume in the right ventricle (Bullock and Henze, 2000)
  - Right ventricle cannot pump and there is a backlog of blood that occurs in the right atrium and vena cava
  - The venous system becomes congested
  - Blood pools in the systemic circulation leading to peripheral oedema
- *Clinical features*
  - Increase in breathlessness
  - Due to the raised pressure in the systemic veins oedema forms
  - Weight gain
  - Distended jugular veins may be visible
  - Fall in cardiac output results in salt and water retention by the kidneys
  - Ascites (fluid accumulated in the peritoneal cavity) may occur
  - Pleural effusion (fluid in the pleural space) may add to the breathlessness
  - All the abdominal organs are engorged with blood and in the liver this may cause abdominal pain
  - Loss of appetite
  - Lethargy and fatigue, muscle weakness
  - Mental changes:
    - Irritability
    - Reduced attention span
    - Restlessness

- *Treatment and drug therapy*
  - Breathlessness
    - Sit upright in bed or in a chair. Some patients even to prefer sleep sitting in a chair
    - Oxygen should be administered, 2 L at the outset, prescribed oxygen titrated to oxygen saturation
  - Oedema
    - An accurate record of fluid intake and output is kept
    - Assessment of the oedema, daily weighing may be done
    - Diuretics will be prescribed – examples are Frumil or, if the oedema is not so severe, bendrofluazide
    - Reduced salt intake
    - Fluid restriction may become necessary if diuretics fail
  - Fatigue
    - The patient will feel tired as the heart cannot respond to any increased demands made upon it
    - Rest is important to reduce the strain on the heart
  - Abdominal discomfort
    - Venous congestion can cause problems throughout the GIT
    - Loss of appetite and constipation are common
    - Straining to go to the toilet should be avoided
    - Congestion of the liver may lead to slight jaundice
  - Administration of medication (NICE, 2003)
    - Diuretics are essential to help to reduce the oedema
    - Digoxin may be prescribed to increase the force of the cardiac contractions
    - ACE inhibitors such as captopril are now commonly used help to take the strain off the heart by causing vasodilation
    - Anticoagulants, e.g. heparin, may be ordered for some clients if the risk of thromboembolism is assessed as severe.

Cardiomyopathy

Cardiomyopathy is a disorder of the cardiac muscle that can be acute, subacute or chronic (Edwards and Coyne, 2013). It is often of an unknown aetiology but can occur at birth or in childhood.

Aetiology

- Idiopathic
- Familial and/or genetic – the condition appears to be a common genetic malformation of the heart affecting 1 in 500 of the population
- Viral and immune

- Alcoholic/toxic
- Associated with recognised cardiovascular disease in which the degree of myocardial dysfunction is not explained by the abnormal loading conditions or the extent of ischaemic damage.

Pathology

- Dilated cardiomyopathy
  - Characterised by dilatation and impaired contraction of the left ventricle or both ventricles
- Hypertrophic cardiomyopathy
  - Characterised by left and/or right ventricular hypertrophy, which is usually asymmetric and involves the intra-ventricular septum
  - The left ventricular volume is normal or reduced
  - Systolic gradients are common
  - Arrhythmias and premature sudden death are common
  - There are 4 main abnormalities found:
    - Ventricular hypertrophy
    - Rapid contraction of the left ventricle
    - Impaired relaxation
    - Intracavity systolic gradients
- Arrhythmogenic right ventricular cardiomyopathy (ARVC)
  - Characterised pathologically by right ventricular myocardial atrophy and fibro-fatty replacements
  - ARVC changes are frequently transmural
  - ARVC is a progressive heart muscle disease that with time may lead to more diffuse right ventricle involvement and left ventricular changes leading to heart failure
  - Can be difficult to diagnose as the patient may be asymptomatic until the first presentation with cardiac arrest, heart failure or ventricular arrhythmias.

Clinical features

- Asymptomatic
- Palpitations
- Atrial fibrillation
- Syncope
- Lethargy/fatigue for many months or years before diagnosis
- Chest pain on exertion
- Dyspnoea, paroxysmal nocturnal dyspnoea, orthopnoea
- Cyanosis

- Systolic murmur
- Pulmonary oedema
- Chest pain.

Investigations

- Routine medical screening
- 12 lead ECG, but this can be normal
- Chest X-ray may reveal an enlarged heart
- 24-hour ambulatory electrocardiographic monitoring
- Echocardiogram can confirm diagnosis
- Exercise testing
- Medical, family and drug history
- Cardiac catheterisation can diagnose the cause of the cardiomyopathy
- Viral serology
- First degree relatives of an affected person are offered cardiac screening and evaluation.

Treatment/drug therapy

- To control symptoms
- Prevent disease progression and complications such as progressive heart failure, thromboembolism and sudden death
- Diuretics such as spironolactone
- Digoxin, isosorbide dinitrate to produce dilation and to relieve chest pain
- Beta-blockers e.g. verapamil, diltazem
- Anti-arrhythmics e.g. amiodarone to control arrhythmias
- ACE inhibitors to reduce afterload
- Anticoagulants
- Heart transplant
- Multisite ventricular pacing
- Cardioversion to treat atrial fibrillation (AF)
- Implant cardioverter-defrillator to correct ventricular arrhythmias
- Left ventricular assist device (VAD) if resistant to medical therapy.

Cardiogenic shock

In cardiogenic shock the heart is unable to deliver adequate amounts of oxygen to the peripheral tissues the body demands (Josephson, 2008).

Aetiology

Extensive MI, but has been observed in patients with a smaller infarction (O'Donovan, 2011).

- Complications of MI:
  - Mitral valve regurgitation
  - Rupture of the inter-ventricular septum
  - Left ventricular failure/heart failure
- Cardiac tamponade
- End stage cardiomyopathy
- Septic shock.

Pathology

- There is a marked decrease in stroke volume and cardiac output, due to myocardial ischaemia or necrosis
- The ventricular pump fails, with an increase in filling pressures through all chambers, with pulmonary and systemic oedema
- Coronary artery perfusion decreases, decreasing oxygen delivery to the myocardium
- Heart rate increases, blood pressure drops
- Several compensatory mechanisms are activated to maintain blood pressure, but as the condition progresses they become maladaptive and can serve to worsen the situation (O'Donovan, 2011)
- Evidence of tissue hypo-perfusion, despite an adequate blood volume
- The condition is further compromised and the ischaemia worsens
- The myocardial oxygen demands cannot be met (Figure 8.8).

Clinical features

- Hypotension systolic blood pressure less than 90 mmHg
- Arrhythmias
- Delayed capillary refill
- Decreased urine output
- Confusion, disorientation
- Cool extremities
- Coughing up of pink and frothy sputum
- Raised jugular venous pressure
- Chest pain
- Breathlessness, use of accessory respiratory muscles, reduced oxygen saturation.

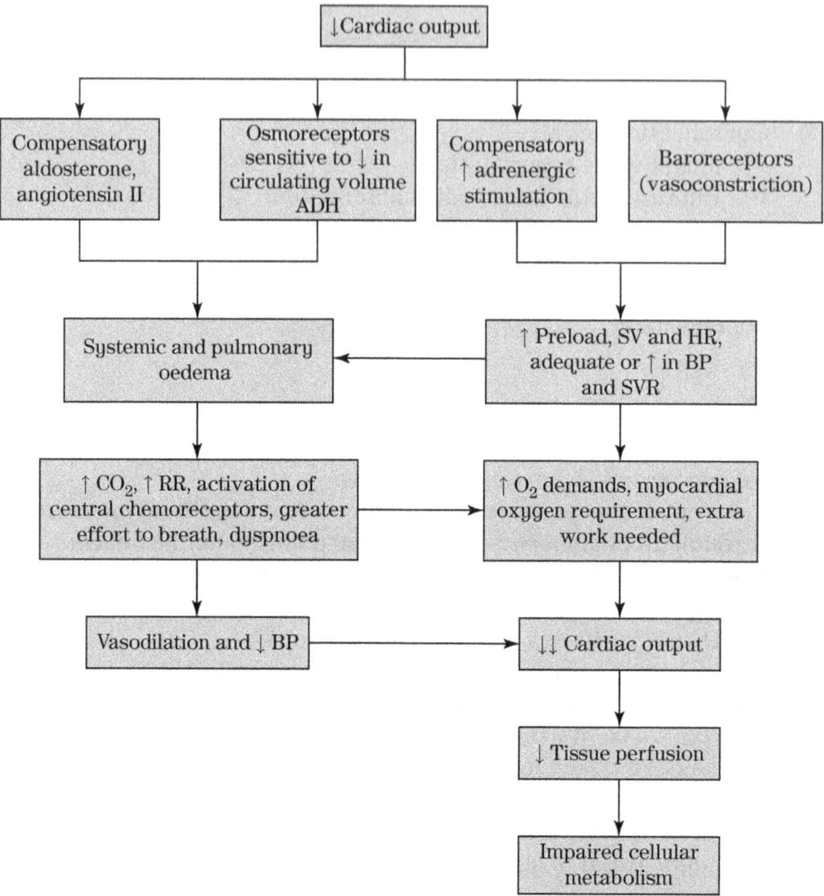

Figure 8.8 Cardiogenic shock

Investigations

- Arterial blood gases to exclude hypoxia or acidosis as the primary cause of the shock
- Chest X-ray
- ECG to rule out other causes and disease
- Blood tests FBC
- Cardiac enzymes
- Echocardiography is central to the diagnosis of cardiogenic shock (O'Donovan, 2011)
- Haemodynamic monitoring e.g. CVP, oesophageal Doppler, vital signs.

Treatment and drug therapy

- Inotropic support e.g. dopamine, dobutamine, noradrenaline
- Maintaining blood glucose level has shown some benefits in cardiogenic shock (Josephson, 2008)
- Ventilation support to maintain oxygen supply
- Intra-aortic balloon pump (IAPB)
  - Inserted into the femoral artery into the thoracic aorta to give circulatory support
  - The IABP has a 40 ml balloon catheter
  - The function is counter-pulsation
    - When the heart is in systole, the balloon is deflated
    - When the heart is in diastole the balloon is inflated increasing perfusion through the coronary and renal arteries
- Revascularisation methods:
  - Left ventricular assist device (LVAD) has many side effects and is not usually the method of choice
  - Percutaneous coronary intervention (PCI) can be successful when carried out within 6 hours
- Thrombolysis e.g. streptokinase or alteplase is controversial in cardiogenic shock, as thrombolysis is less effective when compared to PCI, but is indicated when PCI is impossible (O'Donovan, 2011).

DISORDERS OF ELECTRICAL ACTIVITY: ARRHYTHMIAS

Sinus bradycardia

In sinus bradycardia (Figure 8.9a) the heart rate falls below 60 bpm, but maintains a regular rhythm and originates from the sino-atrial node.

- *Aetiology*
  - It can be normal, for example in athletes or during sleep
  - An increase in vagal tone and a decrease in sympathetic stimulation
  - An inferior MI due to right coronary artery disease
  - Drugs
- *Clinical features*
  - On ECG reading:
    - P waves: upright, normal in shape
    - PR interval: 0.12–0.20 seconds
    - QRS interval: 0.14–0.12 seconds
- *Treatment/drug therapy*

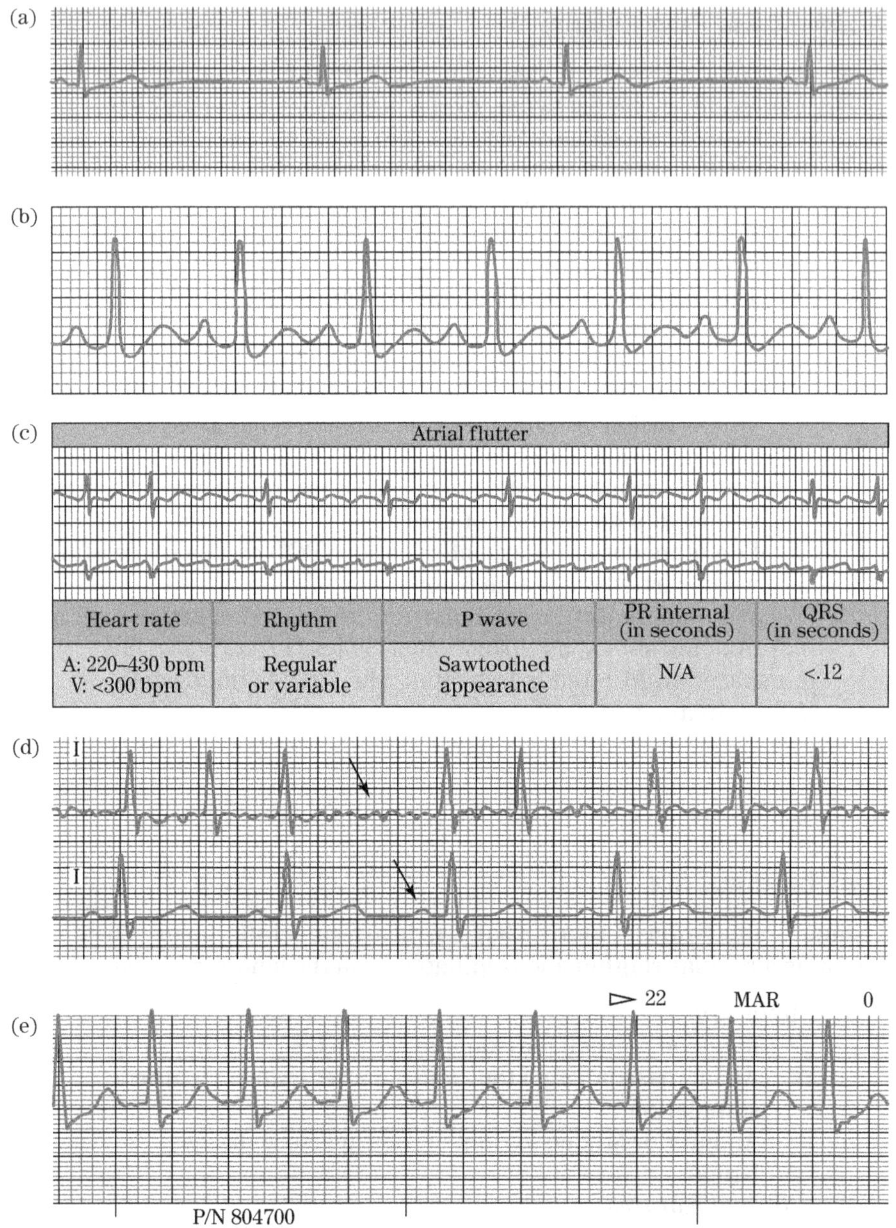

Heart rate	Rhythm	P wave	PR internal (in seconds)	QRS (in seconds)
A: 220–430 bpm V: <300 bpm	Regular or variable	Sawtoothed appearance	N/A	<.12

Figure 8.9 (a) Sinus bradycardia; (b) Sinus tachycardia; (c) Atrial flutter; (d) Atrial fibrillation; (e) Atrial tachycardia/SVT

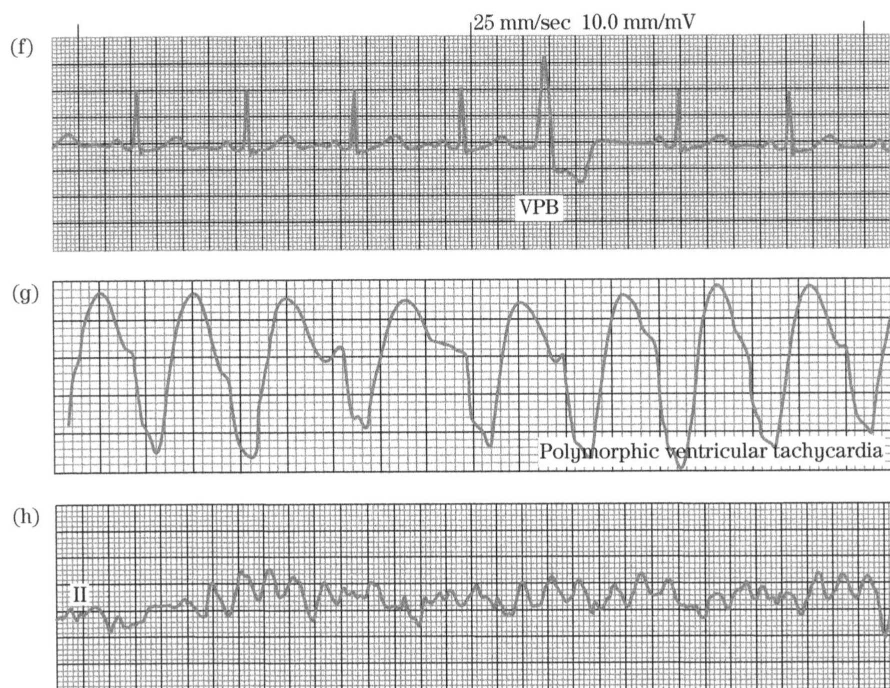

Figure 8.9 (Continued) (f) Premature ventricular contractions; (g) Ventricular tachycardia; (h) Ventricular fibrillation

- If the bradycardia continues to drop e.g. to 45 bpm patient can show signs of reduced cardiac output, hypotension, dizziness, confusion
- Nothing if fit young person
- Atropine
- Internal pacing wires if history of an MI
- Can trigger more serious arrhythmias such as ventricular tachycardia/fibrillation, ectopics.

Sinus tachycardia

A sinus tachycardia (Figure 8.9b) is identified as a heart rate above 100 bpm.

- *Aetiology*
  - It is a normal response to exercise
  - Anxiety, stress and emotions
  - Normal homeostatic compensation for nearly all conditions e.g. hypovolaemia, cardiac failure
  - High temperatures

- *Pathology*
  - Maintains a regular rhythm
  - The pacemaker site is the SA node
- *Clinical features*
  - On ECG reading:
    - P waves: upright, normal in shape
    - PR interval: 0.12–0.20 seconds
    - QRS interval: 0.14–0.12 seconds
- *Treatment/drug therapy*
  - None required, normal compensatory mechanism to stress
  - Long-term sinus tachycardia can lead to hypertension and ACS
  - Can result in decreased cardiac output, increases myocardial oxygen demand
  - If the heart needs to be slowed down, drug therapy is beta-adrenergic blockers or calcium channel blockers.

Atrial flutter

Atrial flutter (Figure 8.9c) is very fast with an atrial rate than can reach 150–350 + bpm.

- *Aetiology*
  - Rapid re-entry focus
  - The impulse fails to conduct through AV node
  - Seen in middle age to older adults, with advanced cardiovascular disease e.g. cardiomyopathy, hypertrophy, heart failure, cardiac infections
- *Pathology*
  - The beat originates from a single ectopic focus within the atria,
  - Instead of flowing through the AV node the electrical impulse continues around the atria in a re-entry circuit
  - The atrial rate is regular, but is not always followed by a QRS wave
- *Clinical features*
  - On ECG reading:
    - P waves: 'sawtooth' pattern:
      - Unless in 2:1 block conduction when difficult to see – can appear to be sinus rhythm
      - Easier to spot if 3:1 or 4:1
    - PR interval: usually constant
    - QRS: 0.04–0.12 seconds
- *Treatment/drug therapy*

  - Usually well tolerated if reasonable ventricular rate, but may ultimately reduce cardiac output
  - Treat underlying cause
  - Digoxin, amiodarone
  - Synchronised cardioversion.

Atrial fibrillation

Atrial fibrillation (Figure 8.9d) chaotic, irregular heart beat than can be 350–700 bpm, with a varying ventricular rate.

- *Aetiology*
  - Following cardiac surgery
  - Drugs such as aminophylline
  - More often chronic, associated with heart failure, cardiac disease, may be on digoxin, calcium channel blockers or beta-blockers
- *Pathology*
  - Multiple areas of ectopic pacemaker cells in the atria originating outside of SA node
  - AV conduction becomes random
  - Sometimes the atrial rate cannot be counted
  - The rhythm is irregular
- *Clinical features*
  - On ECG reading:
    - P waves: not visible, fibrillation waves
    - PR interval: none
    - QRS: 0.04–0.12 seconds as long as not ventricular conduction disturbances
  - Cardiac output reduced by up to 15%, may precipitate angina, MI, cardiac failure
  - Palpitations and an irregular heart beat, as in the case of Jerico:

Case study 8.2

Jerico is a 58-year-old male patient who had gone to his GP complaining of palpitations, which were concerning to him as he was usually 'healthy'. An irregular pulse rate was subsequently detected and he was referred as an outpatient to discover the reason behind this. At his outpatient appointment Jerico underwent various tests. He was diagnosed with atrial fibrillation. He was admitted to the ward for stabilisation, observation, monitoring and possibly cardioversion. Jerico's condition remained stable and his wife and elderly parents have been contacted and informed of his admission following his outpatient appointment.

- *Treatment and drug therapy*
  - May not require treatment if tolerated
  - If haemo-dynamically unstable will require:
  - Cardioversion
  - Drug therapy
    - Amiodarone
    - Beta blockers
    - Digoxin
    - Anti-coagulants.

Atrial tachycardia or supraventricular tachycardia (SVT)

SVT (Figure 8.9e) is identified as a heart rate of 150–250+ bpm, which originates from an ectopic focus above the ventricles, but remains in or close to the atria.

- *Aetiology*
  - Occurs at any age
  - Rare in patients with MI
  - Can be precipitated by stress, tobacco, caffeine etc.
  - Digoxin toxicity
  - An overactive thyroid
  - Electrolyte imbalance
  - Hypoxia
- *Pathology*
  - The rapid rate shortens the diastolic time e.g. the time the heart has to fill
  - Leading to a reduced cardiac output, and coronary perfusion
  - Can lead to more serious arrhythmias
- *Clinical features*
  - On ECG reading:
    - Rhythm: usually regular
    - Pacemaker site may vary from SA node to AV node
    - P waves may be upright, normal if pacemaker at SA, inverted if near AV junction
    - PR interval: usually shortened, possibly normal
    - QRS interval 0.14–0.12 seconds
  - Accompanied often by palpitations, dizziness, anxiety and nervousness.
- *Treatment and drug therapy*
  - Can occur in healthy hearts, can be well tolerated
  - Cardiac output can be compromised

- May increase myocardial ischaemia
- Vagal stimulation such as the valsalva manoeuvre or carotid sinus massage can reduce heart rate, but should only be undertaken by a qualified HCP
- Drugs such as
  - Adenosine
  - Amiodarone
  - Verapamil
- Synchronised cardioversion
- Atrial overdrive pacing can be used to stop the arrhythmia.

Premature ventricular contractions (PVC)

A premature ventricular contraction (Figure 8.9f) is defined as an early ectopic beat, which follows an abnormal conduction pathway leading to an abnormal ECG trace.

- *Aetiology*
  - Electrolyte imbalance:
    - Hypokalaemia and hyperkalaemia
    - Hypomagnesaemia and hypocalcaemia
  - Changes in acid base e.g. metabolic acidosis
  - Hypoxia
  - Myocardial infarction, heart failure
  - Drug toxicity e.g. cocaine, amphetamines and tricyclic antidepressants
  - Increased sympathetic stimulation
  - Stimulants e.g. alcohol, sympathetic drugs
- *Pathology*
  - PVCs ectopic pacemaker site (or sites) that originates from ventricles
  - Occurs in many underlying rhythms
  - Alters sequences of ventricular depolarisation
  - The PVC is often followed by a compensatory pause
  - PVCs may be:
    - Unifocal (from one ectopic site)
    - Multifocal (from several ectopic sites) are more dangerous than unifocal due to the risk of R on T phenomenon
- *Clinical features*
  - On ECG reading:
    - Rate: depends on underlying rhythm and number of PVCs
    - Rhythm: when a PVC present, irregular

        - Pacemaker site: ectopic focus in ventricles/bundle
        - P waves: present in normal beat, undetectable in PVCs
        - PR interval: none in the PVC, present if interrupted by normal rhythm
        - QRS: equal or greater than 0.12 seconds, wide and bizarre
        - T wave after the PVC may be deflected in opposite direction due to altered depolarisation sequence
    - This can get serious and lead to worsening arrhythmias e.g. ventricular tachycardia (VT) and ventricular fibrillation (VF)
    - Usually significant if appear in runs of 5 or more, hypotension, poor output, may present as a pre-arrest rhythm
- *Treatment and drug therapy*
    - Oxygen
    - Anti-dysrhythmics, possibly lidocaine, possibly amiodarone
    - Check potassium and magnesium levels
    - Treat and correct the cause.

Ventricular tachycardia

VT (Figure 8.9 g) is when 3 or more consecutive ventricular complexes occur together at rate over 100, which override the primary pacemaker. Usually triggered by PVC, but the atria and ventricle activity asynchronous.

- *Aetiology*
    - Cardiac ischaemia
    - Hypoxia
    - Electrolyte imbalance
    - MI, heart failure, cardiac valve disease, cardiomyopathy
    - Drug toxicity e.g. digoxin
    - Sympathetic drugs
    - Stimulants
- *Pathology*
    - Occurs due to myocardial instability
    - Does not occur in healthy individuals
    - It is unpredictable and can lead to death
    - Can last for short periods and revert back to the patient original rhythm or can be sustained and require life saving interventions e.g. CPR, as there can be rapid deterioration
- *Clinical features*
    - On ECG reading:

    - PR interval: none in the PVC, present if interrupted by normal rhythm
    - Rate: 100–250
    - Rhythm: regular or slightly irregular
    - Pacemaker site: ventricles
    - P waves: not related to QRS (if seen)
    - PR interval: none
    - QRS complex: wide and bizarre greater than 0.12 seconds
- *Treatment and drug therapy*
  - Life-threatening management:
    - Follow the ABCDE of life support interventions
    - Early defibrillation
    - Administration of oxygen
    - Anti-dysrhythmics
    - Possibly lidocaine, amiodarone
    - Check potassium levels
    - If pulseless treat as VF.

Ventricular fibrillation

VF (Figure 8.9 h) is characterised by chaotic ventricular rhythm resulting in quivering ventricular movements and pulseless.

- *Aetiology*
  - Coronary artery disease
  - Ischaemia, MI
  - Hypoxia
  - Acidosis
  - Electrical injury
  - Electrolyte imbalance
  - Hypothermia
  - Shock
  - Drugs and toxicity
- *Pathology*
  - Do not allow sufficient mass of myocardial muscle to fully depolarise and repolarise
  - Organised ventricular contraction does not take place
  - Most common presenting rhythm in cardiac arrest
- *Clinical features*
  - On ECG reading:
    - Rate: not determined
    - Rhythm: not determined

        - Pacemaker site: numerous in ventricles
        - P waves: not determined
        - PR interval: not determined
        - QRS complex: wide and bizarre and not determined
        - A lethal dysrhythmia, with light-headedness, followed by loss of consciousness and cessation of circulation and breathing
- *Treatment and drug therapy*
    - An emergency
    - Follow CPR and BLS
    - Defibrillation
    - Administer oxygen
    - IV cannula insertion for drug administration.

Asystole

Asystole is the absence of all ventricular activity. The patient is unresponsive, with no cardiac output, which can quickly become irreversible.

- *Aetiology*
    - May be primary event in cardiac arrest or subsequent to VT, VF, PEA arrest
    - Associated with global myocardial ischaemia and necrosis
    - Electrolyte disturbances
    - Electric shock
    - Shock
    - Drug intoxication
    - Acid base balance disorders
- *Clinical features*
    - On ECG reading:
        - Rate: none
        - Rhythm: none
        - Pacemaker site: none
        - P waves: none
        - PR interval: none
        - QRS complex: none
    - A lethal dysrhythmia, with a poor prognosis
    - Should be confirmed by a 3 lead ECG rhythm. Check patient and connections!
- *Treatment and drug therapy*
    - Basic Life Support (BLS)
    - Administer oxygen
    - Adrenaline
    - Possible pacing.

Electromechanical disassociation

Electromechanical disassociation (EMD) is when there is no electrical activity without any resulting mechanical output.

- *Aetiology*
  - The 4 Hs
    - Hypoxia
    - Hypothermia
    - Hypovolaemia
    - Hypo/hypercalcaemia
  - The 4 Ts
    - Tension pneumothorax
    - Tamponade
    - Toxins
    - Thromboembolic disturbances
- *Pathology*
  - Prognosis is poor
- *Clinical features*
  - Rhythm can be any, but often bradycardia
- *Treatment and drug therapy*
  - CPR, adrenaline, atropine if slow rate, treat reversible causes.

Heart block

Heart block occurs when there is an interruption in the conduction of impulses between the atria and the ventricles (Carlene, 2010). The blocks can be simply a delay in the electrical impulse or partial or total block. The block can occur in the AV node, the bundle of His or the bundle branches.

1st degree AV block

1st degree heart block (Figure 8.10a) is a delay in conduction at the AV node, within an underlying rhythm.

- *Aetiology*
  - Associated with myocardial ischaemia, MI
  - Increased vagal tone
  - Digoxin toxicity
- *Clinical features*
  - On the ECG reading
    - Rate: generally sinus or rate of underlying rhythm
    - Rhythm: regular or that of underlying rhythm
    - Pacemaker: SA node
    - P waves: normal

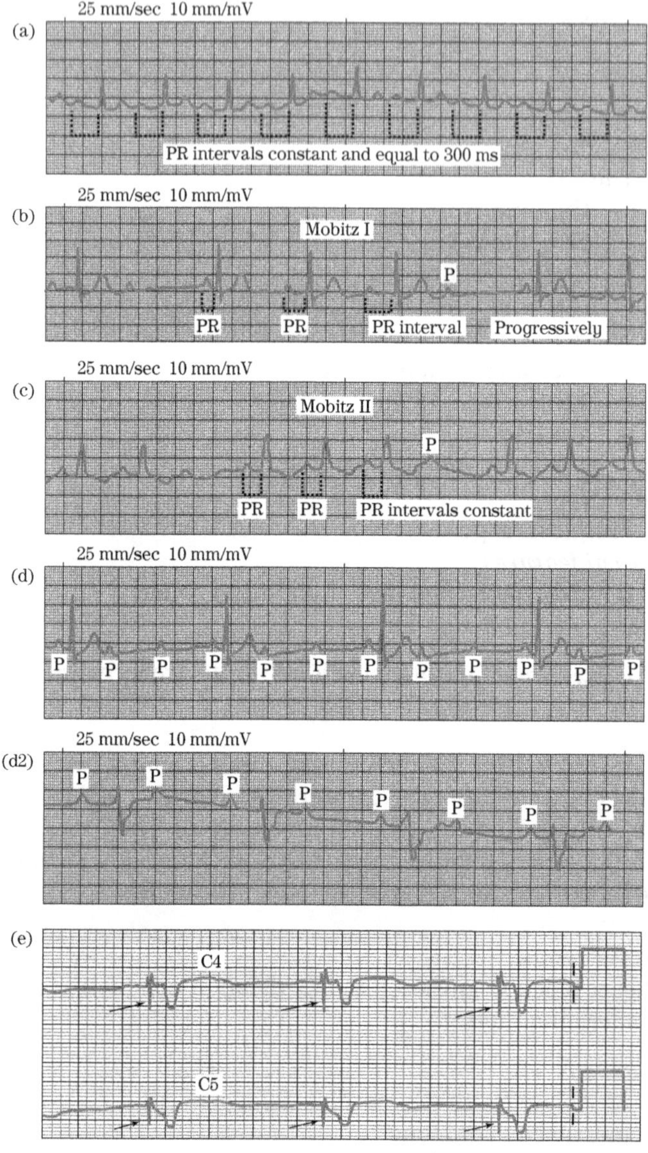

Figure 8.10 (a) 1st degree heart block; (b) 2nd degree heart block, type 1 Wenckebach; (c) 2nd degree heart block, mobitz type 2; (d) 3rd degree heart block (the block is high in the AV node, the QRS appears normal); (d2) 3rd degree heart block (2) (the block is low in the AV junction and the QRS complexes are wide and bizarre) (I put the (2) in to distinguish between the two Figures 8.10d); (e) Pacing spikes shown on an ECG (defined by the arrow)

    - PR interval: prolonged greater than 0.20 seconds
    - QRS: usually normal
  - May progress to other AV blocks
  - Many patients are asymptomatic
- *Treatment and drug therapy*
  - Generally none required
  - Close monitoring to check worsening condition.

2nd degree AV block, Mobitz type 1 (Wenckebach)

2nd degree AV block type 1 (Figure 8.10b) is intermittent block at the level of the AV node. There is conduction delay shown by a lengthened PR interval increasing until conduction is blocked and a beat is missed.

- *Aetiology*
  - Occurs often in MI and myocarditis
  - Increased vagal tone
  - Ischaemia
  - Drug toxicity
  - Electrolyte imbalance
- *Clinical features*
  - On ECG reading
    - Rate: atrial rate is that of underlying sinus or atrial rhythm, ventricular rate is normal or slow but slightly less than atrial rate
    - Rhythm: atrial rhythm is regular, ventricular rhythm is irregular
    - Pacemaker: SA node
    - P waves: normal
    - PR interval: progressively lengthens before non-conducted P wave
    - QRS: usually normal
  - Usually transient and reversible
  - Can develop into more serious block
  - If dropped beats are regular, patient may become haemodynamically unstable
- *Treatment and drug therapy*
  - If asymptomatic no treatment may be given
  - If symptoms give atropine
  - Temporary pacing for short term, but if persists then a permanent pacemaker can be inserted.

2nd degree AV block, Mobitz type 2

2nd degree AV block type 2 (Figure 8.10c) is intermittent block whereby the AV node does not conduct the electrical impulse but there is normal conduction, followed by a non-conducted impulse. The ratio of conducted to non-conducted is usually constant. Usually occurs below the bundle of His.

- *Aetiology*
  - Usually associated with MI
  - Septal necrosis
  - Does not result solely from increase parasympathetic tone or drug
- *Clinical features*
  - On ECG reading
    - Rate: atrial rate is unaffected, that of underlying rhythm ventricular rate less, may be bradycardic
    - Rhythm: regular or irregular, depending on whether conduction ratio is constant or variable
    - P waves: upright and uniform, some P waves not followed by QRS complexes
    - PR interval: usually constant for conducted beats and may be greater than 0.20 sec
    - QRS: may be wider than normal due to bundle branch block
  - A serious dysrhythmia, may be sufficiently severe as to compromise the haemodynamic state of the patient
  - A risk of progression to a more severe form of heart block
- *Treatment and drug therapy*
  - If symptomatic atropine
  - Pacing.

3rd degree AV block (complete heart block)

3rd degree AV block (Figure 8.10c) is complete block at AV node or complete AV disassociation; SA node activates atria and ectopic pacemaker serves ventricles. Atrial and ventricular electrical activity completely unrelated.

- *Aetiology*
  - Increased septal necrosis
  - Acute myocarditis
  - Digoxin overdose
  - Beta blocker or calcium channel blocker
  - Vagal tone
  - Electrolyte imbalance
- *Clinical features*
  - On the ECG reading
    - Rate: atrial rate of underlying atrial or sinus rhythm, ventricular rate 40–60 typically if in junction, may be lower if in ventricles.
    - Rhythm: atrial and ventricular rhythm regular but independent of each other

    - P waves: present, unrelated to QRS complexes
    - PR interval: no relationship between atrial and ventricular activity
    - QRS: usually wide and bizarre especially if pacemaker site in ventricles, occasionally normal duration
    - A severe bradycardia and cardiac compromise may be very unstable and is potentially lethal
  - *Treatment and drug therapy*
    - Pacing (Figure 8.10e) there are two types:
    - Internal pacing wires are temporary; usually inserted following cardiac surgery or following a right coronary artery MI, bradycardia, heart block
    - External pacing wires are permanent; usually undertaken to maintain a regular rhythm.

VASCULAR SYSTEM DISORDERS

Vascular disorders affect arteries and veins or can occur in both types of vessels (Carlene, 2010).

Varicose veins

- *Aetiology*
  - Trauma of the saphenous veins of the legs causing damage to one or more valves
  - Standing for long periods of time
  - Wearing constricting garments
  - Crossing of legs or knees
  - Underlying deep vein thrombosis (DVT)
- *Pathology*
  - Trauma leads to blood pooling in the legs due to damaged valves
  - Normal venous pressure cannot be maintained
  - Hydrostatic pressure in the veins increases
  - Can progress to chronic venous insufficiency (CVI), leading to:
    - Cellular and tissue hypoxia (Figure 2.2)
    - Inflammation and ulceration (Figure 2.3)
- *Clinical features*
  - Swelling
  - Unsightly raised areas along the veins of legs, which can bulge out
  - Pain

- *Investigations*
  - Doppler
- *Treatment and drug therapy*
  - Leg elevation
  - Compression stockings
  - Physical exercise
  - Endovascular ablation or removal of the varicose veins by surgical procedure
  - Surgical vein stripping.

Deep vein thrombosis (DVT)

DVT can be a silent killer and a threat to recovery from surgery. A DVT is a venous thrombosis (blood clot) that forms in a vein (Welch, 2006), accompanied by an inflammatory response in the vein wall (Quigley *et al*, 2012).

Aetiology

- Varicose veins and CVI
- Problems with circulation
- 3 factors can lead to DVT known as the Virchow triad:
  - Venous stasis
  - Venous endothelial damage
  - Hyper-coagulation states
- Recent orthopaedic surgery
- Spinal cord injury
- Obstetric or gynaecological condition.

Pathology

- There are 3 pathophysiological processes referred to as Virchow's triad:
  - Venous trauma
  - Venous stasis
  - Hypercoagulability.

Clinical features

- Pain in the arm or legs, which can be relieved by elevating the leg
- Intermittent claudication, cramp during walking or on exertion
- Swelling, redness and tenderness in the calves, legs or feet
- Unequal calf measurements
- Cold, numbness or pallor in the legs.

Investigations

- Risk assessments for the development of DVT have been devised e.g. McCaffrey *et al* (2007) and Auter (2003)
- Comparison of arm and calf measurements – one is usually larger than the other
- Radial pulse (arm), femoral and foot pulses (leg), skin colour
- D-dimer blood test:
  - When increased can indicate a rise in fibrin degradation products (clots broken down and loose in the blood stream) and so can be raised in DVT (Welch, 2006)
  - Not always reliable as blood clot fragments can increase after:
    - Operation
    - Injury
    - Inflammation due to infection or disease
- Additional tests need to be performed to confirm DVT such as:
  - Contrast venography but is expensive and invasive
  - Ultrasound but this again is not always conclusive or can give a false negative result
  - Doppler to measure ankle-brachial index (ABI) and toe brachial index (TBI) to asses lower extremity arterial blood flow (Bonham, 2006)
  - Computed tomography (CT scan)
  - Magnetic resonance imaging (MRI)
  - Due to the unreliability of these investigations combinations are usually performed.

Treatment

- Prevention with the use of elastic stocking, mobility and anti-coagulant therapy
- If DVT occurs:
  - Low molecular weight heparin (LMWH)
  - Heparin
  - Warfarin should continue for at least 3 months or sometimes longer
  - Fibrinolytic therapy, but there is a risk of bleeding
- Observation and monitoring for signs of pulmonary embolism (see chapter 9).

Arterial and venous leg ulcers

There is a difference between arterial and venous leg ulcers, which can be observed by understanding the two conditions.

Aetiology

Arterial and venous leg ulcer can occur in a variety of conditions:

- Heart failure
- Peripheral vascular disease
- Diabetes mellitus
- Varicose veins and CVI.

Pathology

- Arterial leg ulcers
  - Lack of blood supply to the lower limbs leads to slow cell and tissue death
- Venous leg ulcers
  - There is poor venous return of blood from the lower limbs due to damage of the veins and valves, leading to congestion and build up of fluid.

Clinical features

- Arterial leg ulcers
  - There is intermittent claudication and pain at rest
  - Pulses are hard to palpate or sometimes absent
  - Skin colour is pale and then later becomes red
  - There is loss of hair over the area and toe nails become thickened and hard
  - The ulcer often appears on toes or feet
  - There is tissue ischaemia giving ulcers a black necrotic appearance and gangrene can be associated with arterial leg ulcers (Quigley *et al*, 2012)
- Venous leg ulcers
  - The ulcers can be painful, but are more likely to ache usually at the end of the day, when pain increases to become chronic; this can effect quality of life (Quigley *et al*, 2012)
  - Venous congestion and increase in hydrostatic pressure
  - Pulses are normal, but sometimes difficult to feel through the swelling and oedema
  - Colour can appear normal, but later brown pigmentation appears on the skin
  - The leg(s) are swollen and can be severe, leading to skin breakdown that is often yellow, with redness, scaling and pruritus; gangrene is rare (De Araujo *et al*, 2003)
  - The ulcer usually appears on the ankles.

For investigations and treatment see chapter 16 section on wounds.

Aortic aneurysm

An aneurysm is a bulge or dilation in the vessel wall usually due to atheroma. It is a weak point and the danger is that it will leak or rupture. Aneurysms usually occur in the thoracic or abdominal aorta.

Aetiology

A thoracic or abdominal aneurysm can occur for a number of reasons:

- Can be related to age e.g. sluggish circulation, immobility, dehydration
- Chronic hypertension
- Smoking
- Atherosclerosis as the plague erodes the vessel wall
- Systemic lupus erythematosus (SLE)
- Diabetes mellitus
- Trauma to the chest or abdomen
- Marfan's or Turner syndromes
- Pregnancy.

Pathology

- An aneurysm occurs from a defect in the middle layer of the arterial wall (tunica media or medial layer)
- The middle layer becomes damaged and loses some of its elasticity and the wall thins
- If hypertension is present this leads to stretching of the wall further weakening the vessel
- Blood begins to flow through the weakness, pushing blood into the inner layer of aorta or blood vessel
- A bulge may form, out from the aorta (thoracic or abdominal) filled with stagnant blood, which can contain clots and press on surrounding tissue or organs.

Clinical features

- Thoracic aortic aneurysm
  - Early symptoms:
    - It may be asymptomatic and found as a pulsatile mass on examination or as calcification on an X-ray
    - A dissecting (splitting) aortic (thoracic) aneurysm usually starts in the ascending aorta and pain is severe and central, often radiating to the back
    - It may feel similar to a myocardial infarction
    - Breathlessness

        - Dysrhythmias
        - Heart murmur
        - Different blood pressure and pulse reading when done on both arms
    - Progression and growth of the aneurysm:
        - Severely elevated blood pressure
        - Mental changes
        - Jugular vein distension
        - Tracheal deviation
        - Signs of MI and/or heart failure
        - Rupture causes intense pain in the back and the patient is shocked due to blood loss
- Abdominal aortic aneurysm
    - Constant abdominal pain
    - Back pain in the lower lumbar region that is not affected by movement
    - Feeling of fullness
    - Palpable abdominal mass in the umbilical area.

Investigations

Usually found following a routine examination or testing for other medical conditions

- Blood tests are not diagnostic but might help e.g. haematocrit and FBC
- An ultrasound will show how large the aneurysm is and if a leak has occurred
- Echocardiography to determine location and blood flow pattern
- Trans-oesophageal echocardiography (TOE) allows visual examination of the aneurysm, combined with Doppler flow studies
- X-rays of the chest or abdomen
- CT scan or MRI may give information about the aneurysm's effect on other organs.

Treatment/drug therapy

If the aneurysm is large, producing symptoms and/or there is a risk of rupture, emergency surgery resection of the aneurysm and grafting of the aortic section may be necessary.

- Rupture of an aneurysm requires emergency interventions:
    - Immediate transfer to theatre
    - Fluid and blood replacement
    - Drugs to reduce myocardial contractility e.g. labetalol and blood pressure e.g. nitroprusside

    - Pain relief
    - Arterial line to monitor arterial blood gases (ABG) and urinary catheter to measure urine output
- Surgery may be delayed if the aneurysm is small and its growth monitored using physical examination or ultrasound
- Medications are required to control blood pressure, control any pain and to relieve any anxiety.

Hypertension

A blood pressure of 130/85 bpm or below is regarded as normal by the WHO any increase above the normal is termed hypertension. Hypertension can include high reading for both systolic and diastolic or isolated to just one. Hypertension is the *most important risk factor* for diseases of the cardiovascular system e.g. stroke, ACS and peripheral vascular disease.

Aetiology

- Hypertension with no definite cause is *essential, idiopathic* or *primary hypertension.* risk factors:
    - Genetic factors
    - Low birth weight
    - Physical inactivity, obesity
    - Smoking
    - High salt intake, low potassium intake
    - High alcohol intake
    - Stress
- Secondary hypertension is where a definite cause can be found:
    - Atherosclerosis
    - Diabetes
    - Kidney disease
    - Others are mostly endocrine and include:
        - Phaeochromocytoma (tumour of the adrenal medulla)
        - Conn's syndrome (hyperaldosteronism)
        - Cushing's disease (overactivity of the adrenal cortex or due to administration of long-term steroids)
        - Hyperthyroidism, hyperparathyroidism
        - Renal hypertension
- Malignant hypertension

    - Lifestyle changes may be recommended first:
        - Weight loss
        - Reduction in salt intake

    - Safe exercise
    - Stopping smoking
    - Stress reduction.

Pathology

- Primary hypertension
  - There is a combination of genetics and environment:
    - Prolonged stress stimulates the sympathetic nervous system, increases heart rate, blood pressure, and the release of renin angiotensin aldosterone system
    - A diet high salt diet that increases blood volume and a reduced excretion of salt in urine
    - Leading to a sustained increase in blood pressure
    - The increased pressure on endothelial cells contributes to the thickening of arterial blood vessel walls
    - Thickening reduces their ability to respond to SNS response when blood pressure increases
- Secondary hypertension
  - If the cause of the hypertension is removed blood pressure can return to normal, before irreversible damage occurs
- Complicated hypertension
  - The walls of arteries and arterioles undergo hyperplasia and hypertrophy
  - This can lead to complications such as:
    - Left ventricular failure
    - Acute coronary syndromes
    - Sudden death
    - Aneurysms (aortic and cerebral)
    - Renal insufficiencies
    - Retinal vascular sclerosis
    - Stroke
    - Confusion and mental deterioration
- Malignant hypertension
  - A dangerous form of accelerated hypertension, which is life threatening and a hypertensive emergency (McCance *et al*, 2010)
  - BP rises rapidly and diastolic BP is >120 mmHg
  - May lead to progressive:
    - Encephalopathy
    - Cerebral oedema
    - Loss of consciousness
    - Kidney failure
    - Retinal haemorrhages

    - Heart failure
    - Stroke
- If treatment not given less than 20% survive after 1 year.

Clinical features

- Diseases of the CVS kill more people in Britain than all other causes of death (NICE, 2003) – known as the 'silent killer':
  - Patients may have no symptoms but the raised BP may be slowly damaging their bodies
  - Many have had raised blood pressure for many years.
  - The risk rises progressively as the BP rises
  - Control can lead to the prevention of CVS complications
- Approximately 30% of those over 50 in the UK have hypertension.

Investigations

- A single increased BP measurement is not a diagnosis of hypertension
- If diagnosis is confirmed:
  - Complete medical history
  - Assessment of lifestyle
  - Physical assessment
  - Ambulatory blood pressure measurement over a period of 24 hours
  - Blood tests:
    - Haematocrit
    - Urinalysis
    - Biochemical analysis e.g. cholesterol, sodium and potassium.

Treatment and drug therapy

- Guidelines given by the British Hypertension Society (BHS) and National institute for Health and Care (NICE) (www.nice.org.uk)
  - Younger than 55 years:
    - Angiotensin-converting enzyme (ACE) inhibitors – these drugs block the angiotensin converting enzyme preventing the formation of angiotensin II from angiotensin I manufactured from renin, produced by the kidney e.g. ramipril, captopril, lisinopril and enalapril
  - For those over 55 yrs:
    - Diuretics e.g. bendrofluazide – these drugs increase excretion of water and sodium, decreasing blood volume and

    peripheral resistance and so reducing blood pressure (Whittaker, 2004)
  - Diuretics and calcium channel-blockers are the first line of therapy. Calcium channel blockers act by inhibiting the transfer of calcium ions into cells e.g. nifedipine or they can be more selective to specific areas in the heart such as verapamil or diltiazem
  - If the hypertension is not controlled, further drugs are added e.g. ACE inhibitors, a diuretic and a calcium channel blocker
  - If still not controlled than an alpha-blocker such as doxazosin or a beta-blocker (should not be given to patients with airway obstruction) such as atenolol are added to the drugs already taking
- In malignant hypertension managed with:
  - Rapid infusion of vasodilators e.g. nitrates
  - BP should be controlled slowly and should not be given drugs to act quickly by IV route
  - The aim is to reduce the BP 10% to 25% within 2 hours.

Hypotension

Hypotension is a fall in blood pressure that is significant, leading to changes in haemodynamic state (see chapter 4).

Aetiology and clinical features

- Depletion in blood volume
  - Blood loss
  - Dehydration
  - Loss of serous fluid from severe burns
- Pump failure
  - Myocardial infarction
  - Pulmonary embolism (if very large)
  - Depression of the myocardium acidosis/sepsis
  - Drugs e.g. beta-blockers
- Large fall in peripheral resistance
  - Septic shock
  - Peritonitis
  - Pancreatitis
  - Anaphylactic shock
  - Neurogenic shock.

Pathology

- A low blood pressure (hypotension) will:
  - Lead to reduced tissue perfusion throughout the body
  - Reduce the blood supply to the heart
  - Reduce renal blood flow and thus reduce urine output
  - Reduce blood flow to the brain and eventually lead to unconsciousness
- Postural hypotension
  - Drop in systolic and diastolic BP of at least 20 mmHg on standing
  - Normal reflex actions compensate BP when and individual moves from a lying or sitting position to standing
  - In the elderly this does not function well and this response may not occur
  - May occur in pregnancy, or because of vasodilator drugs, immobility, low blood volume
  - Accompanied by dizziness, blurring or loss of vision, fainting.

Treatment and drug therapy

- Hypotension
  - Record observations of BP, HR and RR
    - When BP is low, the HR will usually be increased (*tachycardia*)
    - RR may also be increased
  - Fluid replacement may be commenced IV
  - If blood lost blood sent for group and cross-match for transfusion
  - Monitor urine output (UO) as can lead to impaired renal function, catheterise if UO falls – it should remain above 30 ml per hour
  - Oxygen may be prescribed
  - The patient may be anxious and will need reassurance
  - Investigations such as an ECG, chest X-ray and blood cultures
- Postural hypotension
  - Liberal use of salt intake
  - Raising the head of the bed
  - Compression stockings
  - Increase in fluid intake
  - Vasoconstrictor or mineralocorticoid drugs.

CONCLUSION

The heart is a double pump that propels blood through the major arteries and veins and around the body, and is essential for life. The numerous dysfunctions associated with the heart can develop over time; others can appear as life-threatening conditions that require immediate interventions. The HCP's role is to recognise signs of deterioration and take prompt action to prevent further complications.

SELF-ASSESSMENT QUESTIONS

1. Provide an outline of the structure, chambers and valves, of the heart the cardiac cycle and coronary arteries.
2. Describe the electrical conduction, depolarisation and repolarisation and the normal electrocardiograph.
3. Identify the nervous control of the heart, cardiac output, blood flow and blood pressure.
4. Explain some of the common cardiac, rhythm and vascular disorders.
5. Describe the aetiology, pathology, clinical features, investigations and treatments commonly used for cardiovascular disease.

REFERENCES

Alexander, M.F., Fawcett, J.N., Runciman, P.J. (eds) (2006) *Nursing Practice Hospital and Home: The Adult,* 3rd edn, Edinburgh: Elsevier.

Auter, R. (2003) The management of deep vein thrombosis: the Auter DVT risk assessment scale re-visited, *Journal of Orthopaedic Nursing,* 7, 114–124.

Bonham, P.A. (2006) Get the LEAD out: non-invasive assessment for lower extremity arterial disease using ankle brachial index and toe brachial index measurements, *Journal of Wound Ostomy Continence Nursing,* 33(1), 30–41.

Bullock, B.A. and Henze, R.L. (2000) *Focus on Pathophysiology,* Philadelphia: Lippincott.

Carlene, C.L. (2010) *Cardiovascular Care Made Incredibly Easy,* Philadelphia: Lippincott Williams & Wilkins.

De Araujo, T., Valencia, I. and Federman, D. (2003) Managing the patient with venous ulcers, *Annals of International Medicine,* 138(4), 326–334.

Edwards, S. and Coyne, I (2013) *A Survival Guide to Children's Nursing,* Edinburgh: Churchill Livingstone Elsevier.

Josephson, L. (2008) Cardiogenic shock, *Dimensions of Critical Care Nursing,* 27(4), 160–170.

Lemone, P. and Burke, B. (2004) *Medical and Surgical Nursing–Critical Thinking in Client Care,* New Jersey: Pearson Education.

McCaffrey, R., Bishop, M. and Adonis-Rizzo, M. (2007) Development of and testing of a DVT risk assessment tool: providing evidence of validity and reliability, *Worldviews on Evidence Based Nursing,* 4(1), 1–20.

McCance K.L., Huether, S.E., Brashers, V.L., Rote, N.S. (2010) *Pathophysiology: The Biologic Basis for Disease in Adults and Children*, 6th edn, Edinburgh: Mosby Elsevier.

NICE (National Institute for Health and Clinical Excellence) (2003) *Chronic Heart Failure,* National Clinical Guidelines for diagnosis and management in primary and secondary care, Guidelines No. 5, London: NICE.

Nicholas, M. (2004) Heart failure: pathophysiology treatment and nursing care, *Nursing Standard,* 19(11) 46–53.

O'Donovan, K. (2011) Cardiogenic shock complicating myocardial infarction: an overview, *British Journal of Cardiac Nursing*, 6(6), 280–285.

Quigley, B.H., Palm, M.L., Bickley, L. (2012) *Bates' Nursing Guide to Physical Examination and History Taking*, Philadelphia: Wolters Kluwer/Lippincott Williams & Wilkins.

Richards, A. and Edwards, S. (2012) *A Nurse's Survival Guide to the Ward*, 3rd edn, Edinburgh: Churchill Livingstone Elsevier.

Waugh, A. and Grant, A. (2010) *Ross and Wilson Anatomy and Physiology in Health and Illness,* 11th edn, Edinburgh: Churchill Livingstone.

Welch, E. (2006) The assessment and management of venous thromboembolism, *Nursing Standard,* 20(28), 58–64.

Whittaker, N. (2004) *Disorders and Interventions*, Basingstoke: Palgrave Macmillan.

9 The respiratory system

Sharon Edwards

RESPIRATORY ANATOMY

All of the body's cells require a supply of oxygen; as cells use oxygen they produce carbon dioxide. It is the function of the respiratory system to supply the body with oxygen and dispose of carbon dioxide. To accomplish this, 4 processes are required:

1. Pulmonary ventilation
2. External respiration
3. Transport of respiratory gases
4. Internal respiration.

FUNCTIONAL ANATOMY

The respiratory system is confined within the thoracic cage or bony thorax and includes (Figure 9.1):

- The nose and nasal cavity
- Pharynx, larynx, trachea
- Bronchi, and smaller branches known as bronchioles
- 2 lungs:
  - Right lung has 3 lobes
  - Left lung has 2 lobes
- Terminal sacs or alveoli are where gas exchange takes place; the alveoli:
  - Provide structure
  - Secrete surfactant:
    - A lipoprotein that coats the inner surface of the alveolus
    - Facilitates expansion during inspiration
    - Lowers alveolar surface tension at the end of expiration
    - Prevents lung collapse
- Respiratory muscles (diaphragm and intercostal muscles).

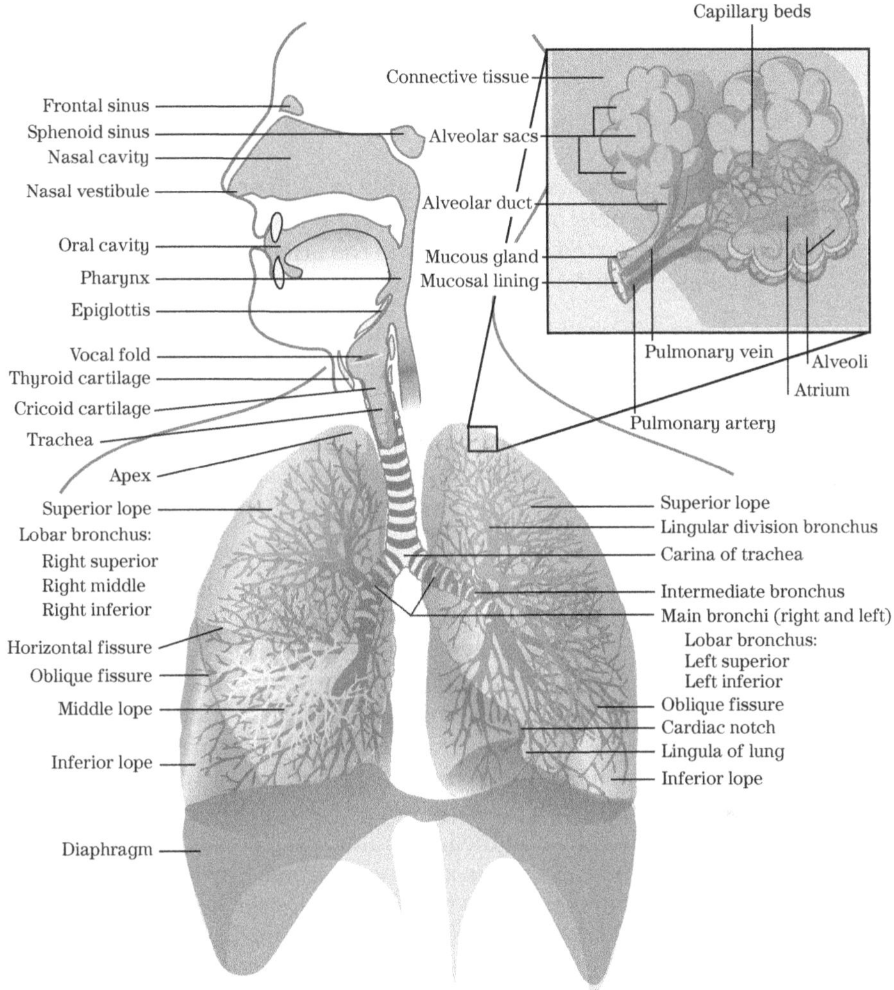

Figure 9.1 The respiratory system

The mechanics of breathing

The basic rhythm of respiration is generated by the cyclical nerve impulses that pass from the respiratory centre of the medulla, down the intercostal and phrenic nerves to the intercostal muscles and diaphragm. This results in the cyclical expansion and relaxation of the thoracic cage, which causes air to be drawn into the lungs (inspiration) and expelled from the lungs (expiration).

Respiratory pressures

To understand respiratory anatomy it is necessary to know a little about the pressure of gases:

- The movement of gases occurs along a pressure gradient and is called bulk flow
- The movement is always from an area of high pressure to one of lower pressure until an equilibrium is reached
- The pressure exerted by the gases in the atmosphere at sea level is 101 kiloPascals (kPa) or 760 millimetres of mercury (mmHg).

The pressure of a gas is always described relative to atmospheric pressure:

- A negative pressure (e.g. 0.5 kPa), indicates that the pressure is lower than atmospheric pressure by 0.5 kPa
- Positive pressure is higher than atmospheric pressure
- Respiratory pressure of zero is equal to atmospheric pressure.

Intrapulmonary (alveolar) pressure

- The respiratory muscles cause pulmonary ventilation by alternatively compressing and distending the lungs, which in turn causes the pressure in the alveoli to rise and fall
- During inspiration the intrapulmonary pressure becomes slightly negative with respect to atmospheric pressure, normally less than –0.5 kPa e.g. air moves from a higher atmospheric pressure to a lower intrapulmonary pressure, and this causes air to flow inward through the respiratory passageways
- During normal expiration the intrapulmonary pressure rises to approximately + 0.5 kPa, e.g. air moves from a higher intrapulmonary pressure to a lower atmospheric pressure, which causes air to flow outwards through the respiratory passages.

Intrapleural pressure

- The pressure within the pleural cavity
- Fluctuates with breathing
- Always about 0.5 kPa less than alveolar pressure – always negative relative to atmospheric and intrapulmonary pressure.

Compliance in the lungs

- Compliance refers to the lungs, which allows them to expand very easily, determined by:
  - The elasticity of the lung tissue and surrounding thoracic cage
  - The surface tension in the alveoli

  - These are often reduced in lung disease such as pulmonary fibrosis and can reduce total lung pulmonary compliance
  - When compliance is low more energy is needed to breathe
- Airway resistance
  - Gas flow changes inversely with resistance, if resistance increases, gas flow will decrease
  - The greatest resistance occurs in the medium size bronchi
    - Smooth muscle of the bronchi wall is sensitive to neural and other controls such as chemicals
    - Parasympathetic stimulation causes bronchial constriction and reduces air passage; strong bronchial constriction in an asthma attack can stop pulmonary ventilation completely
    - Local mucous infectious material and solid tumours are also possible sources of resistance
  - To overcome increased resistance, airway movements become more strenuous
- Recoil tendency (opposing forces)
  - The lungs have a continual elastic tendency to collapse, called the recoil tendency of the lungs, caused by:
    - Elastic fibres found throughout the lungs that are stretched by lung inflation and are continually attempting to shorten once stretched
    - Surface tension of the fluid lining the alveoli also causes a continuous elastic tendency for the alveoli to collapse
    - This process is facilitated by surfactant:
      - A lipoprotein secreted by special cells which are component parts of the alveolar epithelium
      - Reduces the surface tension preventing alveoli from completely collapsing to their smallest size
  - Neither force wins as fluid in the pleural cavity creates a surface tension holding the two layers together, they can slide but not separate.

Pulmonary ventilation

The lungs can be expanded and contracted in two ways:

- By downward and upward movement of the diaphragm to lengthen or shorten the chest cavity
- By elevation and depression of the ribs to increase and decrease the antero-posterior diameter of the chest cavity.

The chief muscles of ventilation are:

- The diaphragm is supplied by the phrenic nerve
- The intercostal muscles, which are supplied by the thoracic intercostal nerve
- During inspiration
  - The diaphragm moves downwards pulling the lower surfaces of the lungs downwards
  - The rib cage moves upwards and outwards to expand the lungs
  - Together these increase the volume of the thoracic cavity by almost half a litre
  - The attachment of the lungs to the inside of the chest cavity causes lung volume to increase further
  - Pressure drops in the pleural cavity air flows into the lungs until the pressure equalise
- During expiration
  - The diaphragm and intercostal muscles relax
  - The elastic recoil of the lungs, chest wall and abdominal structures compresses the lungs and the ribs slant downwards
  - The chest cavity and the size of the lungs reduce, the pressure in the pleural cavity increases, the gases leave the lungs until the pressures equalise
  - At the end of expiration there is a slightly negative intrapleural pressure of –0.5 kPa, which is transmitted to all other structures including the heart and aids venous return by exerting a slight 'sucking' force.

Laws applied to respiration

- Boyle's law
  - The volume of a gas is directly proportional to its absolute temperature, assuming that the pressure remains constant
- Dalton's law
  - Each gas in a mixture of gases exerts its own pressure as if all the other gases were not present
- Henry's law
  - The quality of a gas that will dissolve in a liquid is proportional to the partial pressure of the gas and its solubility co-efficient, when the temperature remains constant.

Pulmonary volumes and capacities

Pulmonary volumes

- Tidal volume (TV) – the volume of air inspired or expired with each normal breath = 500–800 ml
- Inspiratory reserve volume (IRV) – extra volume that can be inhaled forcefully after the end of tidal inspiration = 3000 ml
- Expiratory reserve volume (ERV)- the air that can be exhaled forcefully after the end of a normal tidal expiration = 1100 ml
- The residual volume (RV) – the volume of air still remaining in the lungs after the most forceful expiration = 1200 ml.

Pulmonary capacities – combinations of volume

- Inspiratory capacity (IC) – tidal volume + inspiratory reserve volume e.g. maximum amount of air that a person can breathe in = 3500 ml
- Vital capacity (VC) – inspiratory reserve volume + tidal volume + expiratory reserve volume e.g. maximum inspiration followed by maximum expiration = 4600 ml
- Functional residual capacity (FRV) – expiratory reserve volume + residual volume e.g. the amount of air that remains in the lungs at the end of normal expiration = 2300 ml
- The total lung capacity (TLC) – maximum volume to which the lungs can expand.

Alveolar ventilation

- The ultimate importance of the pulmonary ventilatory system is to renew the air in the gas-exchange areas of the lungs where the air is in close proximity to the pulmonary blood
- These include the:
  - Alveoli are the primary gas-exchange units of the lungs
  - Alveoli sacs lead from the alveoli ducts
  - Alveoli ducts are found at the end of bronchioles
  - Respiratory bronchioles walls are very thin
- The rate at which new air reaches these areas is called alveolar ventilation
- Dead space (DS) is the air that does not contribute to gas exchange = approx. 150 ml
- Alveolar ventilation per minute is the TV of air entering the alveoli areas each minute

    - Alveolar ventilation (V_A) per minute = respiratory rate (tidal volume – DS) or RR(TV – DS))
    - e.g. RR = 12, TV = 500, DS = 150–12(500–150) = 12(350), therefore, V_A = 4200 ml
- When the TV falls to equal the DS volume no new air will enter the alveoli with each breath, and the alveolar ventilation/min (V_A) will become zero however rapidly the person breathes
- Alveolar ventilation is one of the major factors that determines the concentrations of O_2 and CO_2 in the alveoli
- All discussions of gaseous exchange emphasise alveoli ventilation
- The RR/TV/MV are of importance only in so far as they affect alveoli ventilation.

The respiratory system is one of the major organs of the body (Marieb, 2012). Therefore, any disorders to the respiratory system can severely affect normal functioning of other organs.

RESPIRATORY PHYSIOLOGY

The main functions of the lungs are to provide continuous gas exchange between inspired air and the blood in the pulmonary circulation. Survival depends upon this process being reliable, sustained and efficient.

Gas exchange in the body

Dalton's Law of Partial Pressures (PP)

- Each gas in a mixture of gases exerts its own pressure as if all the other gases were not present
- Atmospheric pressure
    - Is 101 kPa
    - 21% of air is oxygen
- Contents of air:
    - Nitrogen 78.6% of air
    - Oxygen 20.9% of air
    - Carbon dioxide 0.04% of air
    - Water vapour 0.5%
- Partial pressure of oxygen (O_2) in atmospheric air is:

$$\frac{21}{100} \times 101 \text{ kPa} = 21.2 \text{ kPa}$$

- Gas will move from an area of high PP to an area of lower PP until equilibrium is reached
- Constant consumption of oxygen and production of carbon dioxide in the alveoli means that there is a PP gradient both in the lungs and at tissue level.

Composition of alveolar air

- The gaseous makeup of the atmosphere is quite different from that in the alveoli:
  - O_2 is 14%
  - CO_2 is 6%
  - Nitrogen is 80%
- Partial pressure of oxygen (O_2) in alveolar air is:

$$\frac{14}{100} \times 101 \text{ kPa} = 14.1 \text{ kPa}$$

- Alveolar air contains much more carbon dioxide and water vapour and much less oxygen due to:
  - Gas exchanges occurring in the lungs
  - Humidification of air by the conducting passages
  - The mixing of alveolar gas that occurs with each breath.

Internal and external respiration

External respiration

- The movement of oxygen and carbon dioxide across the respiratory membrane from lungs to blood, influenced by:
  - Partial pressure gradients and gas solubility
  - Structural characteristics of the respiratory membrane
  - Functional aspects, such as the matching of alveolar ventilation and pulmonary blood perfusion.

Internal respiration

- Gaseous exchange between the systemic capillaries and the tissue cells

External and internal respiration take place by simple diffusion driven by the partial pressure gradients of oxygen and carbon dioxide that exist on the opposite sides of the exchange membranes (Figure 9.2).

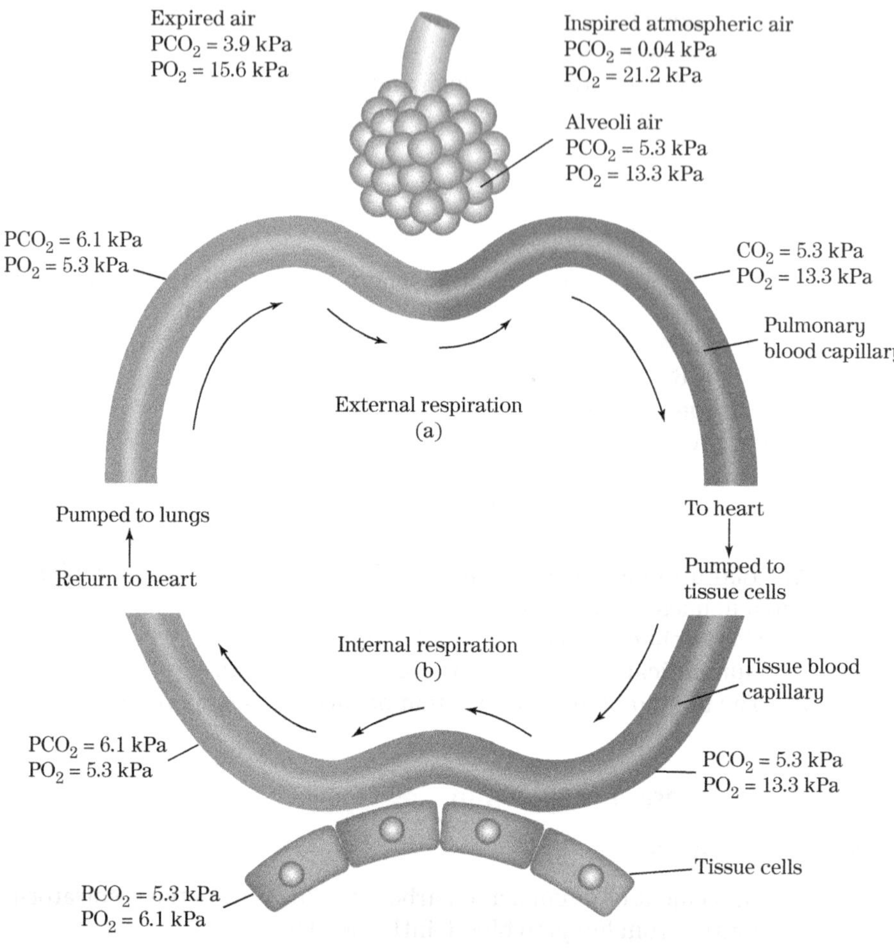

Figure 9.2 Internal and external respiratory processes

Transport of respiratory gases

Oxygen transport

- Blood carries oxygen (O_2) in two ways:
  - 3% dissolved in plasma.
  - 97% bound in haemoglobin within the red blood cells
- Haemoglobin
  - Is made up of protein, globin, bound to iron containing pigment–haem

    - The oxygen diffuses into the blood and binds with the haemoglobin – oxyhaemoglobin – HbO_2
- Association of oxygen and haemoglobin
    - Each haemoglobin molecule can combine with four molecules of O_2:
        - After the first molecule of oxygen binds the haemoglobin molecule changes shape
        - The change of shape allows haemoglobin to take up 2 more molecules of oxygen more readily; uptake of the fourth is further facilitated
        - When all four molecules of oxygen are bound to haemoglobin, it is fully saturated
        - When only 1, 2, 3 molecules of oxygen are bound to haemoglobin, it is partially saturated
        - The unloading of 1 oxygen molecule enhances the unloading of the next, and so on.
    - When oxyhaemoglobin saturation is plotted on a graph against the PP of oxygen an S-shaped curve results known as the oxygen disassociation curve (Figure 4.4), which determines the relationship between:
        - The amount of O_2 bound to Hb (oxygen saturation)
        - The PO_2 of the blood
        - It is not linear because of the association of oxygen to haemoglobin
    - The shape of the curve means that a fall in PO_2 from the normal arterial value will have little effect on the Hb saturation (and oxygen content) until the steep part of the curve is reached 8 kPa
    - Once the PO_2 has reached this level, a further decrease in PO_2 will result in a dramatic fall in the Hb saturation
- The Bohr effect
    - When conditions within the body are normal, the bond between Hb and O_2 is stable
    - However, in certain conditions the bond between the Hb and O_2 bond is either weakened or strengthened:
        - Is weakened in acidosis, high temperatures and reduced pH – oxygen unloading is accelerated where it is most needed
        - Is strengthened in alkalosis, low temperatures and increased pH – oxygen unloading is slowed down and the O_2 remains attached to the Hb.

Carbon dioxide transport

- Blood carries carbon dioxide (CO_2) in 3 ways:
    - 7% dissolved in plasma

    - 20–30% bound to haemoglobin in red blood cells (carbaminohaemoglobin)
        - Rapidly dissociates from Hb in the lungs where the PCO_2 of alveolar air is lower than that in the blood
        - Deoxygenated Hb combines more readily with CO_2 –the Haldane effect
    - 60–70% of CO_2 is converted to bicarbonate ions and transported in plasma
        - Diffuses into RBC and combines with water to produce carbonic acid (H_2CO_3)
        - This is unstable and quickly dissociates into hydrogen ions and bicarbonate ions
        - This also occur in plasma but is a thousand times faster in the RBC due to the presence of carbonic anhydrase – an enzyme that reversibly catalyses the conversion of carbon dioxide and water to carbonic acid
        - Hydrogen ions released bind to Hb to produce the Bohr effect. Thus oxygen release is triggered by carbon dioxide loading
        - The bicarbonate ions diffuse quickly from the RBCs and into the plasma where they are carried to the lungs
        - To counteract this rapid movement of negative ions from the RBC, chloride ions move from the plasma into the erythrocyte (the chloride shift)
- The Haldane effect is when carbon dioxide transported in blood is affected by oxygenation of the blood:
    - The lower the PO_2 and the Hb saturation with oxygen, the more carbon dioxide can be carried in blood
    - Reflects the ability of reduced Hb to form carbaminohaemoglobin and to buffer H^+
    - Encourages CO_2 exchange in both tissues and lungs.

Carbon dioxide and blood pH

- Bicarbonate ions in the plasma act as an alkaline reserve and form part of the carbonic acid–bicarbonate buffer system of the blood
- If the hydrogen ion concentration of the blood starts to rise, excess H^+ is removed by combining with HCO_3^- to form carbonic acid

$$CO_2 + H_2O \rightleftharpoons \text{Carbonic acid} \rightleftharpoons H^+ + HCO_3^-$$

- If HCO_3^- concentration falls, carbonic acid dissociates, releasing hydrogen ions and lowering pH again
- Changes in respiratory rate and depth can produce dramatic changes in blood pH

- Respiratory ventilation can provide a fast-acting system to adjust blood pH
- If HCO_3^- concentration falls, carbonic acid dissociates, releasing hydrogen ions and lowering pH again.

Ventilation perfusion

- Ventilation (V) and perfusion (Q) are not distributed evenly throughout the lungs;
- The bases of the lungs receive substantially more of both than the apices
- Perfusion:
  - Largely due to gravity
  - Perfusion pressure in the base of the lung is greater than in the apices
- Ventilation
  - The bases also receive a greater degree of ventilation.

Neurochemical control of breathing

The mechanisms that control breathing are complex; for more information see chapter 10.

Voluntary and involuntary ventilation

- Involuntary ventilation is observed when a person holds their breath; homeostatic mechanisms that control ventilation rate and volume adjust to the needs of the body; triggered by chemoreceptors
- Voluntary ventilation is necessary for talking, singing, laughing and holding your breath.

Chemoreceptors

Chemoreceptors monitor changes in pH, partial pressure of arterial carbon dioxide (PaCO2), hydrogen ions (H^+) and reductions in oxygen (O_2); they are split into 2 types:

- Central chemoreceptors
  - Changes in cerebral spinal fluid (CSF) pH and hydrogen ion concentration are sensed by central chemoreceptors, located near the respiratory centre in the brain stem, which monitor very small increases or decreases in pH, partial pressure of carbon dioxide in arterial blood ($PaCO_2$) and hydrogen ions (H^+)

    - When a person holds their breath $PaCO_2$ increases and CSF senses the change in pH and increases rate and depth of breathing
    - If hypoventilation is long term e.g. in chronic obstructive airways disease (COPD) the central chemoreceptors become insensitive to small changes in $PaCO_2$ and regulate ventilation poorly
- Peripheral chemoreceptors
    - Are located in the aortic arch and the carotid bodies near the baroreceptors
    - Peripheral chemoreceptors are sensitive to reductions in O_2 levels in arterial blood (PaO_2)
    - The PaO_2 must drop quite significantly before the peripheral chemoreceptors have influence on ventilation
    - The peripheral chemoreceptors are the major stimulus for breathing when central chemoreceptors become insensitive to increases in PaCO2 e.g. in COPD.

Lung receptors

- There are receptors situated in the lungs constantly sending impulses to the respiratory centre in the brain stem. There are 3 groups:
    - Irritant receptors: sensitive to irritates e.g. dust and when activated stimulate the cough reflex, bronchoconstriction and increase respiratory rate
    - Stretch receptors: sensitive to increases in volume and size of the lungs, when stimulated decrease the respiratory rate and volume (the Hering-Breuer expiratory reflex) and protect against excess lung expansion
    - *J*-receptors: sensitive to increases in pulmonary capillary pressure and will initiate hyperventilation, hypotension and bradycardia.

RESPIRATORY PATHOPHYSIOLOGY

This chapter has so far covered the normal anatomy and physiology for the respiratory system. We now turn to the pathophysiology of this system and outline the key alterations that occur.

The main functions of the lungs are:

- To provide continuous gas exchange between inspired air and the blood in the pulmonary circulation

- Supply oxygen and remove carbon dioxide, then cleared from the lungs by expiration.

Survival depends upon these processes being reliable, sustained and efficient. A good understanding of these processes is essential to better place healthcare professionals to manage any resulting problems efficiently and effectively.

Asthma

Asthma is a response to an antigen resulting in an abnormal stimulation of the inflammatory immune response. The antigen irritates the airway epithelial cells and stimulates cell-mediated T-helper cells to stimulate B-cell activation to produce antigen-specific IgE. IgE leads to mast cell degranulation with the release of large amounts of inflammatory mediators e.g. histamine, prostaglandins and leukotrienes. This process contributes to difficulty in breathing out, and becomes an active rather than passive process (Figure 9.3a). This is demonstrated in the following case study:

Case study 9.1

Ella is a 55-year-old woman who is a known asthmatic since childhood. For the past 14 years she has been well and coping with her asthma. Yet over the last 4 years her condition has worsened, and her attacks have been becoming more frequent, with recurrent chest infections, 2 of which have required admissions to hospital, with intensive courses of antibiotics. Since the last admission, just 2 months previously, Ella feels that she was not allowed time to fully recover and because of this a repeat of the same infection has emerged. Her husband David continues to work, but does spend time during the morning and evening at home with Ella.

A neighbour who is concerned about Ella calls an ambulance. An attack started 30 minutes ago, and the symptoms were not relieved by her usual medication. Ella had a nebuliser containing salbutamol and Atrovent and oxygen administered in A&E. Ella's vital signs are:

Pulse oximetry SaO2 90%
Heart rate 145 bpm
Blood pressure 155/92
Respiratory rate 30 bpm

On the ward Ella continues to struggle to breathe, is finding it hard to speak and appears blue in colour.

Aetiology

- Precipitating factors are exercise, house dust mites, pollen and spores, pets, smoke, chemicals, certain foods, drugs, emotional factors
- Extrinsic asthma
  - Childhood asthma
  - Identifiable factors provoke wheezing e.g. allergy
  - Associated with hay fever and eczema
  - Nocturnal cough (only a symptom)
- Intrinsic asthma
  - Begins in adult life, obstruction more persistent
  - Obvious stimuli other than respiratory tract infection (RTI).

Pathology

- Is an inflammatory condition of the airways mediated by a wide range of stimuli; the inflammation may lead to obstruction of airflow

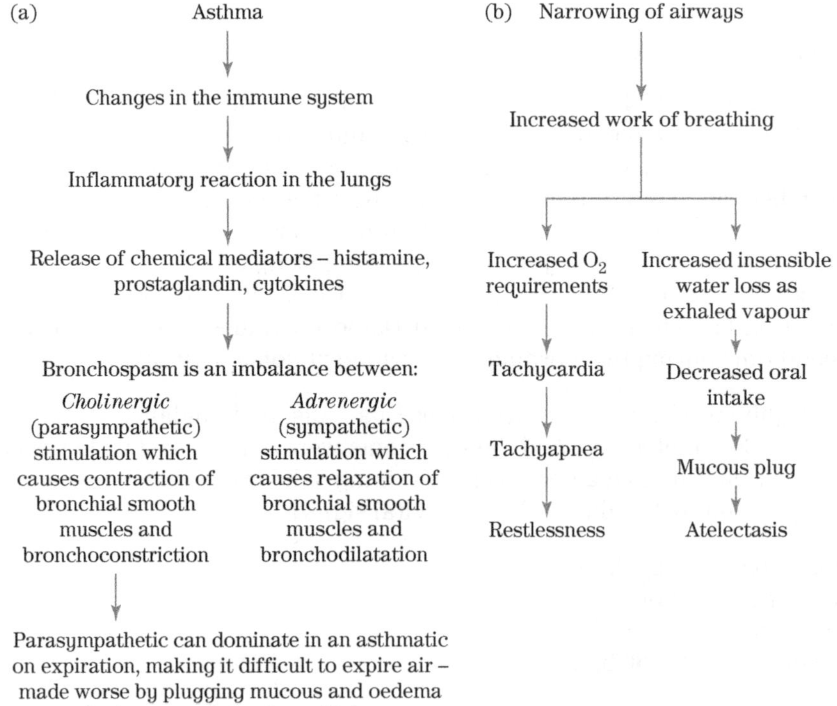

Figure 9.3 (a) Sequence of events leading to asthma; (b) Sequence of events leading from asthma to hypoxaemia

- Bronchoconstriction is an abnormal narrowing of the airways caused by bronchospasm, mucosal oedema and increased secretion of mucus (Figure 9.3b)
- Bronchospasm is an imbalance between (Figure 9.3a):
  - Cholinergic (parasympathetic) nervous system activity
  - Adrenergic (sympathetic) nervous system activity
- In many patients airway resistance can be overcome by homeostatic mechanisms:
  - Maintain oxygen levels by central chemoreceptor response leading to a hyperventilation and a respiratory alkalosis (see Figure 4.7)
  - When the effort of breathing leads to exhaustion, homeostasis can no longer be maintained, oxygen levels decrease and carbon dioxide levels rise leading to a respiratory acidosis (Figure 4.7) and hypoxia (Figure 9.3b)
- As asthma attack worsens:
  - Normal passive expiration is not enough to promote adequate excretion of CO_2
  - The patient has to resort to forcing air out of the lungs during expiration
  - Generating high intrathoracic pressures that force smaller airways to close, leading to atelectasis.

Clinical features

- Asymptomatic between attacks and pulmonary function tests are normal
- At the beginning of an attack:
  - Chest constriction – feeling of tightness
  - Expiratory wheeze, with prolonged expiration, making it difficult to breath out
  - Dyspnoea – cannot complete a sentence in one breath
  - Non-productive cough
  - Tachycardia: an increase in heart rate
  - Tachypnoea: an increase in respiratory rate (hyperventilation)
- Severe attacks involve:
  - Use of assessor muscles to breathe
  - Wheezing can be heard or silent
  - A pulsus paradoxus (decrease in systolic blood pressure during inspiration of more than 10 mmHg)
  - Weak and feeble respiratory effort
  - Cyanosis (a bluish discolouration of the skin and mucous membranes caused by increasing desaturation)

  - Bradycardia or hypotension
  - Confusion, exhaustion or coma.

Investigations

- Peak expiratory flow rate (PEFR) useful in determining the severity of the attack and is less than predicted for age, sex and height
- Search for the trigger to the attack, as avoidance can then be instigated
- Chest X-ray
- Vital signs
- Pulse oximetry measurements
- Arterial blood gas (ABGs) alterations:
  - Respiratory alkalosis: normal physiological process homeostasis maintained expected early in the course of an acute attack:
    - Dyspnoea ↑ respiratory rate
    - End tidal carbon dioxide ($ETCO_2$) normal or low (hyperventilation)
    - Cough/wheezing
  - Respiratory acidosis: indicates Ella may not be maintaining homeostasis and signals the need for mechanical intubation and ventilation
    - Worsening wheeze
    - ↑ Respiratory rate >30/min
    - Cyanosis/tachycardia >110/min
    - Peak flow <33%.

Treatment and drug therapy

- Remain calm and reassuring
- Sit the patient in an upright position supported with pillow; this will open the airways and facilitate breathing
- Administer oxygen to maintain oxygen saturation, but in the instance of signs of deterioration oxygen saturation is not a good indicator (Clarke *et al*, 2006)
- Drug therapy to alleviate dyspnoea:
  - Selective $beta_2$ agonists e.g. salbutamol and terbutaline inhaler on demand/nebuliser and longer-acting $beta_2$ agonist (salmeterol)
  - Atropine analogues – ipratropium bromide (Atrovent) nebuliser
  - Inhaled short-acting steroid (beclomethasone, budesonide, fluticasone)
  - Long-acting preparations such as aminophylline IV in 5% dextrose
  - Hydrocortisone IV hydrocortisone or oral prednisolone may be added

  - Antibiotics IV may shorten exacerbation
  - Small dose of magnesium sulphate may be administered IV if not responding to treatment (Richards and Edwards, 2012)
- Compliance with drug therapies and steroid inhalers is imperative to reduce and in some instances prevent further attacks.

Practice point

The seriousness of an asthma attack should not be underestimated. An asthma attack can be life threatening.

Chronic obstructive pulmonary disease (COPD)

Terms also used are chronic airflow limitation (CAL) and chronic obstructive airways disease (COAD), however chronic obstructive pulmonary disease (COPD) is now more commonly used. Albert is suffering from COPD:

Case study 9.2

Albert is a vigorous 62-year-old and a heavy smoker. He smokes over 20 cigarettes a day and has done so for 40 years. He has had chronic obstructive pulmonary disease for 6 years and has been to see his doctor with recurrent exacerbations of his condition on at least 3 occasions this year. He has over the last 6 days been coughing up thick yellow sputum. Albert's GP visited him at home and diagnosed an acute chest infection and a consequent exacerbation of his COPD. The GP prescribed him antibiotics.

Over the next 2 days Albert's condition worsens, he is breathless on the slightest of exertion and his wife calls an ambulance. He is admitted to your ward via A&E for management and observation. Albert arrives to your ward with a persistent cough productive of yellow sputum; he is prescribed intravenous (IV), apically, 24% oxygen, salbutamol (Venation) and ipratropium bromide (Atrovent) nebulisers and paracetamol. A specimen of sputum is obtained and sent to the laboratory for microscopy, culture and sensitivity (MC&S). His observations on admission are as follows:

BP = 150/90 mmHg
Pulse =115 beats / min
Temperature = 38.4 °C
Respiration =32 breaths / min
Oxygen saturation 92%

Aetiology

- Cigarette smoking, both active and passive, has been highlighted as a cause of COPD
- Occupational exposure to harmful substances e.g. chicken faeces, asbestos
- Air pollution.

Pathology

- COPD is characterised by restricted airflow into the lungs that is irreversible and progressive
- Associated with an abnormal inflammatory response of the lung to continuous exposure to harmful elements or gases
- Incorporates two similar but distinct conditions: chronic bronchitis and emphysema:
  - Chronic bronchitis
    - Productive cough for most days of 3 consecutive months for more than 1 year
    - Characterised by excessive mucous production, as a result the bronchi become blocked, causing inflammation, thickening of the bronchial wall leading to airway obstruction
  - Emphysema
    - Permanent enlargement of the air sacs within lung tissue and destruction of the alveolar wall
    - Destruction of pulmonary tissue is by (Hogg and Senior, 2002):
      - Proteases: destructive enzymes released during infection
      - Alpha 1 antrysin counteracts the destructive action of proteases
      - Smoking reduces the effect of alpha 1 antrysin and proteases are allowed to continue to destroy the alveoli unabated
      - As a result there is a loss of elastic recoil.

Clinical features

- The condition develops over many years, but rarely occurs before middle age
- A morning cough, with the production of little sputum may be the first sign, which does not improve

- Wheezing and breathlessness on exertion gradually increases and in the later stages dyspnoea occurs at rest
- If bronchitis predominates periodic chest infections occur causing an exacerbation of COPD
- Cyanosis due to hypoxia may occur
- If emphysema predominates extreme breathlessness often not cyanosed – the retention of carbon dioxide in arterial blood (hypercapnia) may occur and the skin may appear pink
- A wheeze can be heard
- The patient uses their accessory muscles of respiration to breathe
- This leads to extreme anxiety during very breathless periods
- Changes occur to acid base balance to maintain body pH:
  - Respiratory acidosis (PCO_2 > 5.7 kPa; pH < 7.4)
  - Metabolic alkalosis (HCO_3^- > 26 mmol/l; pH > 7.40).

Investigations

- Evidence of airway obstruction is shown on spirometry:
  - Early in the disease shows airway obstruction e.g. decrease forced expiratory volume in one second (FEV_1)
  - Later in the disease forced vital capacity (FVC) and FEV_1 become markedly reduced and comparing the FEV1: FVC ratio usually >80% is an indication of airway obstruction
  - Forced residual capacity (FRC) and residual volume (RV) are increased as airway obstruction and air trapping become more pronounced
- Peak expiratory flow rate (PEFR) measures the force of expiration in litres per minute; can be a quick and simple assessment of airways obstruction
- Copious amounts of sputum are produced
- Chest X-ray
- ABGs and white blood cell count
- Sputum specimen
- Haemoglobin levels may show polycythaemia (increase in erythrocytes) to maintain oxygen levels.

Treatment and drug therapy

- Focused on self-management e.g. recognition of exacerbations and symptom control (NICE, 2004)
- Oxygen therapy should be administered with care

Practice point

COPD patients (late in the disease process) do not have a normal physiological response to breathing e.g. increase in CO_2 via central chemoreceptor response. Over time the chemoreceptors cease or reduce their response and fail to stimulate breathing and increase respiratory rate. The peripheral chemoreceptors, sensitive to reductions in oxygen, become the patient's stimulus to breath. High concentrations of oxygen can reduce the patient's stimulus to breath.

- Drug therapy
  - Bronchodilators:
    - Salbutamol, terbutaline
    - Atropine analogues – ipratropium bromide (Atrovent)
    - IV aminophylline is only used in serious cases as has serious side effects, plasma concentration levels are required (BNF, 2014)
  - Corticosteriods
    - Oral prednisolone
    - Inhaled steroids prescribed if improvement in lung function of at least 15%
  - Antibiotics used but some bacteria resistant to ampicillin
  - Diuretics can be added if right sided heart failure is present
  - A new class of drug called phosphodiesterase E4 (PDE4) inhibitors may be beneficial in selected patients (Boswell-Smith and Spina, 2007)
- Chest physiotherapy deep breathing and postural drainage
- Respiratory hygiene is important during exacerbations due to chest infections e.g. recognition of early signs, techniques to relieve dyspnoea, and covering mouth when coughing and sneezing to prevent spread
- May require non-invasive ventilation (NIV).

Pneumonia

Pneumonia is an infection of the alveoli and small airways leading to an acute inflammation of the substance of the lungs (Dunn, 2005).

Case study 9.3

Nina is a vigorous 62-year-old who is a heavy smoker. She smokes over 20 cigarettes a day and has done so for the past 40 years. She generally suffers from a chesty cough most winters, but is usually treated in the community by her GP. Her GP visited her at home and prescribed her antibiotics. However, on this occasion her 'chesty cough' did not improve and over the last 2 days she began to cough up thick 'rusty' coloured sputum and became breathless on the slightest exertion. Her husband was concerned and contacted the GP who visited her at home again and diagnosed her with pneumonia, possibly exacerbated by her smoking and the cold weather.

Her GP could not control her infection, and she was referred to A&E for admission for further investigations, observation and management. Nina arrived on your ward with a persistent productive cough and expectorating rusty coloured sputum; she is prescribed intravenous (IV) cefuroxime, oxygen, salbutamol (Ventolin) and ipratropium bromide (Atrovent) nebulisers and paracetamol. A specimen of sputum was obtained and sent to the laboratory for microscopy, culture and sensitivity (MC&S). Her observations on admission were as follows:

BP = 150/90 mmHg
Pulse =115 beats / min
Temperature = 38.8 °C
Respiration =32 breaths / min
Oxygen saturation 92%

Practice point

Pneumonia leads to stimulation of the inflammatory immune response and is what leads to some of the clinical features observed and dictates some of the interventions required.

Aetiology

- Pneumonia can be community or hospital acquired
- The most common bacteria that lead to pneumonia are:
  - *Streptococcus pneumonia*
  - *Mycoplasma pneumoniae*
  - *Haemophilus influenza*
  - *Staphylococcus aureus*
  - *Legionella pneumophilia*
  - *Myobacterium tuberculosis*
- Pneumonia can also be due to any of the following:

    - Chemical causes e.g. carbon monoxide poisoning
    - Aspiration of oropharyngeal secretions
    - Radiotherapy
    - Allergic mechanism (asthma)
- Pneumonia in the immuno-compromised patient:
    - More common with the emergence of HIV
    - Opportunistic infections
    - Rapid pneumonias extensive and life threatening
    - Viral, fungal, protozoal or bacterial in origin
    - Pneumocystis carinii is the commonest.

Pathology

- The most common cause of pneumonia is aspiration of oropharyngeal secretions
- Pneumonia can arise from the inhalation of microorganisms released into the air when an infected person sneezes, coughs and talks or from contaminated respiratory therapy equipment (McCance *et al*, 2010)
- Usually held in check by innate immunity in the upper and lower airways (see chapter 5).

Clinical features

- Cough can be productive or non-productive
- Pyrexia, chills
- Dyspnoea
- Malaise
- Pleuritic chest pain, a pleural rub may be heard over the painful area
- Inspiratory crackles.

Investigations

- History of an upper respiratory infection
- Physical examination
- Close monitoring of vital signs (British Thoracic Society, 2004)
- White blood cell count usually elevated or reduced if the patient is immunosuppressed
- Sputum specimen and characteristics (colour and odour)
- Blood cultures
- Chest X-ray shows infiltration, single lobe or more diffuse establishing the extent of infected lung tissue
- If condition does not respond:

- Bronchoscopy
- Lung biopsy.

Treatment and drug therapy

- Establish adequate oxygen and ventilation to correct hypoxaemia
- Temperature management e.g. anti-pyretic drugs
- Maintain hydration IV fluid therapy if required (Dunn, 2005)
- Chest physiotherapy, deep breathing, coughing
- Positioning of patient in the upright position
- Antibiotics; multiple drug therapies may be necessary if resistant strain or opportunistic micro-organisms are the cause
- Patients with underlying lung disease may require non-invasive ventilation or mechanical ventilation.

Aspiration

Aspiration pneumonia is aspiration of gastric contents into the lungs and can lead to severe illness. It can be fatal, as gastric acid contents in the lungs are very destructive to lung tissue. Aspiration material enters the right lung. This is because the right bronchus has a wider opening and is slightly higher than the left due to the heart on the left side.

Aetiology

- Predisposing factors:
  - Altered consciousness
  - Drug overdose, anaesthesia, epilepsy, CVA, alcoholism
  - Dysphagia, oesophageal disease
  - Stricture, fistula, hiatus hernia, reflux
  - Neurological disorders
  - Myasthenia gravis, motor neurone disease
  - Nasal gastric tubes
  - Terminal illness.

For more information see pneumonia above.

Pulmonary oedema

Pulmonary oedema is fluid in the interstitial and alveolar spaces of the lungs (Figure 8.7b).

Aetiology

The general cause is an increase in hydrostatic pressure within the pulmonary circulation (Figures 4.6 and 8.7b), which can be due to:

- Protein energy malnutrition (see chapter 11)
- Liver failure (see chapter 11)
- Left ventricular failure (see chapter 8)
- Pulmonary hypertension
- Fluid overload (see chapter 4); increased infusions of
  - Crystalloids
  - Colloids
- Myocardial infarction
- Inhalation burns, as in the case of Graham:

Case study 9.3

A 25-year-old male was rescued from a smoke-filled room in his house in the middle of the night. The fire was thought to have started due to a cigarette end being thrown into the kitchen bin not competently extinguished, before going to bed. He was unconscious at the time of rescue. The kitchen was completely demolished.

The patient's name is Graham, and it appears that he has not suffered burns, but he is covered in soot. Examination reveals that he is coughing up black soot and the palate reveals soot particles. Observations:

BP	90/70 mmHg
RR	28 bpm
HR	120 bpm
GCS	11
O_2	100%

He is admitted to the ward with 100% oxygen and the medical team are considering intubating him.

Practice point

Graham has suffered inhalation burns, which stimulate the inflammatory immune response. Figure 2.3 gives an explanation as to why he would develop pulmonary oedema.

For more information see the relevant chapters given above, in relation to the formation of oedema in different circumstances.

Pulmonary embolism (PE)

A pulmonary embolism is an obstruction of one of the pulmonary arteries by a blood clot known as an embolism.

Aetiology

- Patients that are susceptible to PE belong to 3 categories referred to as Virchow's triad:
  - Venous stasis such as slow or stagnant blood flow through the veins
  - Hypercoagulopathy or any disorder that promotes blood clotting
  - Injury to vessels that line blood vessels
- Usually the blood clot originates from a DVT in the leg
- Should be suspected in patients:
  - Who collapse suddenly 1–2 weeks following surgery
  - Who have recently been on a long haul flight, as in the case study of Dick:

Case study 9.4

You are called to see Dick, a 65-year-old man who is complaining of chest pain. He has no previous history of any cardiac illnesses, but it is known from a neighbour that he recently flew back from Australia after visiting his daughter there for 3 months. On initial assessment you find the following:

RR	30/min
Pulse	130/min
B/P	90/70 mmHg
O_2	92%

You decide to undertake a 12 lead ECG on Dick, which shows what you think looks like a right ventricular hypertrophy.

Practice point

A pulmonary embolism can be fatal, and Dick's clinical features, results obtained from investigations and PMH are classic signs that require immediate attention.

Pathology

- A PE is an occlusion of a portion of the blood supply to the lungs by:
  - A tissue fragment
  - Lipids (fats)
  - An air bubble
  - A thrombus or emboli dislodged from the deep veins in the leg
- PE can occur as:
  - Embolus with infarction causing death to a portion of the lung
  - Embolus without infarction; perfusion is maintained and does not cause permanent lung damage
  - Massive occlusion of a portion of the lungs e.g. the main pulmonary artery
  - Multiple PEs
- Stimulates the release of:
  - Inflammatory mediators
  - Neuroendocrine substances e.g. catecholamines, angiotensin II, serotonin
- There is widespread vasoconstriction further reducing blood flow to the lungs
- An increase in pulmonary artery pressure and right-sided heart failure
- Ventilation/perfusion mismatching
- A decrease in surfactant production
- Atelectasis occurs and contributes to further hypoxia.

Clinical features

- If the PE is large it can be a medical emergency – leading to death (Chopra *et al*, 2012).
- Check for source of the PE:
  - Calf tenderness
  - Calf asymmetry
- The clinical features depend on the size of embolism:
  - Sharp, knife-like pain in the chest, well localised in a small embolus
  - If large the pain is more central and as such can be difficult to distinguish from cardiac pain
  - Shortness of breath
  - Unexplained anxiety and distress
  - Haemoptysis
  - Hypotension, tachycardia, pallor

    - Cyanosis (suggests a large embolism)
    - Collapse, cardiac arrest or shock
- If pulmonary infarction of lung tissue occurs:
    - Dysrhythmias
    - Decreased cardiac output
    - Shock and death.

Investigations

- Past medical history
- Symptoms and physical findings
- Chest X-ray can be normal in the first 24 hours
- Arterial blood gases (ABGs) usually show a respiratory alkalosis
- ECG shows right ventricular strain
- D-dimer measure the products of thrombus degradation
- Elevated troponin levels have been used in identifying the severity of PE (Dimarsico and Cymet, 2007).

Treatment and drug therapy

- Prophylactic anticoagulation
- Administration of oxygen
- Haemodynamic stabilisation with fluids, if required
- Continuation of warfarin for weeks or months following insult
- If a severe PE fibrinolytic agents may be used e.g. streptokinase infused through a pulmonary artery catheter
- Percutaneous or surgical embolectomy.

Adult respiratory distress syndrome

Is a form of respiratory failure that is sudden and severe characterised by inflammation and diffuse injury.

Aetiology

- Complication of long-term invasive ventilation
- Can be the result of an injury that is related or unrelated
    - Sepsis
    - Multiple trauma e.g. bruising to the lung, blast injuries, fat embolism, head injury and raised intracranial pressure (ICP)
    - Aspiration of gastric acid, near drowning
    - Inhalation of smoke, corrosive gases, oxygen toxicity
    - Blood e.g. disseminated intravascular coagulation (DIC), massive blood transfusion, post cardiac surgery

- Metabolic acidosis as in renal failure, pancreatitis, liver failure, diabetic ketoacidosis
- Drug abuse such as heroin, barbiturates
- Miscellaneous causes are high altitudes, radiation, eclampsia.

Pathology

- The initial injury to the lungs damages the pulmonary capillary endothelium and stimulates the inflammatory immune response and the release of mediators
- Increased capillary permeability fluid and proteins leak into the interstitial space
- Pulmonary oedema forms and haemorrhage reduces lung compliance and impairs alveoli ventilation
- Pulmonary vasoconstriction leading to pulmonary hypertension, which is variable throughout the lung beds resulting in ventilation/ perfusion mismatch
- Surfactant is inactivated and lungs become less compliant and collapse (atelectasis)
- Fibrosis progressively occludes the alveoli (McCance *et al*, 2010)
- Worsening hypoxaemia and hypercapnia decrease oxygen delivery to tissues leading to organ dysfunction
- Decrease in cardiac output and hypotension leads to death.

Clinical features

- Early features include:
  - Increasing dyspnoea
  - An increased work of breathing
  - Decreased minute volume
  - Tachypnoea an increase in respiratory rate
  - Changes in the chest X-ray
  - Hypoxaemia (a reduced oxygenation of arterial blood)
- As the condition progresses:
  - Pulmonary oedema worsens
  - Hypoxia become resistant to increases in oxygen
  - Respiratory failure occurs
  - Hypercapnia.

Investigations

- History of the insult
- Physical examination
- Arterial blood gases (ABGs)

- Chest X-ray
- Auscultation of the chest crackle are heard throughout the lungs
- Exclusion of cardiac pulmonary oedema
- CT of the chest
- Bronchoscopy.

Treatment and drug therapy

- Early detection
- Supportive therapy and prevention of complications
- Non-invasive ventilation (NIV)
- Mechanical ventilation with positive end expiratory pressure (PEEP)
- High oxygen concentrations
- Steroid therapy is controversial.

Lung cancer

Lung cancer is the commonest cause of cancer deaths in men in the UK, second in women only to breast cancer. There has been minimal improvement in the 5-year survival rate in the past 15 years. Ninety per cent of cases are related to cigarette smoking.

Aetiology

- Cigarette smoking including passive smoking
- Environmental and occupational risk factors for cancer:
  - Mining such as uranium, iron, coal
  - Asbestos
  - Diesel exhaust
  - Air pollution.

Pathology

- Lung cancers arise from the bronchi due to damage of the tissue lining leading to cellular mutations
- The repetitive exposure to cigarette smoke, and eventually epithelial cell adaptations begin to be visible on biopsy
- This is followed by tumour growth, progression, invasion of surrounding tissue and metastasis (brain, bone marrow and liver)
- There are 2 main types:
  - Non-small cell lung carcinoma (NSCLC): 75-80% of all cancers, of which there are 3 common types:
    - Squamous cell arises from central bronchi fairly well localised and do not metastasise; chemotherapy has limited effects, but newer agents have proven to be useful

    - Adenocarcinoma arises from glands, usually small and slow growing, but have an unpredictable pattern of metastasis
    - Large cell undifferentiated carcinoma due to its size can grow to distort the trachea and lead to mediastinal shift
  - Small cell lung carcinoma (SCLC) arise from the central part of the lungs; have a rapid rate of growth.

Clinical features

- In the early stages symptoms are nonspecific and attributed to smoking:
  - Coughing
  - Chest pain that does not radiate down the left arm or improve with rest
  - Sputum production
  - Haemoptysis: coughing up blood
  - Recurrent pneumonia
  - Airway obstruction
  - Pleural effusions: collection of fluid in the pleural space
- By the time the symptoms manifest the disease is usually advanced.

Investigations

- Sputum cytology
- Computed tomography (CT) scan
- Chest X-ray
- Bronchoscopy and biopsy to determine cell type
- Stage the tumour:
  - SCLC is staged as either limited or extensive
  - NSCLC uses the tumour, node metastasis (TNM) classification system in which T denotes the extent of the primary tumour
- Search for metastatic disease.

Treatment and drug therapy

- Drug therapies similar to COPD to open airways and improve obstruction
- Pneumonectomy or lobectomy if appropriate
- Chemotherapy and radiation are used depending on cell type, but are commonly used to reduce the tumour when condition has become palliative
- Pleural effusion, drainage of fluid that can collect in the pleural space as a result of inflammation secondary to the tumour.

Respiratory trauma

Respiratory trauma can manifest itself as either direct or indirect or be unrelated directly to the respiratory system. The effects of direct trauma can be life threatening and need to be identified efficiently and appropriate interventions instigated. Equally, indirect trauma can lead to serious complications and death if not identified early. The manifestations of trauma can occur without the occurrence of any direct or indirect trauma. Knowledge of these areas is imperative to deliver effective interventions.

Direct chest injury

The most common type of respiratory trauma is closed chest injury from a road traffic accident (RTA), with associated extra-thoracic injuries, all of which may be life threatening. Rudolph's case:

Case study 9.5

Rudolph, a 23-year-old student, is found in the local park in the early hours of the morning. He has sustained a number of superficial knife wounds to the anterior chest area and one deep wound to the right axilla, through which a significant volume of blood has been lost. The night has been cold with an average air temperature of 8°C. He is taken to A&E and an underwater seal chest drain is inserted and he is admitted to your ward.

Swift assessment and resuscitation of Rudolph need to be carried out simultaneously. Initial management is directed toward detection and correction of life-threatening effects from the injuries sustained.

Practice point

Normal body homeostatic mechanisms have sustained Rudolph through the night and sustained his major organs.

Aetiology

- Knife wounds
- Injury due to a fall
- Road traffic accidents
- Violent incidents (beatings, boxing)
- Inhalation burns
- Blast injury.

Indirect chest injury

Aetiology

- Pulmonary embolism
  - Dyspnoea of sudden onset
  - Chest pain of substernal or pleuritic type
  - Apprehension
  - Non-productive cough
  - Syncope associated with massive PE
  - Pleuritic pain and haemoptysis not early signs, but present if infarction has occurred
- Carbon monoxide poisoning
- Hanging
- Aspiration pneumonia
  - Occurs due to presence of fluid or food
  - Impaired laryngeal defence
  - Acute aspiration is manifested by a sudden onset of some or all of the following:
    - Cough
    - Dyspnoea
    - Wheeze
    - Tachypnoea
    - Stridor
    - Crepitations
    - Rhonchi
    - Cyanosis
    - Hypotension
    - Tachycardia
    - Pyrexia
- Obstruction
  - The disorders associated with acute upper airway obstruction
  - Abdominal thrust if aspirated foreign body
  - If unsuccessful:
    - Tracheostomy
    - Cricothyrotomy (minitracheostomy)
      - A small diameter endotracheal tube inserted through the midline incision in the relatively avascular cricothyroid membrane
      - Safer procedure for those without surgical training
    - Transtracheal ventilation

        - Large bore intravenous cannula, 3 ml syringe and an endotracheal tube (ETT) adapter connected to an aesthetic bag or oxygen source
        - An effective emergency technique
- Drowning
    - Claims approximately 420 lives each year in the UK (NWSF, 2012)
        - Diving reflex aids survival in cold water e.g. bradycardia and peripheral vasoconstriction
        - Breakpoint – water enters the lungs, gasping occurs, loss of consciousness, respiratory arrest, cardiac arrhythmias, death
    - In fresh water:
        - Water is absorbed from the small intestine into the circulation haemodilution of the blood leads to a reduction in all solutes e.g. electrolytes, other chemicals e.g. hormones, plasma proteins and haemoglobin
        - Surfactant characteristics are altered leading to atelectasis and ARDS
    - In sea water:
        - Hypertonic sea water promotes rapid fluxes of water and plasma proteins into the alveoli, dilutes surfactant, disrupts alveolar capillary membrane
    - Both produce:
        - An inflammatory reaction in the alveolar capillary membrane (pulmonary oedema)
        - Hypoxaemia.

Unrelated injuries

This includes any conditions whereby the demand for oxygen outweighs supply and can lead to unrelated trauma to the respiratory system.

Aetiology

- Stress
- Major trauma
- Hypovolaemia
- Diabetic ketoacidosis
- Myocardial infarction
- Pancreatitis
- Liver/renal failure

- Hyperpyrexia, hyperthermia, hypothermia
- Burns.

Clinical features

Specific thoracic injuries should be excluded, with signs of:

- Ruptured aorta
  - Determined by:
    - Widened mediastinum
    - Left haemothorax
    - Depressed left main bronchus
    - Fractured 1st rib
  - Ruptured diaphragm
    - Due to abdominal compression (risen since seat belts made compulsory)
    - Risk of gut strangulation
    - Left-sided rupture is more common; right difficult to diagnose due to the liver
  - Disruption of major airways frequently determined due to:
    - Respiratory distress
    - Subcutaneous emphysema
    - Haemoptysis
    - If ruptured bronchus, a pneumothorax is common
  - Massive pneumothorax/haemothorax
  - Pulmonary contusion
    - Bruising of the lungs
  - Fat embolism syndrome (FES)
    - Blockage of pulmonary and systemic capillaries with fat or other microaggregates or platelets, red cells and fibrin
  - Contributes to cause of death in multiple injuries (5%)
  - Occurs in multiple fractures, higher incidence in closed fractures
  - Myocardial contusion
    - Common in blunt chest trauma
    - May result in arrhythmias – non-specific T wave changes to pathological Q waves
    - Cardiac failure may be evident – generally should be managed as a myocardial infarction
  - Oesophageal perforation
  - Due to penetrating injury, occurs rarely with closed chest trauma; the patient develops:
    - Restrosternal pain
    - Difficulty in swallowing

    - Haematemesis
    - Cervical emphysema
  - Pulmonary oedema
  - Systemic air embolism
    - More common in penetrating injuries – life-threatening
    - Uncommon, but is thought to generally be under-diagnosed
    - Caused by a broncho-pulmonary vein fistula, an abnormal passage from one tissue surface to another
  - Cardiac tamponade
  - Suspected in a patient with thoracic trauma with a low blood pressure and raised venous pressure
  - Differential diagnosis are:
    - Tension pneumonothorax
    - Severe heart failure
    - Prolonged and inadequate treatment of shock
  - Aspiration of the pericardial sac under ECG control
  - Flail chest:
    - Disruption of the normal structure of the chest due to:
      - Fracture of three or more adjoining ribs in one or more places
      - Rib fractures with costochondral separation
      - Sternal fractures
    - Paradoxical movement occurs
      - On inspiration the intact chest expands, the injured flail segment is depressed
      - On expiration the flail segment bulges outward, thus interfering with exhalation
    - Mediastinal shift occurs (Figure 9.4):
      - During inspiration the increased intrapleural pressures on the unaffected side displace the mediastinum toward it
      - During expiration the negative pressure on the unaffected side is less than on the affected side, and the mediastinum shifts toward the affected side (mediastinal flutter)
  - Changes on inspiration lead to reduced cardiac output.

Pathology

- Cellular hypoxia (see chapter 4)
- Stimulation of the stress response (see chapter 4)
- Stimulation of the inflammatory immune response (see chapter 4)
- Changes in capillary dynamics (see chapter 4)
  - Hydrostatic pressure
  - Colloid oncotic pressure.

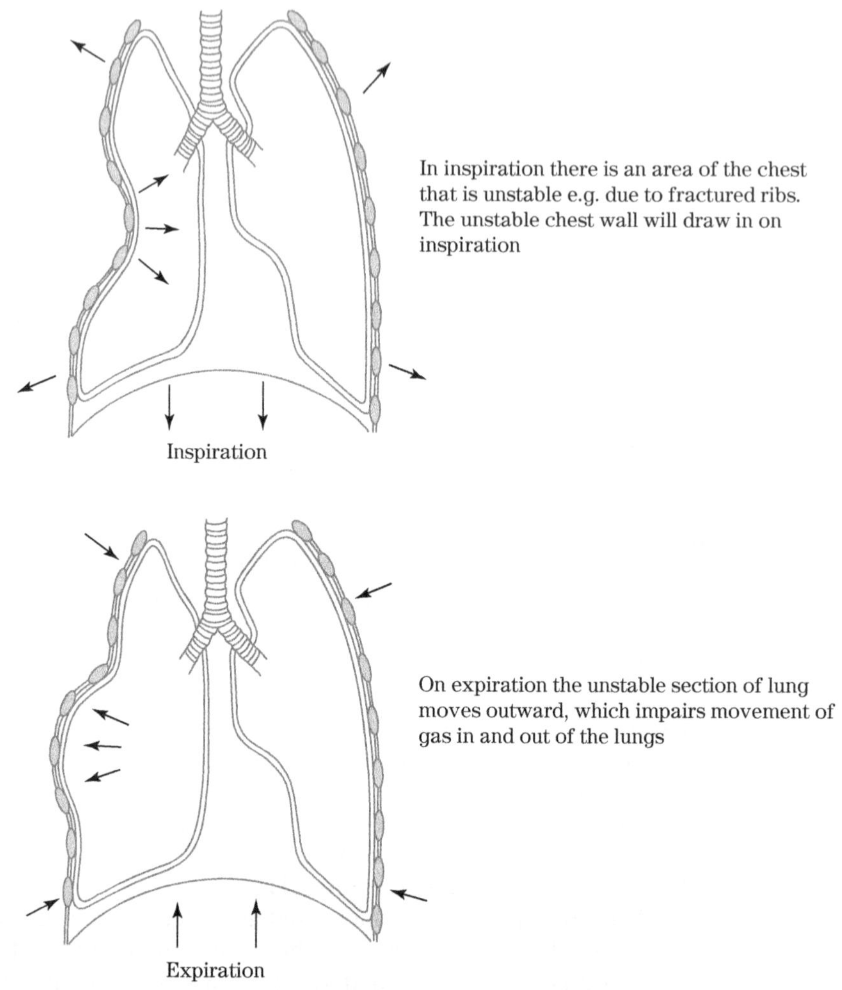

Figure 9.4 Flail chest changes on inspiration and expiration

Investigations

- Chest X-ray to determine fractured ribs, pneumothorax, tamponade
- ABGs to ascertain respiratory acidosis or alkalosis
- Haemodynamic state, respiratory and pain assessment
- Sputum analysis for blood, white/pink and frothy indicating pulmonary oedema

- Oxygen saturation, end tidal CO_2 monitoring ($ETCO_2$)
- 12 Lead ECG.

Treatment and drug therapies

- Pain management, as pain will prevent deep breathing and can lead to serious complications
- Surgical interventions if required
- Pleural effusion to drain excess fluid, or insertion of a chest drain to remove air or fluid from the pleural cavity
- Insertion of an IV cannula for administration of fluids for essential circulatory resuscitation
- Control any bleeding
- Administration of oxygen, saturation or end tidal CO_2 monitoring
- Exclude or treat pneumothorax or haemothorax by insertion of 12 or 14 gauge intravenous cannula inserted percutaneously in dire emergencies
- Assessment of extra thoracic trauma, head, neck and abdominal injuries and significant concealed blood loss must be excluded
- Gastric decompression – risk of regurgitation (vomiting or aspiration)
  - Extremely common in severe cases of chest trauma
- Consider endotracheal intubation, ventilation if:
  - Dangerous hypoxaemia and/or hypercarbia
  - Significant head injury
  - Gross flail segment and/or bruising to the chest, which could effect the lungs and/or myocardium
  - Respiratory distress
- The mortality rates in chest injured patients increases with:
  - Age – over 60 years with respiratory failure, all age groups who require mechanical ventilation
  - Pulmonary contusion and flail chest
  - Often reflecting the severity of the chest injury and the extent of extra thoracic injuries
- Knowledgeable nurses giving efficient and skilled interventions will undoubtedly prevent further complications and improve the chances of survival.

Practice point

Oxygen saturation is not a good indicator of a deteriorating patient, as haemoglobin saturation with oxygen can remain normal despite reductions in oxygen content (measured as partial pressure) due to the oxygen disassociation curve.

CONCLUSION

Respiratory physiology is a complex process by which gas exchange in the body is maintained and regulated (Edwards, 2008). With a fuller understanding of the processes of oxygen and carbon dioxide transport, the oxygen disassociation curve, its relationship to monitoring oxygen saturation and how they might be disturbed, the healthcare professional is better placed to manage any resulting problems logically and effectively. In addition, the multitude of respiratory diseases that disturb homeostasis can present with a variety of symptoms, but whatever the primary cause, pulmonary ventilation and external respiration leading to hypoxaemia and hypoxia and possibly increasing carbon dioxide can result.

SELF-ASSESSMENT QUESTIONS

1. Provide an outline of the respiratory system from the nasal cavity, the pharynx and larynx, trachea, two main bronchi, bronchioles and alveoli.
2. How does gaseous exchange take place between the alveoli and the blood?
3. Discuss the values of respiratory pressures include the intrapleural pressures.
4. Define the pulmonary volumes and capacities.
5. How are oxygen and carbon dioxide carried in the blood?
6. List several changes to respiratory anatomy and physiology that may occur.
7. Define the terms acidosis, alkalosis and pH, and related medical conditions.

REFERENCES AND FURTHER READING

BNF (British National Formulary) (2014) *BNF 66: The Authority on the Selection and Use of Medicines*. London: British Medical Society, The Royal Pharmaceutical Society.

Boswell-Smith, V. and Spina, D. (2007) PDE4 inhibitors as potential therapeutic agents in the treatment of COPD-focus on roflumilast, *International Journal of COPD*, 2(2), 121–129.

British Thoracic Society (2004) *Pneumonia Guidelines 2004 Update*, London: BTS.

Chopra, N., Doddamreddy, P., Grewal, H. and Kumar, P.C. (2012) An elevated D-dimer value: a burden on our patients and hospitals, *International Journal of General Medicine*, 5, 87–92.

Clarke, A.P., Giuliano, K. and Chen, H. (2006) Pulse oximetry revisited 'but his O_2 sat was normal!', *Clinical Nurse Specialist*, 20(6), 268–272.

Dimarsico, L. and Cymet, T. (2007) Pulmonary embolism – a state of the clot review, *Comprehensive Therapies*, 33(4), 184–191.

Dunn, L. (2005) Pneumonia: classification, diagnosis and nursing management, *Nursing Standard*, 19, 50–54.

Edwards, S.L. (2008) Pathophysiology of acid base balance: the theory practice relationship, *Intensive and Critical Care Nursing*, 24, 28–40.

Hogg, J.C., Senior, R.M. (2002) Chronic obstructive pulmonary disease 2: pathology and biochemistry of emphysema, *Thorax*, 57, 830–834.

McCance K.L., Huether, S.E., Brashers, V.L., Rote, N.S. (2010) *Pathophysiology: The Biologic Basis for Disease in Adults and Children*, 6th edn, Edinburgh: Mosby Elsevier.

Marieb, E. (2012) *Essentials of Human Anatomy and Physiology*, 9th edn, San Francisco, CA: Benjamin Cummings.

NICE (National Institute for Health and Clinical Excellence) (2004) *Clinical Guideline 12: Chronic Obstructive Pulmonary Disease, Management of Chronic Obstructive Pulmonary Disease in Primary and Secondary Care*, London: NICE.

NWSF (National Water Safety Forum) (2012) *UK Water Related Fatalities 2010*, Water incident database (WAID) report, www.nationalwatersafety.org.uk.

Richards, A. and Edwards, S (2012) *A Nurse's Survival Guide to the Ward*, 3rd edn, Edinburgh: Churchill Livingstone Elsevier.

10 Neurological disease – the nervous system

Ann Richards

Alongside the endocrine system, the nervous system coordinates the activities of all the other body systems. It is the major communication system of the body and consists of:

- The central nervous system (the brain and spinal cord)
- The peripheral nervous system (the somatic and autonomic nervous systems).

Both the nervous system and the diseases that affect it are extremely complex. Diseases range from tension headaches to life-threatening tumours. The diseases may be acute, for example an infection such as meningitis; or they may be chronic, for example multiple sclerosis.

Functions of the nervous system include:

- Monitoring internal and external environments
- Integrating sensory information
- Coordinating both voluntary and involuntary responses.

THE BRAIN

The brain contains about 35 billion neurons and weighs about 1.4 kg, although this varies depending on body size. It is divided into the cerebrum, the midbrain and the cerebellum.

- The cerebrum is the largest part, receiving and interpreting sensory input and being responsible for motor output
- There are two cerebral hemispheres and they are responsible for some specific functions
- In most people (all right-handed people and also in 70% of those apparently left-handed), the left hemisphere is dominant and contains the speech centre
- It is responsible for language skills, including reading and writing and is also important in decision-making and mathematical skills

- A lesion of one hemisphere shows its effects on the opposite side of the body and so a blood clot affecting the left side of the brain may cause paralysis of the right side of the body and may affect the ability to speak too.

Lesions within the cerebral hemispheres produce abnormalities dependent upon:

- The lobe affected by the lesion
- How large the lesion is
- How deeply it extends into the brain.

The lobes of the brain are shown in Figure 10.1.

- Destruction of the motor area in the frontal lobe produces a *hemiplegia* – paralysis down the opposite side of the body. Vision will be affected by a lesion in the occipital lobe. Sensation on the opposite side of the body will be affected by a lesion in the parietal lobe
- *Dysphasia* is difficulty in speaking and is common following a stroke affecting the left side of the brain

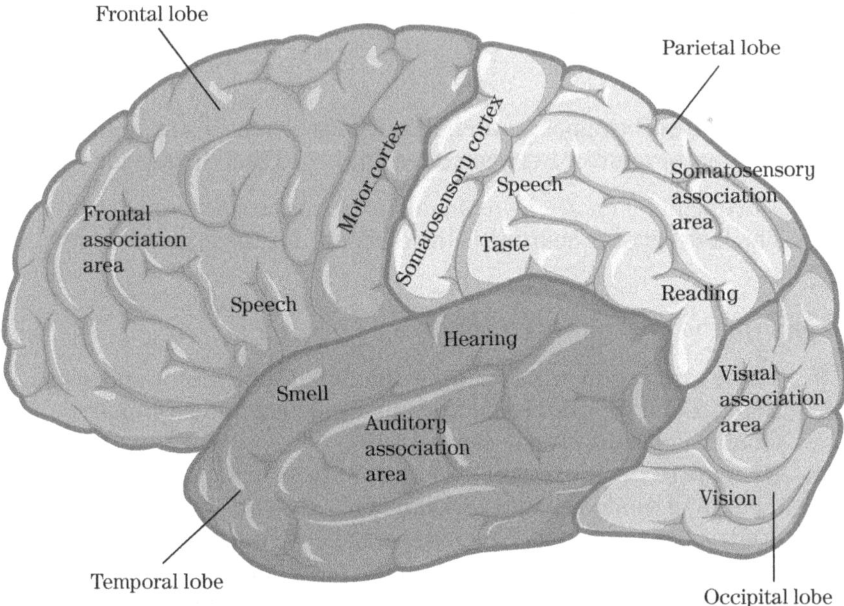

Figure 10.1 The lobes of the brain

- *Aphasia* is loss of or defect in language and is caused by lesions that affect the speech area
- *Dysarthria* is disordered articulation and may occur when there is a problem with facial muscles. It is common in Parkinson's disease, for example
- Convulsions of the opposite side of the body can be caused by an irritative lesion of the cerebral cortex. This may be the first sign of a brain tumour in some patients
- The cerebellum is responsible for maintaining posture and balance. Lesions affect the same side of the body and symptoms may include an intention tremor, decreased muscle tone and marked ataxia (lack of muscle coordination)
- Twelve cranial nerves originate in the brain and neurological disease can affect any of these
- *Papilloedema* is swelling of the optic disc seen through the ophthalmoscope. It may be an early sign of a tumour in the brain but is also seen in oedema of the brain, accelerated hypertension, optic neuritis and subarachnoid haemorrhage
- Destruction of nervous tissue may lead to paralysis or loss of sensation. Damage to the motor system results in weakness or wasting of the muscles. Damage to the sensory system results in tingling or pain.

Motor neurons

Lesions may affect the upper motor neuron, between the brain and spinal cord, or the lower motor neuron, between the spinal cord and the muscle.

- Movement by choice is instigated in the upper motor neurone
- The lower motor neurone is the end path for these movements.

Lesions of the peripheral nerves

- These are mostly mixed nerves that carry both motor and sensory fibres. Each supplies a specific muscle group and has an area of skin from which sensation is carried
- Damage to the nerve will lead to weakness in a group of muscles and a patch of analgesia and anaesthesia
- Sometimes many nerve endings may be diseased together and symptoms will be present in the periphery of all four limbs. This occurs in peripheral neuropathy such as that seen in diabetes.

Lesions of the spinal cord

- The spinal cord extends from the base of the skull to the first lumbar vertebra
- Complete destruction at any point causes paralysis and loss of sensation to all parts of the body supplied by nerves leaving or entering the cord below the level of the lesion
- A lesion in the cervical spine will paralyse the arms, legs and the respiratory muscles if high enough
- If there is partial damage to the cord a variety of clinical features are present affecting both movement and sensation.

Circulation of cerebrospinal fluid (CSF)

CSF is formed by the choroid plexuses in the ventricles of the brain. It circulates in the subarachnoid space, spreading over the surface of the brain and spinal cord, and is reabsorbed into the bloodstream. It is constantly renewed to ensure an approximate volume of 120–150 ml. It protects the brain but also provides nutrients.

- CSF is normally clear and colourless
- A lumbar puncture may be done to obtain a specimen
- The pressure of the CSF is also measured.

Hydrocephalus

This is an increased volume of CSF within the cranial cavity. It can occur when there is an obstruction to the flow of CSF and is very rarely due to an increased production of CSF.

Aetiology

In children it is due to a congenital malformation of the brain, meningitis or haemorrhage.

In adults it may be due to:

- late presentation of a congenital defect
- cerebral tumour
- subarachnoid haemorrhage
- meningitis
- head injury.

Clinical features

- Headache
- Vomiting

- Papilloedema
- All caused by raised ICP
- May also be nystagmus.

If the hydrocephalus is acute and obstructive the excess CSF has to be removed by a drain or shunt.

Raised intracranial pressure (ICP)

- The skull is a rigid bony container after the fontanelles close
- This means that there is little room for expansion of its contents and any increase in volume will lead to an increase in intracranial pressure
- At first it may be possible to reduce the volume of cerebrospinal fluid (CSF) in the ventricles and increase the available space but a point is reached where a further increase in volume will cause an abrupt increase in ICP and a rapid deterioration in the patient's condition
- This is contributed to by any cerebral oedema that is present.

> **Practice point**
>
> Features of increasing ICP:
>
> - Reduced consciousness
> - Dilation of pupil on the other side to the lesion.
> - Bradycardia and increased blood pressure
> - Cheyne-Stokes respiration.

Head injury

The skull provides very good protection for the brain below but a severe blow may cause a fracture.

- The fracture may be simple, compound, comminuted or depressed but the type of fracture is not very important as it is the damage to the brain below that matters
- The main causes of head injury are road traffic accidents, falls, assaults and sports or occupational injuries
- About a quarter of fatal head injuries are not associated with a fracture but there is a high incidence of intracranial haematoma with a fracture.

Intracranial haematoma

- A frequent complication of head injury and the most common cause of death in those conscious after their head injury

- May be extradural, subdural, subarachnoid or intracerebral.

The position of these haematomas is shown in Figure 10.2.

Extradural haematoma (EDH)

- Follows trauma and is due to bleeding from a meningeal (usually the middle meningeal) artery following fracture of the temporal or parietal bone
- There is a collection of blood between the skull and the dura. Usually collects and enlarges fairly quickly, compressing the brain below (Figure 10.2)
- It may follow a mild injury and the patient may be lucid for some hours before developing a headache and becoming drowsy
- Alternatively, the patient may be knocked unconscious and classically recover full consciousness rapidly but within a few hours start to deteriorate.

Other symptoms may include:

- Developing paralysis down one side of the body
- Dilated pupil, one side at first, due to pressure of the expanding haematoma

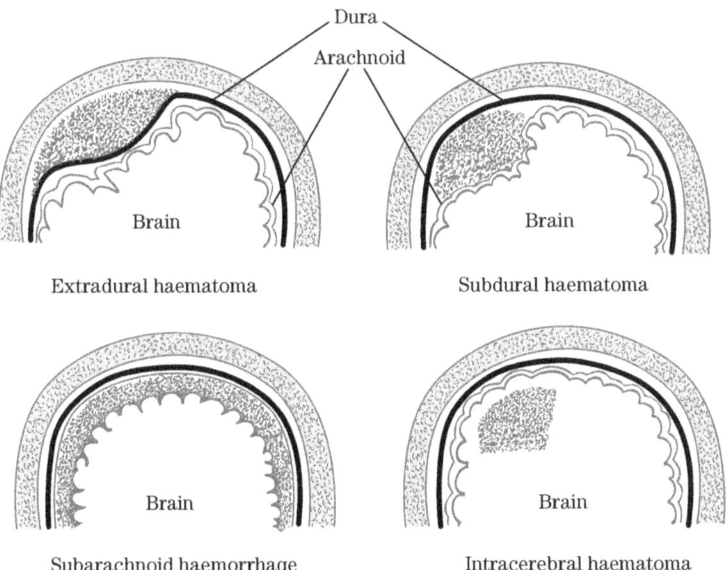

Figure 10.2 Types of intracranial haemorrhage

- Headache
- Nausea or vomiting
- Seizures
- Raised intracranial pressure causing bradycardia and hypertension
- CSF (cerebrospinal fluid) oozing from the nose (rhinorrhoea) or the ear (otorrhoea); this may follow a tear in the dura mater
- Altered level of consciousness and a deteriorating Glasgow Coma Score
- Focal neurological deficits such as aphasia, ataxia or visual field deficits.

If left untreated, the patient may die. A large haematoma requires evacuation. Mortality remains high if the patient in unconscious on admission.

Subdural haematoma (SDH)

- A collection of clotting blood in the subdural space between the dura and the arachnoid mater
- It may result from the rupture of bridging veins in the subdural space or by bleeding from small arteries
- The blood spread diffusely all though the subdural space
- It may be acute and occur 3–7 days after the initial injury, subacute (3–7 days after injury) or chronic (2–3 weeks after injury).

May be caused by a minor head injury that may have been forgotten by the patient. Those at increased risk include:

- Alcoholics – low platelet count and susceptibility to blunt head trauma
- Those prescribed anticoagulation therapy
- The elderly – cerebral atrophy puts tension on the bridging veins.

An acute SDH usually presents soon after a moderate to severe head injury. It is a common finding at autopsy.

A chronic SDH may take 2–3 weeks to present. Blood collects slowly and symptoms tend to be gradually progressive.

- Increasing headache is usually present on presentation
- There may be a history of anorexia, nausea and sometimes vomiting
- An evolving focal neurological deficit may be present e.g. limb weakness
- Personality changes and/or increasing drowsiness or confusion may occur.

Traumatic subarachnoid bleeding

- Bleeding into the subarachnoid space occurs when the vessels between the arachnoid and pia mater are torn

- When the patient recovers consciousness they will have severe headache and stiffness of the neck that gradually improve.

Intracerebral haematoma

- Associated with contusion and usually occurs in the temporal or frontal lobe
- Sometimes there may be small intracerebral haematomas more deeply seated.

Circulatory disturbances

Vascular disease

- A stroke is a sudden disturbance of brain function of vascular origin and strokes are responsible for about 10% of all deaths in the UK. A reduction in cerebral blood flow occurs and may be due to a thrombus, embolus or a bleed. Strokes are described in more detail in chapter 8.

Brain damage due to cardiac arrest

- Nerve cells require a continuous supply of oxygen and glucose and this is dependent upon the functioning of the cardiovascular system and the respiratory system
- Following a cardiac arrest there may be severe and diffuse brain damage with wide death of neurons in the brain.

Spontaneous intracranial haemorrhage

This may be subarachnoid or intracerebral.

Intracerebral haemorrhage

- These are due to the rupture of one of the many microaneurysms found in hypertensive patients
- They usually occur in late middle age and produce a rapidly expanding haematoma
- There is a sudden onset and if the haematoma is large it is rare to survive.

Subarachnoid haemorrhage (SAH)

This is a spontaneous intracranial haemorrhage where the bleeding occurs into the subarachnoid space between the arachnoid and pia mater.

- The mean age is around 50 years and 10–15% die before reaching hospital
- SAH is usually due to a weakness in the vessel wall. An aneurysm or bulge may be present in one of the cerebral arteries in the circle of Willis. It is called a *berry aneurysm* because of its shape and was thought to be congenital
- It is now believed that hypertension and atherosclerosis may play a role in the occurrence of some berry aneurysms
- Risk factors include hypertension, smoking and excessive alcohol intake.

Clinical features

There may be a history of headaches or a rapidly developing devastating occipital headache that spreads down the back of the neck. It may only last a few seconds or a fraction of a second and feels as though the person has been hit on the head. It is the severity of the headache that is typical.

- Vomiting occurs
- *Photophobia* (dislike of the light) is present
- Neck stiffness
- Restlessness and irritability occur
- Seizures may occur
- There is often loss of consciousness
- If small, the blood will be reabsorbed but if large, paralysis and death can follow.

Immediate treatment is aimed at preventing further bleeding and reducing the risk of complications such as cerebral ischaemia.

Infections of the nervous system

The brain and spinal cord are well protected against invasion by microorganisms but if they do gain access to the nervous system they can spread rapidly via the CSF.

Clinical features of acute CNS infection include:

- Headache
- Pyrexia
- Neck stiffness
- Photophobia.

Meningitis

- This is inflammation of the meninges and underlying subarachnoid CSF.

Aetiology

Meningitis may be caused by bacteria or viruses.

Bacteria reach the CNS by direct spread from the ears or nasopharynx, via a cranial injury or by spread in the bloodstream.

Bacteria causing meningitis include:

- *Neisseria meningitidis* (meningococcus)
- *Haemophilus influenzae*
- *Streptococcus pneumoniae*
- *Myobacterium tuberculosis.*

Viral meningitis is more common and usually less serious than bacterial. It is usually a self-limiting disease that lasts 4–10 days. Headache may continue for several weeks but there is no long-term damage.

Meningococcal meningitis is spread by droplet infection from those carrying the bacteria in their nasopharynx. The bacteria spread to the meninges via the bloodstream and fatal meningococcal septicaemia can occur before meningitis is evident. A purpuric rash is a most important early sign.

Occurs in all age groups but more common in infants, young children and the elderly.

Clinical features

- Headache, neck stiffness and fever constitute the meningitic syndrome
- Acute bacterial meningitis has a sudden onset with rigors and a high fever
- Severe headache, photophobia and vomiting are often present
- Consciousness is not usually impaired although the patient may be delirious
- Drowsiness and loss of consciousness may be a sign of complications such as venous sinus thrombosis, severe cerebral oedema or cerebral abscess.

The earlier antibiotics are started, the better the prognosis. Benzylpenicillin is the drug of choice unless the patient is allergic to this.

In fulminant meningococcal septicaemia there are often large ecchymoses (bruises) and gangrenous skin lesions may occur.

> **Practice point**
>
> A generalised non-blanching, petechial rash in an ill child is suggestive of **meningococcal septicaemia.**
>
> If this is present without meningitis, there will be no stiff neck, back rigidity, bulging fontanelle, photophobia or seizures.
>
> There may be cold hands and feet, fever, altered consciousness and skin mottling.

Encephalitis

This is inflammation of the brain and may be caused by a virus or bacterium. Opportunistic organisms (e.g. *Toxoplasma gondii*) are important when HIV infection is present. Occasionally encephalitis may be due to toxins or an autoimmune disorder.

Acute viral encephalitis

Herpes simplex is the most common causal virus in the UK but most viral infections of childhood can cause encephalitis. Examples include herpes zoster (chickenpox), measles, mumps, and the Epstein-Barr virus (glandular fever).

Clinical features

- Flu-like illness
- Headaches and drowsiness
- Some similar symptoms to meningitis – neck stiffness, fever, headache, vomiting
- Occasionally severe with hemiparesis and dysphasia, seizures and coma.

Herpes simplex can be a rapidly fatal necrotising encephalitis and if suspected, is immediately treated with intravenous coordinates.

Anti-convulsants and sedatives may be needed in some cases.

Brain abscess

The abscess consists of pus surrounded by oedematous brain tissue. Intracranial abscesses are uncommon but are life-threatening.

Aetiology

Causative bacteria may be streptococci, staphylococci, *E. coli*, *H. influenzae* and *Proteus*. Sometimes a chronic abscess may be due to tuberculosis.

There are several routes of infection including locally from infection in the skull such as chronic otitis media or chronic mastoiditis. This usually results in a single abscess but multiple abscesses may result from spread in the blood stream from a lung infection or infective endocarditis.

Clinical features

- Fever
- Seizures
- Focal neurological signs
- Raised intracranial pressure.

Diagnosis is by CT or MR scan.

DEMYELINATING DISEASES – MULTIPLE SCLEROSIS (MS)

Myelin forms a fatty sheath around nerve axons and facilitates the conduction of action potentials. The myelin sheath can be destroyed in demyelinating disease but the axon mostly remains intact. The commonest demyelinating disease is multiple sclerosis where lesions develop at different sites within the nervous system at different times, usually with some capacity for regeneration and restoration of function. Remyelination is never complete and the new myelin is thinner than the old.

Aetiology

- MS is a chronic inflammatory disease of the central nervous system with unknown cause. It is believed to be autoimmune with some heritable component
- It is one of the commonest causes of neurological disability amongst people under the age of 50. The onset is usually in early adulthood (20s or 30s) and is slightly commoner in females
- Although not inherited in a simple genetic fashion, genetic factors may be important
- The disease is extremely rare in equatorial regions of the world, being commoner in temperate regions. The highest incidence in the world is in Orkney and Shetland
- Demyelination occurs in multiple foci within the brain and spinal cord
- The sizes of the plaques vary and ongoing disability is variable. Nerve conduction in the affected axon is slow and inefficient
- The disease is chronic but progresses at different rates.

Clinical features

Common presentations include visual disturbance, limb weakness or sensory disturbance.

- Visual disturbance is due to optic neuritis following demyelination of the optic nerve
- This may lead to blurring of vision and pain around the eye
- There may be diplopia (double vision)
- Usually resolves over a period of weeks and there may or may not be some residual visual impairment
- If a lesion affects the spinal cord it most often interferes with the legs and may cause heaviness, dragging or weakness of the arms or legs together with a loss of pain and temperature sensation
- There may be bladder or bowel dysfunction
- Relapses and remissions occur in the early years of MS but each episode tends to lead to increasing disability. The patient may eventually be limited to a wheelchair and sometimes be paraplegic
- Fatigue and depression may become problems but intellectual function is usually preserved.

Investigations

MR imaging may show focal lesions but MS is still difficult to diagnose in the early stages.

Disease modifying drugs can delay the progress of the disease sometimes but cannot cure it.

DISORDERS OF MOVEMENT

There are some diverse disorders in this category where there is a progressive degeneration of neurons in certain regions. The symptoms may be motor or sensory or involve ataxia or dementia. The commonest disorder is Parkinsonism.

Parkinson's Disease (PD)

This is the most common progressive neurological disorder in older patients. As people live longer so the incidence of PD increases.

It is a disorder of movement and the main features are a tremor at rest, muscular rigidity and a slowing of movement (bradykinesia).

Aetiology

- Parkinson's disease occurs due to the progressive destruction of an area of the brain called the substantia nigra within the basal ganglia (an area of the brain that has a role in regulating motor function)

- The remaining cells contain inclusions known as Lewy bodies and these may contribute to dementia in the later stages
- The cells in the substantia nigra use a neurotransmitter called dopamine and in Parkinson's disease there is a reduction in manufacture of dopamine in this area
- Progress of the disease occurs at variable rates and to a variable extent
- Some people may become rapidly disabled in a few years and others may have a mild, slowly progressive disorder that does not need treatment for several years. The majority of cases fall in between these two extremes and the condition slowly becomes more incapacitating over a period of about 10 years
- The prevalence rate is about 1 in 200 over the age of 70 and males and females are equally affected. In two-thirds of cases the first symptoms occur between the ages of 50 and 60 years
- The cause in most cases is not known (idiopathic) but there may be a contribution from some environmental elements such as drugs or toxins, vascular disease or viral infections alongside a genetic risk of developing the disease
- Drug-induced Parkinsonism is caused by drugs that block the dopamine pathway or dopamine receptors. Such drugs are the antipsychotics such as haloperidol and some antiemetics such as *metoclopramide.*

Clinical features

The onset is insidious and there is probably a long presymptomatic phase where dopamine produced by the brain is reduced by about 70–80% before any symptoms appear.

Some features seen in Parkinson's disease are shown in Figure 10.3.

- The tremor is present at rest at first and reduced or eliminated by movement. It usually starts in one hand or arm and takes 2–3 years to spread to the other hand and arm
- The tremor may be described as a 'pill-rolling movement' and is rhythmic. It is absent in sleep but is increased by stress, fatigue and cold. It eventually spreads to include the lips, face, tongue and lower limbs
- Rigidity may occur in virtually all skeletal muscle and throughout the full range of movement of the joints. It affects such movements as turning in bed. Fine movements such as fastening buttons become difficult

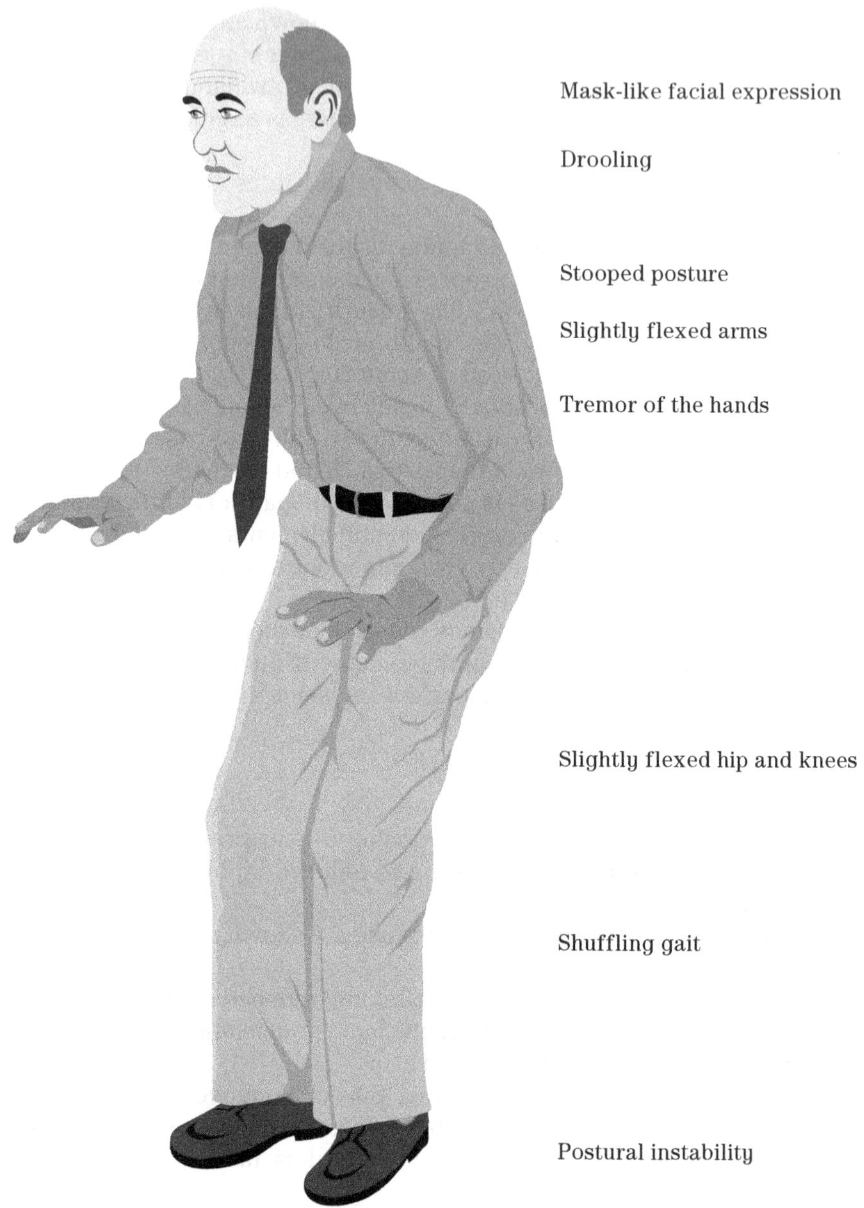

Figure 10.3 Some features seen in Parkinson's disease

- Posture becomes stooped and the body and head are flexed forward as the disease progresses. There is an acceleration in the steps when walking which may lead to falls
- Bradykinesia and akinesia (lack of spontaneous movement) present as a slowness of voluntary movement and reduced automatic movements.

Practice point

Always communicate cheerfully with patients with PD – they may have a mask-like facial expression and never smile but this is because they are unable to do so due to rigidity of the facial muscles. The eyes do not blink and there is a staring expression. Speech is difficult and may be monotone or slurred.

- Remember that it is the same person inside a body that will no longer do what is asked of it.
- The person with Parkinson's disease may have an active mind locked inside a body that will not allow effective communication.

MOTOR NEURON DISEASE

This disease is progressive and relentlessly destroys the upper and lower motor neurons in the brain and spinal cord.

- The sensory system is not involved but it leads to progressive paralysis and eventual death
- Tends to occur in middle and late adult life and the cause is unknown
- There have been links to an abnormality of mitochondrial function and there is one rare familial form of the disease
- The disease has a focal onset but becomes more generalised with time
- Death from respiratory failure usually occurs within 4–5 years.

There are three main patterns of presentation.

Amyotrophic lateral sclerosis

- This is the classical form of the disease and upper motor neurons are affected
- Amyotrophy means atrophy of muscle and the onset is usually in the limbs with one group of muscles affected first

- It is a disease of the lateral corticospinal tracts and produces a spastic paralysis.

Progressive muscular atrophy

- This selectively involves lower motor neurons of the spinal cord and results in weakness and atrophy of affected limb muscles
- Wasting may begin in the small muscles of one hand and then spread through the arm
- May begin unilaterally but soon spreads to both sides.

Progressive bulbar palsy

- This form affects the cranial motor nerve nuclei in the brain stem and causes wasting and fasciculation of the tongue causing dysarthria and dysphagia.
- As the disease progresses, choking and regurgitation of fluids are common symptoms.

The above three variants of motor neuron disease are not totally separate after the early stages. As the disease progresses, dementia is unusual and awareness is preserved. In the late stages there is widespread involvement of motor neurons and remission is unknown. There is progressive respiratory paralysis and, together with aspiration pneumonia, this is the usual cause of death.

BRAIN TUMOURS

- Secondary deposits from a cancer elsewhere are more common than primary brain tumours in adults
- Cancers of the breast, lung, kidney, thyroid, stomach and prostate may all spread to the brain.

There are many different tumours of the nervous system, classified by WHO based on their histology, but most primary brain tumours in the brain come from the glial cells (connective tissue) and are called gliomas.

- They are named according to the tissue they arise from e.g. astrocytoma and oligodendroglioma
- Meninigiomas make up about 20% of intracranial tumours. They arise from the arachnoid mater and compress the brain. They grow slowly and the treatment is surgical removal often followed by radiotherapy
- The commonest early symptoms seen in a brain tumour are headache, seizures or focal neurological deficits which usually occur slowly but sometimes can be sudden and stroke-like

- An intracranial tumour will expand and this expansion is increased by the presence of cerebral oedema, leading to raised ICP. The oedema usually responds dramatically to the administration of corticosteroids (e.g. dexamethasone)
- Some brain tumours are extremely difficult to remove due to their position deep in the brain.

EPILEPSY AND SEIZURES

People who have epilepsy show a tendency to have recurrent seizures due to uncontrolled and excessive activity of neurons in the brain. They have many possible causes.

Seizures are internationally classified into:

1. ***Partial seizures***
   - These are focal and the burst of electrical activity stays in one area of the brain
   - They may be simple (affecting either the motor system or sensory system) or complex (with impaired consciousness)
2. ***Generalised seizures*** (loss of consciousness and both hemispheres involved).

Tonic-clonic (grandmal)

- There may be a warning or aura but many patients do not have this
- The seizure is divided into two phases
- In the tonic phase consciousness is lost and the person may fall to the floor. The muscles tense and contract forcefully. There may be a moan or grunt as air is expelled from the lungs. The body is rigid and arms and legs may be bent or straight. The tongue may be bitten as the jaw clenches. The phase lasts only a few seconds
- In the clonic phase the muscles now contract and relax in turn causing a jerking. The intensity may vary from twitching to violent shaking. This may last from a few seconds to a few minutes
- The breath may be held causing slight cyanosis. The patient may be incontinent of urine
- Following the convulsion there may be a deep sleep with stertorous breathing.

Absence (petit mal)

- Usually occur in children and young adults
- There is no convulsing and the seizures may be undiagnosed

- The child may appear to be just day dreaming and to go into a little trance
- They can occur many, many times a day and interfere with school work
- There is a brief loss of consciousness with a blank expression
- Over very quickly and start and stop abruptly.

3. ***Unclassified seizures***

There are also *febrile convulsions* in children with a high temperature.

Aetiology

Often unknown but include the following:

- Head injury
- Brain infection, e.g. meningitis
- Stroke
- Brain damage – could be birth trauma or hypoxia
- Drugs and alcohol
- Biochemical imbalance
- Hormonal changes
- Cerebral palsy
- Brain tumour.

In a patient with epilepsy seizures may occur due to:

- Forgotten or incorrect medication
- Lack of sleep
- Stress
- Excitement
- Alcohol
- Flashing lights (only 3–5% of people with epilepsy are photosensitive)
- Drugs.

STATUS EPILEPTICUS

This is either when a seizure last for 30 minutes or longer or there are a cluster of short seizures, with virtually no recovery between, and lasting for over 30 minutes.

- It is a medical emergency and there is a risk of cerebral anoxia causing brain damage or death from cardiorespiratory failure

- It is necessary to stop the fitting and rectal *diazepam* or buccal *midazolam* may be used. The rectal route is easier when the patient in convulsing continuously
- In refractory status patients may need to be anaesthetised and ventilated.

DEMENTIA

- This is a progressive and chronic disorder of mental processes due to organic brain disease
- It is marked by a decrease in cognitive functioning such as memory loss, personality changes, impaired ability to reason and disorientation
- The ability to learn new material is decreased and there is a loss of problem-solving skills
- Motor coordination may be affected
- Work is not possible and other social functioning is impaired. Consciousness is not affected
- There are many causes including vascular disease but the commonest cause is Alzheimer's disease, accounting for nearly 70% of cases
- Other causes include cerebral infarctions, alcoholism, hypothyroidism and Parkinson's disease.

Alzheimer's disease

This is a degenerative condition of the brain and the cause is still not known.

Aetiology

- There is a gradual reduction in neurons in parts of the brain and the deposition of amyloid plaques
- Progressive cortical atrophy leads to dilated ventricles within the brain
- There are neurofibrillary tangles in the neurons
- There are plaques and tangles found in the brains of many who have not got impaired cognitive functioning – the positioning of the plaques and tangles is probably important
- There is also a deficiency of a neurotransmitter called acetylcholine in the brain of those with the disease.

Over a quarter of those over 85 years of age in this country have Alzheimer's disease.

Clinical features

- Slow onset that progresses over several years
- Eventually interferes with work and relationships
- Memory loss is usually the first sign
- There is a lack of initiative and repetitive behaviour
- Judgement is impaired and abstract thinking is a problem
- There may be problems with language and word use
- Disorientation to time and place
- Misplacing things – putting things in unusual places
- Changes in mood and behaviour – can show rapid mood swings
- Changes in personality – may become very dependent on one person
- Loss of initiative and desire to do things – may sit for hours in front of the television
- All aspects of cortical function are eventually affected.

There is no cure for Alzheimer's disease but there are drugs available that may slow down the progress of the disease in some cases.

Treatment is usually surgical with the insertion of a shunt to drain the CSF.

DISEASES OF VOLUNTARY MUSCLE

These are the myopathies and weakness is the dominant feature. Some may be congenital, e.g. muscular dystrophy; some are inflammatory and some may be associated with drugs, toxins and endocrine weakness.

Muscular dystrophy

- This is the commonest myopathy
- Duchenne muscular dystrophy is the commonest form of the disease with an onset in childhood
- Weakness occurs in myopathy with reduced muscle strength.

Acquired myopathies

- These are secondary to other diseases especially metabolic or endocrine disease
- Causes include thyroid disease, parathyroid disease, corticosteroids and biochemical causes such as potassium

deficiency (hypokalaemia) may cause a generalised flaccid weakness if severe.

Drug-induced myopathy

- This may occur when the patient is taking statins to reduce their plasma cholesterol.

Myasthenia gravis

An acquired autoimmune disease where antibodies attack and destroy the nicotinic acetylcholine receptors at the neuromuscular junction. This leads to skeletal muscle weakness and fatigue that improves with rest. The thymus gland is enlarged in some cases and a thymic tumour (thyoma) is found in a small percentage of patients.

Clinical features

- Fatigability (weakness of the muscles, worse at the end of the day)
- Proximal limb muscles, eye muscles and muscles of mastication and facial expression are those most commonly involved
- In more than half of cases the eye muscles are the first to be involved.

The anticholinesterase drug pyridostigmine is used in the early stages.

Immunomodulating drugs such as azathioprine and corticosteroids do lead to improvement in some cases.

CONCLUSION

This chapter began by looking at the nervous system in health. This is probably the most complex system in the body and the disorders that may affect it are many. Neurology is the study of the nervous system and the diseases and disorders that affect it. Only the most common disorders have been described in this short chapter but these are the ones that are seen most in nursing practice. The reader should consult one of the many neurology textbooks available for more detailed information on this fascinating subject.

SELF-ASSESSMENT QUESTIONS

1. Describe the divisions of the nervous system.
2. Draw a simple diagram showing the lobes of the brain.

3. Describe the circulation of cerebrospinal fluid within the nervous system.
4. List the symptoms of a subdural haematoma.
5. Describe the possible causes of meningitis and the clinical picture seen.
6. What is meant by a demyelinating disorder?
7. Describe the pathophysiology of Alzheimer's disease.
8. List the signs and symptoms seen in Parkinson's disease.

FURTHER READING

Fuller, G. (2010) *Neurology: An Illustrated Colour Text*, 3rd edn, Edinburgh: Churchill Livingstone.

Ginsberg, L. (2010) *Lecture Notes: Neurology*, 9th edn. Wiley-Blackwell.

Schapira, A. (2010) *Parkinson's Disease*, Oxford: Oxford University Press.

11 The digestive system

Sharon Edwards

FUNCTIONS OF THE DIGESTIVE SYSTEM

The function of the digestive system is to digest nutrients which are required to carry out vital functions to sustain life, to form new body components or to assist in the functioning of various body processes, such as breathing and physical activity. Nutrients such as glucose and vitamins are necessary to combine with oxygen to produce energy in the form of adenosine triphosphate (ATP) for cell, tissue and organ function:

- Respiratory: movement of the diaphragm, stretching of fibres to expand the lungs
- Cardiac: contraction of the heart and circulation
- Kidney: the formation of urine
- Brain: thought process and action potentials (impulses)
- Gastrointestinal tract (GIT)/liver: laying down of reserves of carbohydrates and fats, formation of bile, clotting factors and immunity
- Skin: heat loss, generation of vasoconstriction and vasodilation.

In addition nutrients such as carbohydrates, fats and protein are needed for all body processes.

THE GASTROINTESTINAL TRACT (GIT) ANATOMY

The digestive system is essential for maintaining life and is stimulated by a range of mechanical and chemical processes (Keshav, 2004). There are two main groups of organs:

- The alimentary canal (gastrointestinal tract or GI tract)
- The accessory digestive organs (liver, spleen and pancreas).

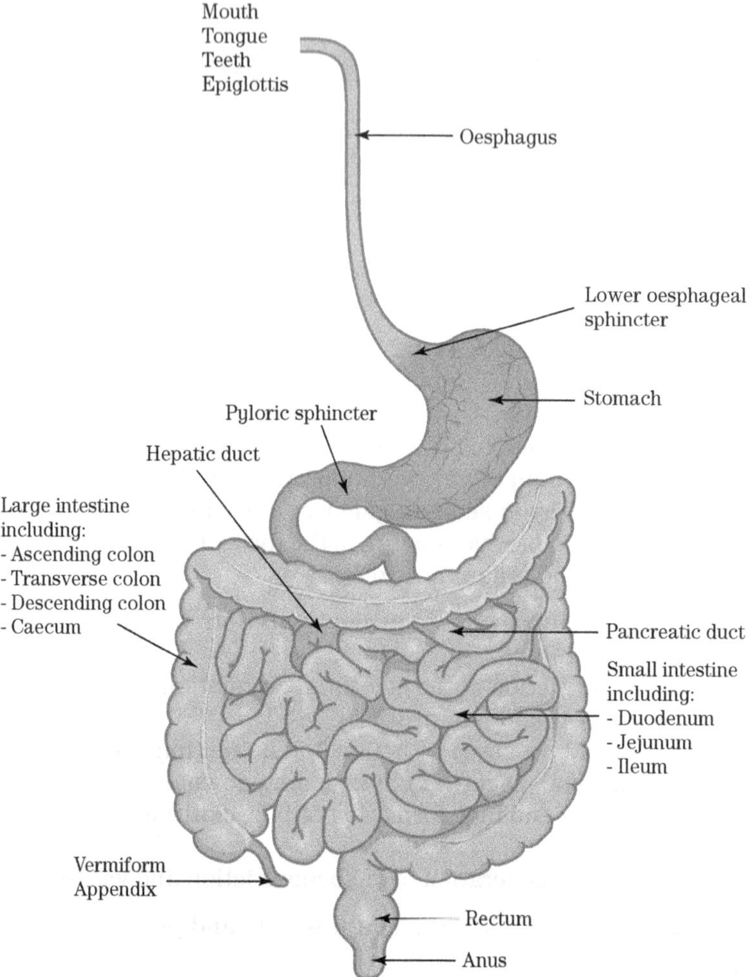

Figure 11.1 The digestive system

The digestive system (Figure 11.1) is made up of the following parts:

- Mouth, tongue, teeth: beginning of the GIT, food is ingested and broken down by chewing and mixing with saliva containing amylase
- Oesophagus: muscular tube which is responsible for peristalsis and the passage of food from the mouth to the stomach by propulsion (Richards and Edwards, 2012). The passage of food is prevented from entering the trachea by the glottis

- Stomach has sphincters on entering (gastro-oesophageal sphincter) and leaving (pyloric sphincter); contracts and churns to break down food into smaller particles (mechanical digestion), mixing with gastric juices (chemical digestion) forming chyme. Gastric juices produce:
  - Pepsinogen (active substance pepsin) – begins the digestion of proteins
  - Parietal cells act to acidify the stomach
  - Intrinsic factor released by the parietal cells necessary to absorb vitamin B_{12}
  - G cells which secret gastrin, which regulates acid secretion
- Small intestine: duodenum, jejunum and ileum
  - Ducts lead into the small intestine from the liver and pancreas to facilitate the breakdown of food
  - The majority of absorption of food takes place in the duodenum
- Large intestine: vermiform appendix, caecum, ascending, transverse, descending, and sigmoid colon
  - Most nutrients have been absorbed
  - Main function is to remove the remaining water, solidifying the material into faeces
  - Contains bacteria to aid digestion
  - The colon intermittently contracts, pushing waste material into the rectum
- Rectum and anus: defecation takes place with the excretion of waste products, and is under neurological voluntary control in adults.

ACCESSORY ORGANS OF DIGESTION

The liver and gall bladder

The liver is covered by the peritoneum and dense connective tissue; there are 4 lobes (Figure 11.2):

- Right lobe is the largest
- Left lobe is smaller and separated from the right lobe by the falciform ligament
- Quadrate lobe
- Posterior caudate lobe.

Functions of the liver

- Manufactures bile salts, which are stored in the gall bladder; bile is part excretory (the removal of bilirubin, the waste product from the

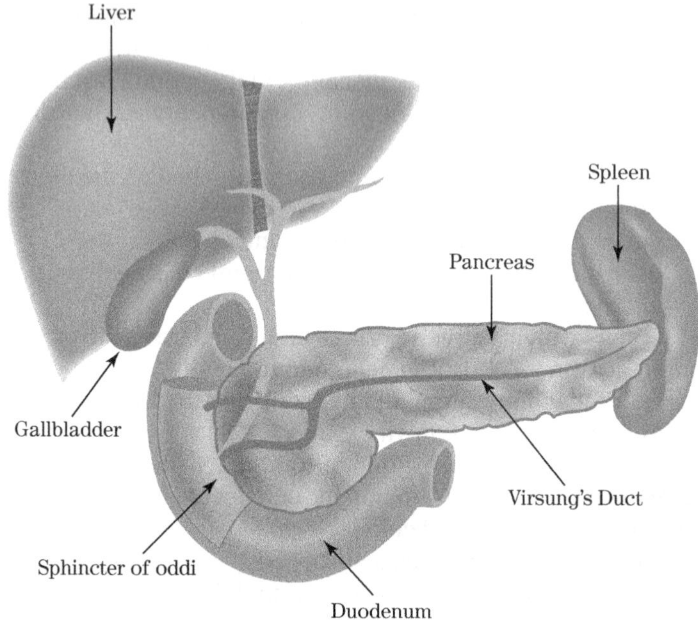

Figure 11.2 The liver, pancreas and spleen

breakdown of red blood cells by the spleen, excreted in faeces) and part digestive (breaks down fat globules). Bile is produced and enters small bile capillaries which empty into small ducts. These all go to:

- Form the right and left hepatic ducts
- Join to form the common hepatic duct
- Eventually joins the cystic duct from the gall bladder
- Becomes the common bile duct
- Joins the pancreatic duct and joins the duodenum at the ampulla vatar

- Newly absorbed nutrients (carbohydrates, fats and proteins) are collected by the liver, metabolised through oxidation processes and the use of co-enzymes (produced by vitamins). See metabolism below.
- Manufactures heparin and other plasma proteins e.g. prothrombin, fibrinogen and albumin:
  - Clotting factors require vitamin K
  - Osmotic pressure in the systemic circulation to hold fluid in the extracellular fluid compartment

- Stores vitamins
- Contains enzymes that breaks down poisonous or harmful substances that enter the body e.g. drugs, foods and transfers them into harmless compounds.

The pancreas

The pancreas has two main functions: endocrine and exocrine (Figure 11.2):

- Endocrine function
  - The islets of Langerhans secrete insulin and glucagon directly into the blood
  - There are three distinctive cells within the pancreas:
    - Alpha 25% secrete glucagon, which increases blood glucose
    - Beta 60% secrete insulin
    - Delta 10% secrete somatostatin which depresses insulin and glucagon secretion and decreases gastrointestinal motility
- Exocrine function
  - Normal digestive and absorptive processes
  - Consists of acinar cells arranged in groups which produce pancreatic juice 3000 ml/day:
    - Trypsin, chymotrypsin, elastase, nuclease (protein metabolism)
    - Amylase (carbohydrate metabolism)
    - Lipase (fat digestion)
    - Bicarbonate ions (neutralisation of acid chyme).

PHYSIOLOGY OF CHEMICAL DIGESTION, ABSORPTION AND METABOLISM

Different segments of the GIT absorb different nutrients. The process of digestion begins in the mouth due to the presence of salivary amylase, in the stomach by hydrochloric acid and pepsin. The stomach produces chyme that passes into the duodenum and meets pancreatic amylase and bile leading to further breakdown of carbohydrates. Fats are mixed and concentrated to fatty acids, through the action of bile and lipase. Proteins are further broken into amino acids and peptides. These are absorbed together with vitamins, minerals and water across the intestinal wall and into blood by active transport, diffusion or facilitated diffusion, with some fatty acids being absorbed into the lymph. The absorption of nutrients ends in the small intestine.

Carbohydrates (monosaccharides)

These account for the majority of the human diet; they include a number of different groups:

- Complex carbohydrates need to be broken down into their simplest form using salivary amylase and pancreatic amylase:
  - Polysaccharides:
    - Starch
    - Glycogen
  - Oligosaccharides:
    - Sucrose (glucose-fructose)
    - Maltose (glucose-glucose)
    - Lactose (glucose-galactose)
- Monosaccharides are absorbed by the intestinal mucosa:
  - Glucose
  - Fructose
  - Galactose.

Proteins

Proteins are the basic structural material of the body.

- Most protein taken in the diet is absorbed
- Absorption begins in the stomach when pepsinogen is activated to pepsin and breaks some amino acid bonds, breaking them into smaller amino acids
- Major protein breakdown is in the small intestine by the pancreatic enzymes trypsin and chymotrypsin
- Some enzymes are pure proteins; some are co-enzymes and derived from vitamins:
  - Collagen: found in all connective tissues for strength of bones, tendons and ligaments
  - Keratin: required for hair, nails, waterproofing of skin
  - Elastin: durability and flexibility of ligaments, and binds bones together
  - Actin and myosin: contractile proteins found in muscle cells, cell division in all cells, and intracellular transport
  - Protein enzymes: essential for every biochemical reaction in the body, such as saliva amylase, starch breakdown, other oxidase enzymes for food
  - Plasma proteins: such as albumin function as acids or bases (buffers) to prevent wide swings in blood pH

  - Hormones: regulate growth and development, insulin helps regulate blood sugar
  - Antibodies: released by the B-cells of immunity and inactivate foreign substances.

Lipids (fats)

Fat is required for cell membranes and organelles, transport and a source of stored energy, insulation and protection.

- Small intestine is the sole site of lipid digestion
  - Emulsification and lipolysis
  - Pancreas is the only source of fat-digesting enzymes or lipases
  - Need to be pre-treated with bile salts
  - Breaks down into:
    - Fatty acids (triglycerides) and glycerol (triacylglycerol)
    - Phospholipids.

Vitamins

Vitamins are needed only in minute amounts. They are not used for energy or as building blocks, but are crucial in helping the body to use nutrients. Without vitamins all carbohydrates, fats and proteins are useless. Vitamins are not made in the body: they must be ingested, with the exception of Vitamin D, B and K. Vitamins are classified as fat soluble or water soluble:

- Fat soluble:
  - A requirement for normal bone and teeth development, an antioxidant for the prevention of cancer and atherosclerosis
  - D used for hormone function
  - E an antioxidant that neutralises free radicals e.g. prevents cell damage and atherosclerosis
  - K is essential for blood clotting
- Water soluble:
  - C is ascorbic acid needed for the formation of connective tissues, enhances iron absorption and the maintenance of homeostasis e.g. vasoconstriction
  - B_1 is thiamine and required for carbohydrate metabolism
  - B_2 is riboflavin required for maintenance of acid-base balance and carbohydrate metabolism to form adenosine triphosphate (ATP)
  - Niacin or nicotinamide is a co-enzyme involved in glycolysis, fat breakdown

- B_8 or pyridoxine involved with amino acid metabolism, glycogenolysis (breakdown of glycogen to glucose), formation of antibodies and haemoglobin
- B_5 or pantothenic acid the formation of ATP in the mitochondria of cells, fatty acid metabolism and synthesis of steroids and haemoglobin
- Biotin is involved in the formation of ATP from glucose and amino acids in the mitochondria of cells
- B_{12} or cyanocolabamin absorbed from the stomach by the intrinsic factor, required by the GIT, nervous system, bone marrow and the replication of DNA
- Folic acid is essential for the formation of red blood cells (RBC), normal development of an embryo and for the use of some amino acids.

Minerals

Minerals are only required in moderate amounts. The major minerals and trace elements are:

- Minerals – most of these are ionised in body fluids or bound to organic compounds:
  - Calcium required for rigidity of bones, membrane permeability, transmission of nerve impulses, muscle contraction, blood clotting
  - Chlorine helps to maintain osmotic pressure and pH of extracellular fluid (ECF) aids in the transport of carbon dioxide (CO_2)
  - Sulphur is needed for insulin formation, and is present in cartilage, tendons and bone
  - Potassium is necessary for responsive muscle cells to stimuli from the central nervous system
  - Sodium is necessary to maintain normal osmolality and water balance
  - Magnesium plays a role in ATP and normal muscle and nerve impulse innervation
  - Phosphorus is a component of bones and teeth, is a buffer for acid and maintains acid base balance, energy storage
- Trace elements:
  - Fluorine important for tooth structure
  - Cobalt combines with vitamin B_{12} for maturation of RBC
  - Chromium required for glucose metabolism, effectiveness of insulin

- Copper required for formation of haemoglobin, manufacture of melanin and myelin and production of ATP
- Iodine is needed for the construction of thyroid hormones to regulate cellular metabolic rate
- Iron is essential for haemoglobin
- Manganese acts in fatty acid, cholesterol, urea and haemoglobin synthesis, needed for neural function and so carbohydrates and proteins can be used by the body
- Selenium is an antioxidant, a constituent of enzymes, and conserves vitamin E
- Zinc is a constituent of enzymes, required for normal growth, wound healing, taste, smell and sperm production.

METABOLISM

During metabolism, substances are constantly being built up (anabolic) and torn down (catabolic). Cells use the energy to drive their activities; even at rest the body uses energy.

Metabolic process

- Anabolism: larger molecules or structures are built from smaller ones e.g. the bonding of amino acids to make proteins and cell membranes
- Catabolism: the breakdown of complex structures to simple ones. Hydrolysis of foods in the digestive tract is catabolism. Cellular respiration during which food is broken down within cells and some of the energy released is captured to form ATP
- Oxidation-reacts:
- Is where the energy-yielding ATP reactions within cells
- Oxidation is the combination of oxygen with other elements e.g. via the gain of oxygen but also the loss of hydrogen.
- Whenever one substances loses electrons another substance gains them oxygen-reduction (O-R)
- Enzymes: the reactions given above are catalysed by enzymes, which remove hydrogen ions; specifically called dehydrogenases and transfer oxygen oxidases derived from the B vitamins.

Carbohydrate metabolism

All carbohydrates are eventually transformed to glucose metabolism. Glucose enters the cell by facilitated diffusion and is increased in the presence of insulin.

- Glucose catabolism
  - Glucose breakdown (glycosis) is a complex process and involves a number of pathways before energy is produced:
    - Acetyl coenzyme A: pyruvic acid from glycolysis is converted to acetyl CoA by thiamine derivative vitamins B1 and B2 riboflavin
    - Krebs cycle: acetyl CoA enters the Krebs cycle and is broken down by mitochondrial enzymes and consists of 8 steps. Other products can be converted to enter the Krebs cycle to produce energy e.g. fats and proteins
    - Electron transport train: the energy produced is harvested and combined with oxygen along a chain, the process requires riboflavin
    - ATP production: in the presence of oxygen cellular respiration if efficient and equates to an energy capture of 40% more efficient than any machine at 10–30%
- Glucose anabolism
  - Glucose storage: glycogenesis, when there is an increase level of production of ATP, glucose catabolism is inhibited and additional glucose is stored as glycogen in the liver or skeletal muscles or as fat. More fat than glycogen can be stored
  - Glucose release: glycogenolysis is when blood levels of glucose decrease and glycogen lysis occur to break it down to enter the Krebs cycle
  - Formation of glucose from proteins or fats: gluconeogenesis is when too little glucose is available, and glycogen stores are almost depleted. Consequently fats and then proteins are used as a source of energy. The use of protein as a source of energy is rare except in malnutrition states e.g. protein energy malnutrition. The heart is entirely muscle protein and when severely catabolised death ensues.

Lipid metabolism

This is the most concentrated source of energy. It contains very little water and energy yield is approximately twice that gained from glucose or protein.

- Lipid catabolism
  - Neutral fats only oxidised for energy; catabolism of these fats involves the separate oxidation of the two different building blocks, glycerol and fatty acid chains:

        - Glycerol: most body cells convert glycerol to glyceraldehydes phosphate, which then flows in the Krebs cycle
        - Fatty acids chains: these are broken apart into two carbon acetic acid fragments, and reduced co-enzymes are produced. Each molecule is fused to co-enzyme A forming acetyl CoA.
- Lipid anabolism
    - When glycerol and fatty acids are not immediately needed for energy they are stored for later. Stored fats are broken down and released to the blood when blood glucose level drops
        - From glucose to fats by the liver (an important function) – lipogenesis occurs when blood glucose is high; 50% ends up in subcutaneous tissue converted into triglycerides and stored. Glucose is easily converted into fats, even if diet is poor
        - From fat to glucose by the liver: lipolysis is the conversion of stored fats into glycerol and fatty acids e.g. lipogenesis in reverse; depends on the availability of oxaloacetic acid to act as the pickup molecule which is converted to glucose when carbohydrates are deficient (for the brain). Without oxaloacetic acid fat metabolism is incomplete; acetyl CoA accumulates and liver converts it to ketones or ketone bodies, which differ from keto acids.
- Synthesis of structural materials
    - All body cells use phospholipids and cholesterol to build their membranes:
        - Phospholipids: are important components of myelin sheath of neurones, the liver synthesises lipoproteins for transport of cholesterol, fats, tissue factor and clotting factors
        - Cholesterol: used to make bile salts; endocrine organs (testes, ovaries, adrenal cortex) use cholesterol as a basis for synthesising steroid hormones.

Protein metabolism

Proteins are broken down into amino acids and replaced. Ingested amino acids are transported in blood and taken up by cells and used to replace tissue proteins. When more are available they can be used as energy or converted to fat.

- Oxidation of amino acids
    - Transamination is the transfer of amino groups to become a keto acid through oxidative deamination
    - Oxidative deamination are part of the amino group glutamic acid to form keto acid and is removed as ammonia combined with carbon dioxide yielding urea and water

    - Keto acid modification molecules are produced and can be oxidised into the Krebs cycle from keto acids to produce energy
- Synthesis of proteins
    - Amino acids are the most important anabolic nutrient and form all protein structures, they occur on ribosomes, controlled by hormones (growth hormone, thyroxin, sex hormones and others)
    - For adequate nutrition a full set of amino acids are required.

THE EFFECT OF STRESS ON THE GIT

Stress is initiated by the nervous and endocrine systems, which stimulates the sympathetic nervous system (SNS), promoting:

- Suppression of reproduction, growth, and thyroid hormones
- The medulla of the adrenal gland releases catecholamines into the blood stream e.g. adrenaline and noradrenaline.

Adrenaline (epinephrine) and noradrenaline (norepinephrine)

Adrenaline (epinephrine) mobilises glycogen from the lever to increase blood glucose levels. Noradrenaline (norepinephrine) acts on the GIT by acting on alpha two (α_2) adrenergic receptors found in the GIT and lead to GIT relaxation, inhibiting GIT activity. It is noradrenaline that has the major effect on the GIT.

The adrenal cortex

- The adrenal cortex is also activated in long term stress:
    - Release of cortisol
    - Affects carbohydrate, protein and fat metabolism resulting in an increase in blood glucose
    - Maximises the action of catecholamines
    - GIT effects of cortisol:
        - Promotes gastric secretion
        - May be enough to cause ulceration of gastric mucosa
- Metabolic effects of cortisol:
    - Circulates in plasma
    - Mobilises substances needed for cellular metabolism
    - Affects carbohydrate, protein and fat metabolism
    - Cortisol increases blood glucose level

- Circulatory effects of cortisol:
  - Maximises the action of catecholamines
  - Maintains normal BP and CO
- GIT effects of cortisol:
  - Promotes gastric secretion
  - May be enough to cause ulceration of gastric mucosa.

The net result

The result of the release of adrenaline, noradrenaline and stimulation of the adrenal cortex is:

- GIT relaxation
- Inhibiting GIT activity and absorption
- May be significant to cause ischaemia to the stomach and duodenal mucosa
- Stress ulcers:
  - To accompany severe illness
  - Systemic trauma
  - Neural injury
  - Generally in the stomach and duodenum
- And/or ischaemic ulcers:
  - Can occur within hours of an event due to
    - Haemorrhage
    - Multisystem trauma
    - Severe burns
    - Heart failure
    - Sepsis
  - Cause ischaemia to the stomach and duodenal mucosa, decreasing gut motility even if nutrition is restored
  - As a result of burns injury frequently called Curling ulcer.

PATHOPHYSIOLOGY OF THE GIT

Nutrients are required in health and even more so during illness. Yet the majority of patients in hospital and in the community suffer from stress and malnutrition which can lead to complications of the GIT such as ulceration and hypoxia (Edwards, 2000). The combination of a reduction in the ingestion of nutrients, stress and malnutrition prevent the replenishment of energy sources (direct and indirect) and complicate a patient's illness and thus recovery. In addition, patients can suffer from conditions related directly to the GIT and/or to the accessory organs of digestion.

Clinical features of GIT disease

There are certain clinical manifestations of GIT conditions that are common to many of the diseases identified below:

- Dysphagia – difficulty in swallowing caused by:
  - Neuromuscular disease
  - Cerebral vascular accident (CVA)
  - Obstruction of the upper GI tract
- Dyspepsia – refers to a combination of symptoms e.g. heartburn, acid regurgitation, pain
- Achalasia is failure of peristalsis in the lower two thirds of the oesophagus resulting in dilatation of the lower oesophagus
  - Symptoms:
    - Dysphagia (difficulty in swallowing)
    - Halitosis (foul-smelling breath)
    - Regurgitation of food
    - Symptoms similar to gastro-oesophageal reflux (see below)
  - Diagnosis
    - Endoscopy to exclude tumour
    - Barium swallow
  - Treatment
    - Dilatation of oesophagus
    - Surgery
    - Bland diet
    - Heller xylotomy (reduces lower oesophageal pressure)
    - Anticholinergic
    - Calcium channel blockers
- Heartburn – acid regurgitation from the stomach, causing a burning sensation in the centre of the chest, can be confused with chest pain caused by a heart condition
- Abdominal pain/acute abdomen
- Loss of weight due to symptoms of other conditions e.g. cancer or GIT condition
- Anorexia due to the lack of desire to eat
- Flatulence (excessive passing of wind) e.g. belching or from abdominal pain caused by trapped air e.g. flatus
- Haematemesis is vomiting blood and may differ in colour or texture:
  - Bright red fresh blood
  - Dark brown with clots or have the appearance of partially digested food and resemble coffee grounds
- Melaena is the passage of black or dark brown faeces, indicates a bleed in the GIT

- Constipation is an accumulation of hard faeces which are hard to pass
- Steatorrhoea is fatty stools that often are pale, usually float and are difficult to flush down the toilet
- Nausea is the conscious desire to vomit
- Vomiting is the ejection of food through the mouth from the upper GI tract. Characteristics:
    - Regurgitation of food: it will be/look like partially digested food
    - Projectile vomit is forceful expulsion of food without nausea
    - Faecal/intestinal vomit can be the result of obstruction
    - Colour of vomit can be either:
        - Coffee ground appearance – may indicate bleeding from the stomach
        - Dark brown appearance – may indicate blood and bleeding somewhere in the GIT; the blood changes vomit to dark brown as a result of interaction with hydrochloric acid in the stomach
        - Bright red indicates active bleeding in the GIT
        - Green indicates the presence of bile
- Diarrhoea – the passing of loose or semi-solid or liquid faeces, passed at frequent intervals, is generally due to a problem of the GIT.

Case study 11.1

A 35-year-old nurse is admitted to your ward with no previous history of illness, having had a 3-day history of vomiting and diarrhoea, abdominal pain, and progressive confusion. On examination, he is apyrexial, unkempt with signs of urinary incontinence and a strong-smelling odour on his breath. Further examination revealed:

RR 35 bmp
HR 120 bmp
BP 80/40 mmHg
O_2 94%

Neurologically he is unreadable, but has normal flexion to pain with a GCS of 6. His jugular venous pressure was not seen. His extremities are cyanosed and cool to touch.

- Causes of diarrhoea are usually:
    - Food poisoning
    - Inflammatory bowel disease such as ulcerative colitis or Crohn's disease

- Broad spectrum antibiotics
- Other drugs such as laxatives, antacids or digoxin
- Diverticular disease
- Malabsorption conditions
- Faecal impaction with overflow
- Tropical diseases

- Investigation might involve the examination of stool specimen for:
  - Melaena
  - Steatorrhoea
  - Diarrhoea
  - Constipation
  - Flatulence
  - Stool type, colour, smell, formation, size.

If the patient's diarrhoea and vomiting, described above, is prolonged, this can lead to:

- Dehydration
- Water, electrolyte loss
- Loss of extracellular fluid leading to circulatory collapse
- Metabolic alkalosis due to the gastric loss of HCL
- Metabolic acidosis if small intestine contents lost (less common).

DISORDERS OF NUTRITION

Starvation and malnutrition

This is due to inadequate food intake or dietary imbalance, leading to a reduction in the formation of energy required to meet the metabolic demands of body systems.

Aetiology

- Low intake of nutrients
- High calorie demand by the body e.g. in shock
- Poor absorption of nutrients or vitamins from the GI tract
- Underlying illness or disease e.g. cancer, Crohn's disease
- Older adults due to inactivity
- Families living in poverty
- Patient suffering from a disability or is infirm due to an underlying pathology e.g. arthritis
- Unconscious patients

- Chronic disease e.g. renal or cardiovascular disease, COPD
- Loss of appetite e.g. due to chemotherapy treatment or liver disease
- Psychological disturbances e.g. anorexia nervosa, bulimia, loss of job, bereavement, depression.

Pathology

- The post-absorptive state is a period whereby the GIT is emptying and the body is being supplied by body reserves. This is to maintain blood glucose levels. Fasting should be no more than 12 hours, as after this time:
  - Glycogenolysis in the liver and skeletal muscles – the liver stores are the first line of glucose reserves, then skeletal muscle stores (transported to the liver) – glycogen is mobilised quickly and efficiently until stores are nearly used up
  - Lipolysis in adipose tissues and the liver – glycerol is converted to glucose by lipolysis then continued as gluconeogenesis by the liver. Fat begins to be broken down before all stores of glycogen have been used, so the remainder can be conserved for the brain (only uses glucose as a source of energy)
  - Catabolism of cellular protein – occurs when fasting is prolonged and glycogen and fat stores are depleted.
- The effects of poor nutrition
  - Nutrients are required to produce adenosine triphosphate (ATP) in cells; if muscle cells have insufficient energy they will become weak, this can lead to:
    - Chest infections and possibly pneumonia
    - Decreased muscle strength and weakness leading to immobility and the potential of complications e.g. deep vein thrombosis (DVT) and pulmonary embolism (PE), pressure ulcer development
  - With a lack of nutrients there become insufficient proteins to build white blood cells (WBC) of innate immunity and the immunoglobulins (Ig) of specific immunity. This can lead to an impaired immune response and an increased susceptibility to hospital-acquired infection (HAI)
  - A reduction in protein, carbohydrates and fats, iron and zinc, vitamin K, A, C and E can lead to delays in wound healing, pressure ulcer development and tissue viability issues
  - Protein energy malnutrition
    - Classification of protein energy malnutrition is determined by body mass index (BMI in kg/m^2):

20–25	Acceptable/desirable range
17–18.4	Moderate protein-energy malnutrition
16–17	Moderately severe protein-energy malnutrition
<16	Severe protein-energy malnutrition

    - BMI = weight (kg)/height^2(m)
  - There are two extreme forms of protein energy malnutrition:
    - Marasmus is protein-calorie malnutrition leading to progressive muscle wasting due to:
      - Disorders of appetite
      - Anorexia nervosa
      - Bulimia
      - Malabsorption
      - Food intolerance and allergy
      - Cachexia due to cancer
    - Kwashiorkor is severe protein deficiency in children, resulting in:
      - Mental retardation and failure to grow
      - Reduced plasma proteins decreases colloidal oncotic pressure (COP) leading to oedema (Figure 11.3)
- Effects on nutrients during shock
  - The loss of lean body mass is different in shock and trauma to that of malnutrition
  - In malnutrition protein is preserved until the final stages
  - In multiple trauma or shock hyper-metabolism occurs e.g.
    - ↑ Metabolic rate
    - ↑ Oxygen consumption
    - ↑ Production of carbon dioxide and heat
  - Mixed fuel sources are used, and all potential glucose sources are mobilised
  - Resulting in a hyperglycaemia
  - Fat deposits accumulate in the liver; can lead to liver failure
  - Protein levels reduce, resulting in decreased colloidal oncotic pressure
  - All cause a reduction of energy stores and sources, depriving cells/tissues/organs of nutrients reducing their function
  - The process of malnutrition due to illness or reduced food intake and nil by mouth (NBM) practices in hospital, combined with stress can lead to the translocation of bacteria (Figure 11.4).

Clinical features

- A reduced BMI over a period of time from mild–severe malnutrition

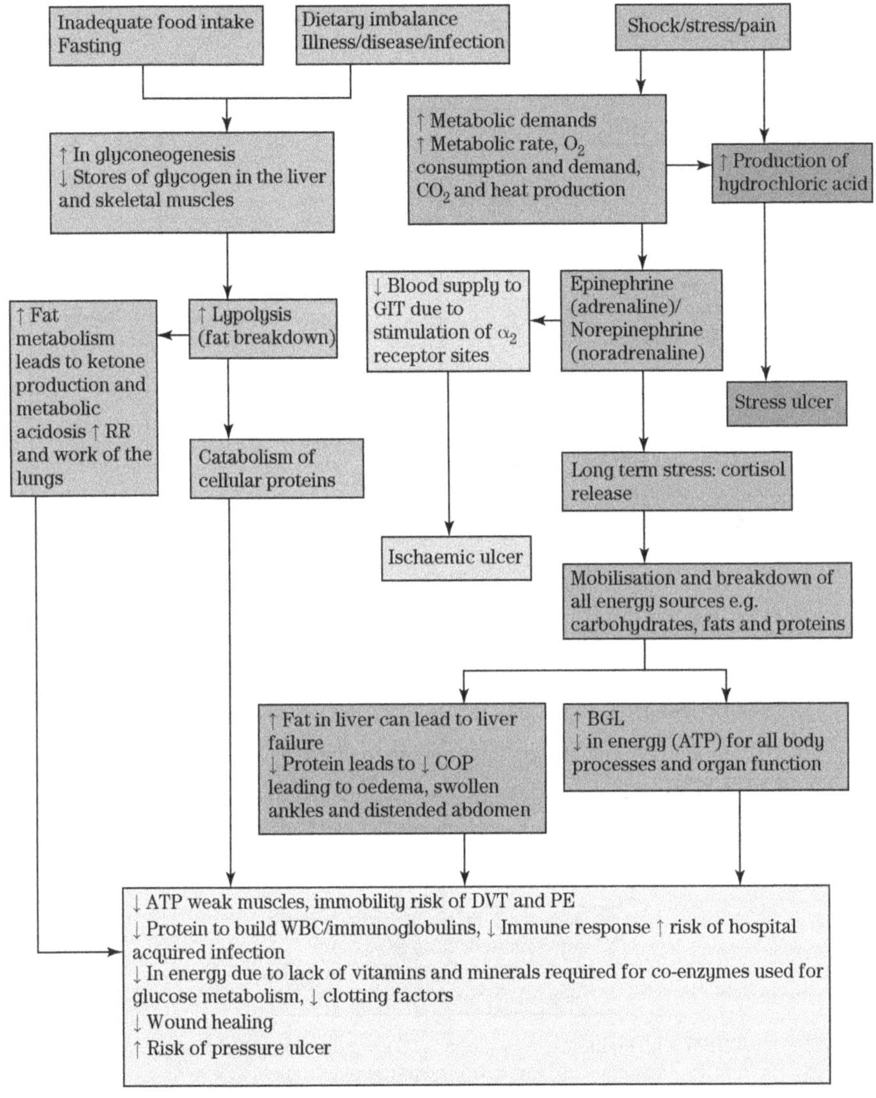

COP = colloidal oncotic pressure; BGL = blood glucose level; ATP = adenosine triphosphate; RR = respiratory rate; CO_2 = carbon dioxide; DVT = deep vein thrombosis; PE = pulmonary embolism

Figure 11.3 The effects of malnutrition on body process

- Muscle wasting as the body will break down muscle and protein as a source of energy
- Distended abdomen and swollen ankles due to reduced oncotic pressure in blood vessels leading to leakage of fluid into the interstitial space

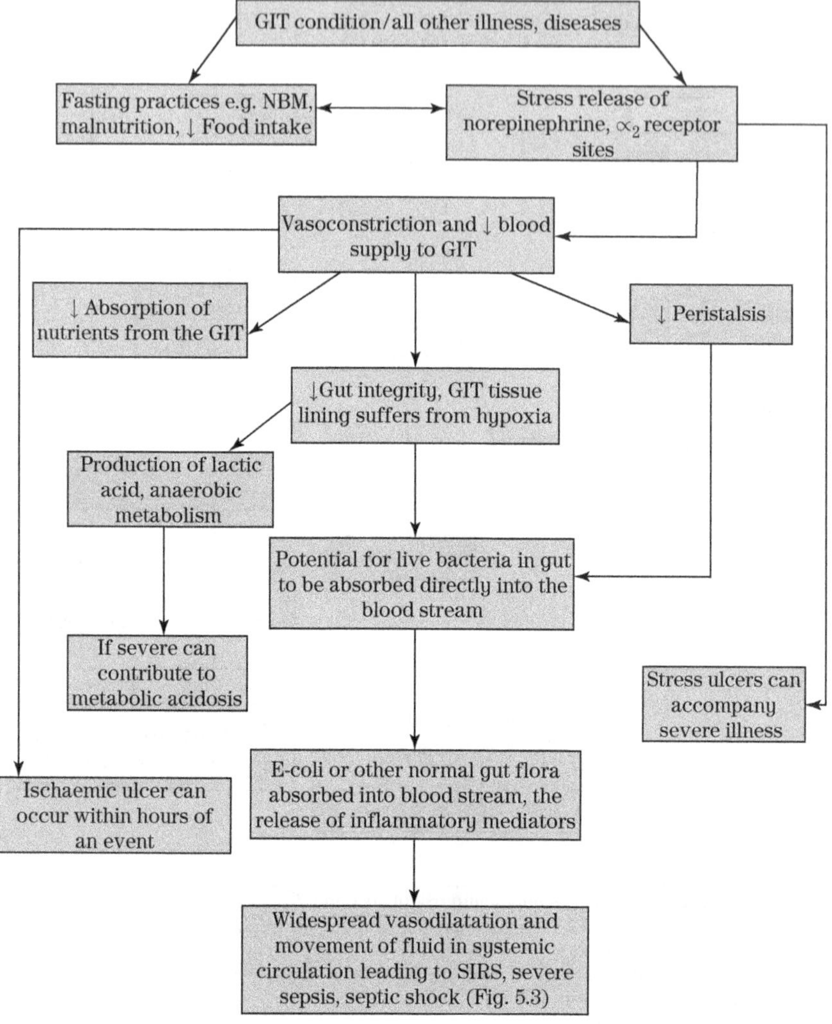

NBM = nil by month; a_2 = alpha 2; GIT = gastrointestinal tract; SIRS = systemic inflammatory response syndrome

Figure 11.4 The formation of translocation of bacteria

- Increased ketones can lead to metabolic acidosis, increase in respiratory rate in an attempt to maintain homeostasis.

Investigations

- Past medical history
- Nutritional assessment is undertaken to identify those at risk from developing malnutrition and those patients with malnutrition

- A full nutritional assessment using appropriate tools e.g. BMI, malnutrition universal screening tool (MUST) (MAG, 2003)
- Body fat content
- Anthropometric measures to determine muscle mass
- Blood tests e.g. serum albumin, serum transferrin and serum haemoglobin
- Urinalysis for ketones.

Treatment and drug therapy

- Early instigation of feeding in conditions such as shock or post-operative
- Adequate ingestion of food, with consideration to vitamins and minerals, as many of these are required for the production of co-enzymes, a necessity for the absorption and breakdown of nutrients
- Behavioural therapy or psychiatric involvement if due to mental ill health
- Food diary
- If unable to take oral diet:
  - Enteral feeding via a tube in the GIT
  - Parenteral nutrition.

> **Practice point**
>
> To prevent malnutrition healthcare professionals need to pay attention to nutritional needs, maintain privacy and ensure patient mealtimes are not disturbed.

Obesity

Obesity is an increase in body fat mass in relation to height, weight, gender and ethnicity. The incidence of obesity has increased significantly over the last decade (McCance *et al*, 2010).

Aetiology

- Excess ingested calories originating from the individual (exogenous) with low physical activity
- In stress individuals can over eat e.g. bereavement, low self-esteem
- Steroid therapy
- Metabolic problem originating from within the individual (endogenous)

- Is associated with the three leading causes of death:
  - Cardiovascular disease due to hypercholesterolaemia and hypertension
  - Type 2 diabetes mellitus
  - Cancer
    - In women breast, cervical, endometrial and liver cancer
    - In men prostatic, colon and rectal cancer.

Pathology

- Classified as either hyperplastic when there is a greater than normal number of fat cells or hypertrophic when there is a greater than normal size of fat cells.
- The fat cell theory is excessive number of fat cells.
- Lipoprotein-lipase (LPL) promotes fat storage – obese people are thought to have elevated levels of LPL in their fat cells.
- Reduced number of brown fat cells – release excess energy through heat production instead of converting energy to fat.
- Reduced level of adenosine triphosphatase (ATPase) pumps in cells leading to less energy release and obesity.
- Psychological causes that may encourage the patient to eat more, stimulated by external cues e.g. sight, smell and taste rather than internal e.g. hunger.

Clinical features

- Accumulation of fat around waist, thighs and hips
- Reduced high-density lipoprotein
- Increase in low-density lipoprotein
- Hypertension
- Insulin resistance in cells
- Pulmonary function compromised
- Sleep apnoea
- Exercise intolerance
- Pain in fingers and joints.

Investigations

- There is no specific measure for obesity, but the following are used:
  - BMI greater than 25 kg/m^2 is overweight and obesity is greater than 30 kg/m^2
  - Body fat mass
  - Anthropometric measurements.

Practice point

BMI is not always an accurate measure of obesity. Muscle mass weighs more than adipose tissue, therefore the addition of muscle can appear as an increase in weight in relation to height, but not an increase in fat.

Treatment and drug therapies

- Correction of metabolic disorder
- Weight loss (NICE, 2006) including:
  - Individually tailored weight loss programmes
  - Exercise programmes
  - Combination of both exercise and weight loss programmes
  - Support and self-motivation are essential for the success of these programmes
- Psychotherapy, behaviour modification
- Medications e.g. orlistat which reduces GIT absorption of fatty acids and cholesterol, and increases the elimination of fat in the bowels
- Bariatric surgery such as gastric bypass.

DISORDERS OF THE UPPER GIT

Disorders of the upper GIT involve the mouth, oesophagus, stomach and duodenum.

Oral infections

- Gingivitis is inflammation of the gums, usually caused by poor oral hygiene and stress, first noticed when gums bleed during brushing; pus may be present, and/or loose teeth (periodontitis)
- Vincent's infection is bacteria due to neglected oral hygiene, ulcerations that bleed, with an increase in saliva and a metallic taste in the mouth, halitosis
- Oral candidiasis (thrush) is caused by the candidiasis albicans and immunosupression, white patches in the oral cavity, treated with nystatin and amphotericin B
- Herpes simplex (cold sore on the lips or mouth) can either be type I or II, exacerbated by stress, treated with antivirals e.g. Zovirax

- Aphthous stomatitis (canker sore) is a chronic form of infection secondary to trauma and/or stress, painful ulcer on the lips, treated with topical/systemic corticosteroids or topical antibiotics
- Perotiditis is caused by a staphylococcal or streptococcus infection; pain is felt in the gland or ear; there is a lack of saliva, purulence, and treatment is usually with antibiotics, mouthwashes and lollipops to stimulate saliva production
- Stomatitis is a side effect of chemotherapy, trauma or pathogens; there is an increase in salivation and halitosis and a sore mouth.

Oral cancer

Oral cancer is more commonly found on the lower lip, on the lateral border of the tongue or on the buccal mucosa.

Aetiology

- Tobacco use
- Chronic irritation in the mouth
- UV light such as often observed in cancer of the lip.

Clinical features

- Early:
  - Leucoplakia is a white patch on or in the mouth, which cannot be wiped off and difficult to diagnose; biopsy may show malignant or pre-malignant changes
  - Erythroplakia is a red or purple lesion which often represents malignant change
  - Generally a sore that does not go away
- Late:
  - Pain especially moving the jaw
  - Dysphagia
  - Cancer growth observed on the lip or on examination in the mouth
  - Pain in the tongue when eating.

Investigations

- History and physical examination
- Biopsy of the lesion/cytology
- Toluidine test-blue dye is taken up by the cancer.

Treatment

- Chemotherapy
- Radiation
- Surgery.

Gastro-oesophageal reflux disease

Gastro-oesophageal reflux is not so much a disease, but a syndrome. It is a clinically symptomatic condition resulting in the reflux of gastric contents into the lower oesophagus.

Aetiology

Is generally a combination of factors:

- Hiatus hernia
- Incompetent lower oesophageal sphincter (LOS)
- Decreased oesophagus clearance
- Decreased gastric emptying
- Increased use of non-steroidal anti inflammatory (NSAID) medications such as ibuprofen
- Results in oesophageal irritation and inflammation.

Clinical features

- Heartburn (pyrosis)
- Burning, tight sensation, which can spread to the jaw
- May wake the person up from sleep
- Rule out cardiac causes
- Heartburn can be relieved with milk, or other alkaline substances
- Wheezing, coughing, dyspnoea, hoarseness
- Lump in throat
- Regurgitation; hot, bitter, sour liquid coming from mouth
- Stomatitis.

Investigations

- History and physical examination
- Barium swallow
- Oesophago-gastro-duodenoscopy.

Treatments and drug therapy

- IV therapy
- Weight reduction and/or smoking cessation

- Medication therapy
  - Antacids such as milk of magnesia
  - Histamine H_2-receptor antagonists such as ranitidine (Zantac)
  - Proton pump inhibitors (PPI) such as omeprazole
  - Antiulcer medication
- Surgery such as:
  - Anti-reflux procedures
  - Nissen fundoplication is a laparoscopic procedure that involves suturing of the fundus of the stomach around the oesophagus to strengthen the valve between the oesophagus and stomach; stops acid from backing up into the oesophagus so easily
- Endoscopic therapy:
  - Stretta procedure is the insertion of a stretta catheter into the oesophagus to the valve between the stomach and oesophagus; radiofrequency energy (heat) is delivered to the muscle of the sphincter. Over time this induces collagen formation, which forms a barrier against reflux
- Education about diet:
  - Food to avoid as it decreases lower oesophageal sphincter pressure:
    - Fatty foods
    - Chocolate
    - Coffee
    - Tea
    - Late night snacks
  - Food that might help:
    - Peppermint
    - Milk
    - Small frequent meals
- Prevention of complications
  - Oesophageal stricture due to scarring, which can be treated with:
    - Dilation via endoscopy by passing a bougie or cannula into the anal canal
    - Balloon dilatation
    - Calcium channel blockers can help to relax smooth muscle
  - Barrett's oesophagus – precancerous lesion for oesophageal cancer/adenocarcinoma
  - Bronchospasm
  - Aspiration pneumonia
  - Dental erosion.

Hiatus hernia

This is a herniation of part of the stomach through the diaphragm. It is common and is one cause of reflux oesophagitis.

Aetiology

Factors include:

- Structural changes of the anatomy of the upper abdominal cavity
- Obesity
- Pregnancy
- Heavy lifting.

Pathology

There are two types:

- *Sliding hiatus hernia* – the stomach herniates into the thorax when the patient is in the supine position
  - Standing causes the stomach to slide back into the abdomen
  - Exacerbated by any factors that increase intra abdominal pressure such as coughing, bending, straining and pregnancy
  - Management is via medical weight loss, antacids and sleeping in the sitting position
- *Rolling or para-oesophageal hernia* – the fundus of the stomach herniates through the hiatus alongside the oesophagus
  - Reflux is less common but there is a danger of congestion, constriction and ulcer formation.
  - The hernia may strangulate which is a major complication
  - Diagnosis is by barium studies and endoscopy.

Clinical features

- May be asymptomatic
- Heartburn
- Dysphagia
- Vomiting reflux when lying down and/or after eating
- Pain, burning when bending over.

Investigations

- Barium swallow
- Endoscopy
- Chest X-ray may show protrusion of the stomach into the thorax.

Treatment and drug therapies

- Eating small frequent meals
- Avoid:
  - Lying down after eating
  - Tight clothing
- Weight control if overweight
- Antacids relieve reflux oesophagitis
- Surgical intervention such as a fundoplication if hiatus hernia not managed by medical interventions
- Prevention of complications:
  - Gastro-oesophageal reflux
  - Haemorrhage
  - Stenosis of oesophagus
  - Ulcerations
  - Strangulation of the hernia
  - Regurgitation
  - Increased risk of respiratory disease.

Oesophageal varices

Oesophageal varices are distended collateral veins due to an increased pressure in the liver.

Aetiology

- Secondary to portal hypertension and liver disease
- Caused by portal hypertension leading to distended and tortuous veins and episodes of bleeding.

Pathology

- 70% patients with cirrhosis will develop varices
- Bleeding is likely from large varices observed in severe liver disease
- They are frequently the cause of life-threatening haematemesis when they rupture
- Rupture is due to a combination of further erosion by gastric acid and elevated venous pressure (McCance *et al*, 2010)
- The mortality rate varies between 30% and 60% (Richards and Edwards, 2012)
- Recurrent bleeding from varices has a poor prognosis with most patients dying within a year.

Clinical features

- Anaemia
- Melaena
- Vomiting of dark blood
- Rectal bleeding
- There is usually no pain.

Investigations

- Past medical history of jaundice, hepatitis or alcoholism
- Diagnosis made at the time of the oesophageal bleed
- Confirmed by endoscopy.

Treatment and drug therapy

- Emergency treatment of bleeding varices
  - Prompt correction of hypovolaemia
  - Vasoconstrictor therapy such as vasopressin or Glypressin may be used
  - A Sengstaken–Blakemore tube is usually used
- Beta-blockers can be effective in prevention of bleeding.

Helicobacter pylorus

The organism *Helicobacter pylori* is a Gram-negative spirochaete now known to be involved in gastritis and peptic and duodenal ulcer formation.

Aetiology

- Spirochaetes were first reported in 1893
- *Helicobacter pylori* is the commonest cause of gastritis
- Have been found to have definite links to the development of cancer.

Pathology

- *Helicobacter pylori* is believed to be acquired in childhood
- It survives, as the spirochaete secretes urease that protects it from being destroyed in the stomach by hydrochloric acid
- The mode of transmission is not certain – person to person and water are suspected and the most likely mediums for transmission
- By about 50 years of age, half the population thought to be affected
- The patient may be asymptomatic.

Investigations

- Tests include C urea breath tests – very simple but not always accurate
- Stool test can be done for diagnosis and to check eradication
- Endoscopic musocal biopsy and culture of the organism is the most certain diagnosis.

Treatment and drug therapy

- Resistant to single antibiotic therapy
- The ideal treatment is still not clear but triple antibiotic regimens do provide higher eradication rates:
  - Amoxicillin
  - Flagyl (metronidazole)
  - Tetracycline
  - Biaxin (clarithromycin)
- Eradication of infection commonly results in long-term ulcer remission
- Antacids and H_2 blockers may be added.

Gastritis

This is inflammation of the gastric mucosa (see chapter 2).

Aetiology

Gastritis can be acute or chronic:

- Acute gastritis caused by drugs or chemicals
  - Alcohol, histamine, certain metabolic disorders, e.g. uraemia, can all contribute to gastritis
  - Medications such as digoxin, steroids, non-steroidal anti inflammatory drugs (NSAIDs) such as aspirin
  - Complication of burns, stress, renal failure, sepsis, shock
  - Trauma from gastroscopy or NGT insertion
- Chronic gastritis associated with:
  - *H. pylori* infection, atrophy of the gastric mucosa and is more common in the elderly
  - Autoimmune attack of the parietal cells in the stomach, leading to an inability to secrete intrinsic factor and pernicious anaemia.

Pathology

See the inflammatory immune response in chapter 2.

Clinical features

- Acute gastritis
  - Abdominal discomfort
  - Epigastric tenderness
  - Bleeding
- Chronic gastritis
  - Elevated plasma levels of gastrin
  - Anorexia
  - Gastric bleeding
  - Epigastric pain
  - Feeling of fullness
  - Nausea and vomiting
  - Pernicious anaemia.

Treatment and drug therapy

- Acute gastritis
  - Usually heals spontaneously over a period of days
  - Drugs that could be causing the problem should be discontinued and antacids given to relieve any excess acidity
- Chronic gastritis
  - If found to be *H. pylori* appropriate drug regime commenced
  - Avoidance of NSAIDs and alcohol
  - Administration of vitamin B_{12}.

Gastric cancer

Adeno-carcinoma of the stomach wall is usually found.

Aetiology

- Generally unknown
- Increase in spicy food
- Nonspecific mucosal injury.

Pathology

- Predisposing factors:
  - Gastritis
  - *H. pylori* at early stage
  - Gastric polyps
  - Pernicious anaemia – absence of the intrinsic factor in the stomach
  - Achlorhydria – absence of hydrochloric acid from the stomach

Clinical features

Early

- Signs of anaemia
  - Pallor
  - Shortness of breath
  - Fatigue, weakness and loss of energy
- Symptoms of peptic ulcer disease
  - Burning pain, alleviated by antacids
  - Vomiting
- Weight loss
- Dysphagia, dyspepsia

Late

- A poor prognosis when diagnosed late
- Usually not discovered until late in the disease process
- Palpable mass in abdomen
- Enlarged hard lymph nodes.

Treatment and drug therapy

- Surgical removal of the tumour – often the surgery is palliative
- Chemotherapy/radiotherapy may be given
- Treat symptoms e.g. correct anaemia and relief pain.

Peptic ulcer

Peptic ulcers occur as a result of an excess secretion of acid digestive juices and can lead to ulcer formation:

- Oesophagus due to reflux of acids from the stomach
- Stomach gastric ulcer (GU) – normal or low acid
- Duodenum duodenal ulcer (DU) – excess acid in stomach flowing into the small intestine, now known that *H. pylori* is a factor.

Aetiology

- Family history
- *H. pylori*
- Over-use of medications such as aspirin and NSAIDs
- Certain behaviours can lead to over-secretion of gastric acid and ulcer formation:
  - Smoking
  - Excessive consumption of alcohol
  - Stress

- Zollinger–Ellison syndrome is a tumour of the pancreas that leads to production of gastrin-like hormones, that simulate gastric juices, which can lead to more than one DU.

Pathology

- Aspirin and NSAIDs suppress the inflammatory response and reduce the effect of prostaglandins, which protects the GIT mucosal lining
- *H. pylori* spirochaete destroys the mucosal lining and can lead to death of the epithelial cells in the stomach and duodenum. The presence of cell death and infection stimulate the inflammatory immune response leading to further damage
- Excessive acid secretion in the stomach due to stress, smoking and alcohol consumption leads to GIT mucosal injury
- All lead to the following:
  - Destruction of the mucous membrane of the GIT
  - The lining of the GIT becomes exposed and unprotected
  - Fistulas can form leading to leakage of gastric acid into the peritoneum and peritonitis (Burkitt *et al*, 2002).

Clinical features

- May include differential diagnosis, as the presentation is similar to other acute abdominal problems
- Dyspepsia
- The pain is in the epigastrium and may be intermittent
  - DU eating relieves the pain and so there is no loss of appetite; patient can be overweight and male; associated with stress and smoking
  - GU eating exacerbates the pain, usually felt 1–2 hours after meals – loss of weight, may suffer from nausea and vomiting, patients can be thin and even emaciated.

Investigations

- Past medical history
- Specimen of vomit or stool for blood
- Endoscopy
- Biopsy to check the peptic ulcer is not due to the presence of *H. pylori*.

Treatment and drug therapy

- Most (over 80%) of peptic ulcers will heal with medical treatment:

  - H_2 antagonist, e.g. ranitidine, omeprazole, is used, with this treatment alone relapse is high
  - Treatment for *H. pylori* infection as well has reduced the relapse rate from 80% to 5–10% (Richards and Edwards, 2012)
  - Sucralfate can be used to further protect the GI mucosa
  - If the peptic ulcer does not heal there is a possibility of malignancy
- Surgery
  - Peptic ulcer is successfully treated with medical interventions, and with the addition of keyhole surgery very few cases now require open surgery
  - Occasionally surgery is still needed due to complications such as uncontrolled haemorrhage or perforation
    - Bilroth I partial gastrectomy for a gastric ulcer – removes the area with the ulcer
    - Highly selective vagotomy for duodenal ulcer
    - Gastrectomy – this is removal of the stomach
    - Partial gastrectomy
- Complications
  - Usually due to chronic peptic ulceration
    - Perforation – causing peritonitis
      - Usually a DU commoner in men
      - Sudden and excruciating epigastric pain that rapidly spreads to the whole abdomen, the patient lies very still as any movement causes pain
      - During abdominal palpation the abdomen is hard due to generalised peritonitis
      - Shock – low blood pressure, rapid pulse, cold and clammy to the touch
    - DU bleed may present as haematemesis or melaena or both, the ulcer can penetrate the gastro-duodenal artery
    - Pyloric stenosis due to scar tissue
    - Malignancy (gastric ulcer).

DISORDERS OF THE LOWER GIT

Disorders of the lower GIT generally involve the small intestine (duodenum, jejunum and ileum), the large intestine (ascending, transverse, descending and sigmoid colon) and the rectum. Lower GIT disorders disrupt one or more of its functions and these may be due to:

- Structural and/or neural abnormalities, which are slow to develop but obstruct or accelerate movement of food at any level in the GIT

- Inflammation and ulceration conditions, which disrupt secretion, motility and absorption.

The acute abdomen

Patients admitted via A&E with symptoms that are of acute onset, the most severe being abdominal pain. This can be a life-threatening condition that may require emergency surgery or simply be due to constipation or trapped wind.

Aetiology

- Abdominal pain can be due to a number of GIT and other disorders
- Usually associated with some form of tissue injury, which can be due to:
  - Chemical mediators of inflammation
  - Mechanical injury such as over stretching
  - Ischaemic damage.

Pathology

- The pain can be any of the following:
  - Parietal (somatic) pain is localised
  - Visceral pain is poorly localised, diffuse and vague; arises from the stimulus e.g. stretching and leads to inflammatory mediator release
  - Referred pain is felt at some distance from the affected area
- The pain can occur in any of the 4 abdominal quadrants (Quigley *et al*, 2012), indicating the effected organ, used in conjunction with other clinical features (Table 11.1):

Clinical features

- Non-specific pain that resolves without intervention
- Clinical features can relate to any of the following conditions:
  - Acute appendicitis
  - Acute intestinal obstruction – strangulated hernia, cancer, adhesions, occlusion of the mesenteric artery
  - Peptic ulcer – severe exacerbation of pain or perforation
  - Gallstones – acute cholecystitis
  - Acute pancreatitis
  - Urinary tract infections
  - Renal colic due to stones in the ureter

Right upper quadrant (RUQ)	Left upper quadrant (LUQ)
Ascending colon	Descending colon
Duodenum	Left kidney
Gallbladder	Pancreas (body and tail)
Right kidney	Spleen
Liver	Stomach
Pancreas (head)	Transverse colon
Transverse colon	Ureter (left)
Ureter (right)	
Right lower quadrant (RLQ)	**Left lower quadrant (LLQ)**
Appendix	Bladder
Ascending colon	Descending colon
Bladder	Ovary, uterus, fallopian tube (female)
Caecum	Prostate and spermatic cord (male)
Rectum	Small intestine
Ovary, uterus and fallopian tube (female)	Sigmoid colon
Prostate and spermatic cord (male)	Ureter
Small intestine	
Ureter (right)	
(Quigley *et al*, 2012)	

Table 11.1 The 4 abdominal quadrants crossing the umbilicus

- Retention of urine
- Constipation
- Leaking or ruptured abdominal aortic aneurysm
- Gynaecological emergencies such as ectopic pregnancy.

Investigations and treatment

For further details refer to the relevant chapter related to the above conditions.

Bowel obstruction

A bowel obstruction may be complete or incomplete. It leads to dilatation of the intestine above the obstruction and fluid accumulates (Hughes, 2005).

Case study 11.2

Elizabeth is 85 years old. She lives in a granny annexe attached to her daughter's house and spends much of her day watching TV. Her daughter, Jean, frequently visits her mother and cooks for her. Elizabeth sometimes forgets to eat her meals and sometimes throws away her food untouched. A neighbour notices that Elizabeth has lost weight when she sees her after a 3-month holiday abroad. Jean is beginning to be aware that her mother is becoming increasingly forgetful, and she eventually seeks advice from her GP.

Elizabeth is diagnosed as having pre-senile dementia. One morning Jean takes her mother her breakfast and is disturbed to find Elizabeth very confused and distressed. Jean cannot understand what is wrong and Elizabeth cannot tell her. Elizabeth appears to be in some pain; Jean decides to take her to the A&E department. She is diagnosed with acute constipation, and is admitted to your ward for assessment and treatment. Following nursing assessment your mentor supervises you giving Elizabeth a phosphate enema, which has been prescribed.

Practice point

HCPs should not underestimate the seriousness of constipation; it can lead to an acute bowel obstruction, intestinal rupture and death.

Aetiology

Other causes of bowel obstruction in addition to constipation are:

- Adhesions or bands from previous surgery
- Strangulated hernia
- Tumours
- Abscess
- Haematoma
- Congenital lesions
- Gallstone ileus
- Foreign body e.g. worms
- Inflammatory strictures as in Crohn's disease
- Impacted faeces
- Intussusception (telescoping of the small bowel – common in children).

Clinical features

Elizabeth (case study 11.2) may be suffering from some of these symptoms:

- Vomiting – this may be in large amounts and, depending on where the obstruction is, may be faecal in nature
- Abdominal pain – usually colicky in nature and more severe in strangulation
- Absolute constipation – no flatus is passed rectally. This happens in complete obstruction but not partial obstruction
- Dehydration due to vomiting and a lack of fluid intake
- Abdominal distension due to gas. The lower the obstruction, the more distension will be present
- Abnormal bowel sounds – exaggerated, high pitched and sometimes tinkling but completely absent in some cases.

Investigations

Elizabeth may require these interventions:

- Plain abdominal X-ray will show the gas-filled loop of bowel
- CT scan may help to determine cause of the obstruction.

Treatment and drug therapy

Elizabeth may require all or some of these interventions:

- Nothing is given by mouth; other forms of nutrition may be considered
- Fluid replacement – the volume and type of fluid depends on fluid and electrolyte balance
- If there has been severe vomiting there may be serious fluid depletion
- Nasal gastric tube if vomiting
- Analgesia will be needed
- Large bowel obstruction due to faecal impaction can be relieved by the use of enemas
- Emergency surgery to relieve the obstruction. A resection of the bowel may be necessary
- Strangulation of the bowel segment of bowel becomes trapped, obstructing its lumen and disrupting its blood supply
    - Ischaemia of the bowel and infarction
    - Perhaps leading to perforation
    - Causes
        - External hernia that may be inguinal, umbilical, femoral or incisional. The bowel becomes trapped and undergoes necrosis

- A loop of bowel may become trapped within the abdominal cavity if there are fibrous bands or adhesions.

Colorectal cancer

There are around 35,000 new cases a year in Britain and it is the second or third most common cancer in both sexes (Richards and Edwards, 2012). Colorectal cancer causes about 14,000 deaths every year and about one-third of the cancers start in the rectum.

Aetiology

- Genetic and environmental factors
- Family history
- The presence of polyps which are localised lesions protruding from the bowel wall; they are common in the colon; they are usually benign neoplasms, but have malignant potential. Usually found in routine investigations. There are two types:
  - Hypoplastic – when large they can be associated with cancer
  - Adenomatous – from which most cancers of the bowel arise.

Pathology

- It is usually an adeno-carcinoma, which invades the bowel wall leading to a narrowing of the lumen and obstruction
- Spreads via the lymphatic system into the bloodstream
- At the time of diagnosis 25% already have metastases.

Clinical features

- Symptomless anaemia
- Change in bowel habit
- Rectal blood loss
- Colicky pain
- Malaise, anorexia, weight loss
- Some patients may present with a bowel obstruction.

Investigations

- Sigmoidoscopy and proctoscopy urgently performed
- Barium enema to show any tumours elsewhere in the colon
- CT scan or ultrasound of the liver to check for metastases
- Stool specimen for blood
- Staging of the cancer TNM (chapter 6).

Treatment and drug therapy

- Surgery is always recommended, but radiotherapy may be given prior to shrink the tumour
- Radical surgical resection formation of colostomy or an end-to-end anastomosis
- Chemotherapy has very limited success but may be used especially in an attempt to control painful liver metastases
- Only about 1 in 10 patients with distant metastases at the time of operation survive 2 years
- The metastases are usually in the liver.

Inflammatory bowel disorders

Ulcerative colitis and Crohn's disease are chronic relapsing inflammatory bowel diseases.

Aetiology

- Genetic factors
- Alterations in epithelial cells related to diet, stress or infection
- Immunological abnormalities related to T-cell reactions to normal bowel flora.

Pathology

- Ulcerative colitis
  - Chronic inflammatory disease – inflammation and ulceration of rectum and sigmoid colon
  - Oedema forms (see chapter 4) and narrows the lumen of the involved colon
  - Mucosal destruction and does have links to cancer formation
- Crohn's disease
  - Difficult to distinguish from ulcerative colitis, but in ulcerative colitis inflammation involves all layers of the bowel wall, which leads to oedema and ulcers and granuloma formation
  - The rectum is seldom involved and the formation of cancer rare
  - Can occur in any part of the GIT but usually the small and large bowel are both affected.

Clinical features

- Ulcerative colitis
  - Mucosal destruction causes bleeding, cramping pain, urge to defecate, nausea and vomiting

  - Diarrhoea which can contain blood, pus or mucus
  - Dehydration, malnutrition, weight loss and lethargy
  - A high risk of cancer
- Crohn's disease
  - Few symptoms other than irritable bowel syndrome (IBS), then inflammation, tenderness, weight loss
  - May develop pernicious anaemia, deficiencies in folic acid and vitamin D absorption, hypo-albuminaemia.

Investigations

- Ulcerative colitis
  - Past medical history
  - Ultrasound will show ulceration
  - Radiological assessment:
    - Sigmoidoscopy or colonoscopy
    - Barium enema
  - Blood analysis shows anaemia, hypo-albuminaemia, low potassium levels, raised white blood cell count
  - Stool culture to rule out infection
  - Differential diagnosis for Crohn's disease
- Crohn's disease
  - Similar to those of ulcerative colitis.

Treatment and drug therapies

- Ulcerative colitis
  - The patient will need steroids/analgesia; can be given immunosuppressive and anti-diarrhoeal drugs
  - Periods of remission, with possible surgical resection if therapy unsuccessful
- Crohn's disease
  - Surgery to manage complications such as peritonitis, pelvic abscess, fistula, abscess, relief of obstruction.

Peritonitis

Peritonitis is inflammation of the peritoneal cavity, covering of the bowel and mesentery, the omentum and lining of the abdominal cavity. Perforation of any region leads to peritonitis.

Aetiology

- Appendicitis
- Crohn's disease

- Diverticulitis
- Cholecystitis is the inflammation of the gall bladder as a result of gall stones
- Salpingitis is inflammation of the fallopian tubes
- Pancreatitis is the inflammation of the pancreas
- Perforated ulcer – small intestine contents or stomach acid leak into the peritoneum due to perforation
- Differential diagnosis, blood in the peritoneum causes peritoneal irritation such as in the cases of:
  - Leaking abdominal aortic aneurysm
  - Ectopic pregnancy.

Pathology

- The peritoneal cavity is lined with a serous membrane that lines all the organs in the abdomen
- If there is an abnormal leakage of infected fluid into the peritoneal cavity the inflammatory immune response is stimulated (see chapter 2)
- Fluids and electrolytes are lost from the systemic circulation, leading to dehydration.

Clinical features

- Localised pain to the affected area
- Electrolyte imbalance
- Abdominal guarding is the spasm of abdominal wall, which is tender to touch
- Rebound tenderness is when pain occurs when pressure is released
- Low grade fever
- Malaise
- Nausea and vomiting
- Hard, rigid abdomen
- Paralytic ileus absence of peristalsis of the bowel; may be absent bowel sounds.

Investigations

- Blood analysis for sodium, potassium, chloride and calcium
- Abdominal palpation and ultrasound
- Physical examination of abdomen e.g. swollen, soft, hard
- Listen for bowel sounds
- Abdominal X-ray.

Treatment and drug therapy

- Nasal gastric tube insertion
- Intravenous fluid administration in the case of dehydration
- May need parenteral feeding if unable to take in oral nutrients
- The patient is usually unwell and there is a risk of dying
- High doses of antibiotics for salpingitis or diverticulitis
- If perforation is the cause a laparotomy may be performed to remove the faecal fluid from the peritoneum.

Appendicitis

This is an inflammation of the vermiform appendix, a projection from the apex of the caecum. It is a common surgical emergency, which affects 7–12% of the population.

Case study 11.3

Ted is a 49-year-old man admitted to the ward yesterday after he presented at the hospital with a 3-week history of acute abdominal pain and distension. Abdominal X-ray was inconclusive, but while on the ward he was nil by mouth, and an intravenous infusion of 0.9% normal saline has been running. In addition, he has been prescribed regular analgesia and his observations are taken at 2-hourly intervals. On the evening of Ted's second day his condition deteriorated. His observations were as follows:

BP = 104/70 mmHg
Pulse = 108 beats/min
Temperature = 38.2°C
Respiration = 28 breaths/min
Urine output <30 ml hr

Within 30 minutes these changes had occurred:

BP = 80/52 mmHg
Pulse = 128 beats/min
Respiration = 34 breaths/min
Temperature = 39°C

A call was put out to the medical emergency team (MET); the surgeons were informed. Due to the life threatening nature of Ted's presentation he warranted emergency surgery. Ted was taken to theatre with a possible perforated appendix.

Practice point

Homeostatic mechanisms can maintain BP for many days. It is important to continuously monitor for early signs, patterns in vital signs and investigations to determine deterioration early.

Aetiology

- Obstruction of the lumen with:
  - Stool
  - Foreign bodies
  - Bacterial infection.

Pathology

- Due to the obstruction of the lumen of the appendix:
  - Drainage of the appendix is reduced
  - Increased pressure appendix becomes hypoxic
  - Bacterial microbial invasion
  - Inflammation and oedema
  - Gangrene.

Clinical features

Ted may be suffering from some or all of these symptoms:

- Classic sign is a rebound tenderness but this does not occur in all cases
- There is abdominal pain in the right lower quadrant, but this may be vague at first and increasing over a period of 3–4 hours
- Nausea and vomiting
- Loss of appetite
- Low-grade fever
- Diarrhoea may occur but is not always present.

Investigations

To diagnose Ted's appendicitis some or all of these investigations can be undertaken to determine severity and likelihood of rupture:

- Appendicitis diagnosis can be assisted by abdominal X-ray
- Computed tomography (CT scan)
- Increase in white blood cell count.

Treatment and drug therapy

- Appendicectomy is the treatment for a simple or perforated appendicitis (as in the case of Ted)

- Recovery is generally without complications, but they can occur (Edwards and Coyne, 2012)
- Antibiotics.

GIT disease in combination with stress and malnutrition can lead to a significant reduction in nutrients in many patients. A deficiency in nutrients and malnutrition due to a number of reasons can have serious effects on the body:

- A reduced immune system increases risk of infection
- Reduced vitamins, minerals, nutrients required for healing
- Weakness and lethargy
- Increased mortality.

DISORDERS OF THE ACCESSORY ORGANS

Liver failure

The liver has great power of regeneration, but when it is unable to regenerate cells, liver failure ensues (Heitkemper *et al*, 2007).

Aetiology

- Cirrhosis of the liver is due to alcohol
- Primary biliary cirrhosis – autoimmune condition
- Non-alcoholic fatty liver disease (NAFLD) observed in obesity, diabetes
- Neoplasms
- Liver disease/failure can also occur from:
    - Herpes simplex
    - Varicella zoster
    - Measles
    - Rubella
    - Coxsackie B
    - Adenoviruses
- Post-viral hepatitis (especially hepatitis C), other viruses affect the liver and cause hepatitis, which can lead to liver failure:
    - Yellow fever virus
    - Epstein-Barr virus (EBV)
    - Cytomegalovirus (CMV).

Pathology

The classifications of liver failure are:

- Fulminant liver failure develops in 8 weeks and there is generally an underlying cause, such as hepatitis. There is death of liver cells,

jaundiced appearance, variable mental state ranging from confusion to coma
- Sub-fulminant liver failure – this develops more slowly over 8–26 weeks
- Chronic liver failure.

Clinical features

- Encephalopathy – confusion to unconsciousness
- Jaundiced – yellow pigment in the skin
- Respiratory failure
- Bleeding and bruising – due to clotting factor deficiencies
- Renal failure – may occur as the liver cannot convert waste products of cellular metabolism from ammonia (a strong acid) into urea (a weak acid) for excretion by the kidney
- Metabolic disturbances
- Impaired drug metabolism
- Ascites – fluid in the peritoneal cavity.

Investigations

Blood tests include:

- Serum bilirubin normal value should be <17 μmol/L
- Enzyme levels:
  - Transaminases:
    - Alanine
    - Aminotransferase (ALT) 10-40 U/L
  - Aspartate transaminase (AST) 10-55 U/L
    - Alkaline phosphatase (ALP) W5-3 U/L
- Gamma glutamyltransferase (GGT) M10-55 ULUK
- Serum proteins:
  - Clotting factors
  - Serum albumin
  - Serum globulins
- Transport proteins
- Coagulation screen
  - Prothrombin time to determine vitamin K status
    - Vitamin K is a fat soluble vitamin stored and catabolised by the liver, bind to lipids
- Full blood count (FBC).

Treatment and drug therapy

This depends on the cause:

- If due to alcohol then advice is to discontinue behaviour; withdrawal symptoms may be treated with diazepam

- Prevention of complications:
  - Oesophageal varices
  - Portal hypertension
  - Ascites
  - Hepato-renal syndrome
  - Jaundice is hyper-bilirubinaemia – see below
  - Hepatic encephalopathy:
    - Absent minded, forgetful
    - Drowsy, night to day reversal
    - Semi-conscious, rousable
    - Comatosed
    - Irreversible brain swelling
- See below for treatment of hepatitis, jaundice and ascites.

Jaundice

A yellow discolouration of the skin and whites of the eyes, due to the inability of bilirubin, the waste product of red blood cell breakdown, to be excreted in bile. It does not reach the intestine so levels rise in the blood.

Aetiology

- Gallstones or tumour leading to an obstruction of flow of bile into the small intestine (duodenum)
- Cirrhosis of the liver or hepatitis inflammation of the liver leads to obstruction to the flow of bile or reduced production of bile
- Excessive breakdown of red blood cells.

Pathology

- Bile accumulates in the liver and enters the blood stream causing hyper-bilirubinaemia
- Hepatocellular jaundice is due to liver disease such as hepatitis or cirrhosis and is unable to cope with the bilirubin
- Haemolytic jaundice is due to excessive breakdown of red blood cells leading to an increased production of bilirubin.

Clinical features

- Urine is dark and stools are pale, as bilirubin gives faeces its brown colour (observed in obstructive and hepatocellular jaundice)
- Bilirubin is present in the urine
- Pyrexia and chills
- Pain

- Anorexia, malaise and fatigue
- Yellow discolouration of the eyes before visible to the skin.

Investigations

- Blood tests for conjugated and unconjugated bilirubin in the blood or both
- Unconjugated indicates haemolysis or hereditary disorders of bilirubin metabolism
- Conjugated indicate liver injury or obstruction
- History
- Physical examination
- Laboratory tests e.g. liver function tests (LFTs) may show an underlying condition e.g. alcoholism, hepatitis or gall stones.

Treatment and drug therapy

Usually involves treatment of the underlying cause.

Ascites

Ascites is an accumulation of fluid in the abdominal cavity and has many different causes.

Aetiology

- Cirrhosis of the liver
- Cancers of the GIT and ovaries
- Heart failure
- Hypoalbuminurea.

Clinical features

- Abdominal distension
- Weight gain and fluid retention
- Difficulty in breathing as expansion of the lungs becomes impaired.

Investigations

- Auscultation of the abdomen (requires at least 1500 ml of fluid)
  - Ultrasound is required to detect smaller amounts.

Treatment

- Treat the underlying cause
- Diuretics such as spironalactone for cirrhosis may be combined with furosemide

- Paracentesis is the insertion of a cannula or needle into the peritoneum to drain the excess fluid.

Viral hepatitis

Infectious due to several different viruses, an acute viral hepatitis is a common and sometimes serious infection of the liver.

Aetiology

There are 3 main groups:

- Hepatitis A (HAV) – enteric, faecal oral transmission, incubation is about 28 days, flu-like symptoms, mild jaundice, does not progress to chronic liver disease, no specific treatment needed, improved personal hygiene and hand washing, immunisation if travelling to countries whereby infection is possible
- Hepatitis B (HBV) – blood and sexual transmission, incubation is 70 days with insidious onset, full recovery and become immune but may be a carrier, fulminant hepatitis can occur, can go on to develop cirrhosis or hepatocellular carcinoma, vaccination is available
- Hepatitis C (HCV) – blood borne transfusion and sexual intercourse, incubation 6–9 weeks and can be acute or chronic, drug therapy follows NICE guidelines. There is no vaccination for HCV.

Pathology

- The invasion of the virus leads to:
  - Hepatic cell necrosis
  - Liver scarring
  - Kupffer cell hyperplasia
  - Infiltration of phagocytes
  - Cell injury occurs due to T-cell and natural killer cells
  - Inflammation occurs leading to obstruction and jaundice
  - Liver damage occurs in hepatitis B and C leading to liver failure.

Clinical features

- Rapid onset of liver failure, begins with the incubation phase, then:
- Prodromal phase
  - Fatigue
  - Anorexia
  - Malaise
  - Nausea and vomiting
  - Headache

    - Hyperalgia
    - Cough
    - Low grade pyrexia
- Icteric phase
    - The phase of illness
    - Dark urine positive to bilirubin
    - Clay-coloured stools
    - Onset of jaundice
- Recovery phase
    - Resolution of jaundice
    - Liver remains enlarged and tender, but diminishing
    - Liver function tests (LFTs) return to normal.

Investigations

- LFTs are abnormal with elevated aspartate transaminase (AST) and alanine transaminase (ALT)
- Specific blood tests if hepatitis is suspected
- Urinalysis for bilirubin
- Examination of stool sample.

Treatment and drug therapies

- Hepatitis A – vaccination is available and successful
- Hepatitis B – includes combination therapy and prevention of drug resistance
- Hepatitis C – there is no vaccine and resistance to drug therapy is common, with re-infection rate high.

Gall stones

Gall stones are often referred to as cholecystitis.

Aetiology

- Obesity
- Rapid weight loss
- Middle-aged women
- Oral contraceptives
- High dietary cholesterol.

Pathology

The gall bladder is a muscular sac that stores and concentrates bile, made in the liver. It emulsifies fats prior to their digestion by lipase enzymes. If bile does not arrive in the duodenum:

- Fats are not digested or absorbed
- Loose, foul-smelling, fatty stools are passed (steatorrhoea).
- This leads to a lack of absorption of the fat-soluble vitamins (A, D, E and K)
- Lack of vitamin K leads to inadequate synthesis of prothrombin and problems with blood clotting
- Most gall-stones are cholesterol mixed with bile pigments and calcium salts (75–90%)
  - Some (up to 10%) are pure cholesterol
  - Women are affected four times as often as men.

Clinical features

- Most often the patient presents with pain in the epigastrium or the right upper quadrant. It is often not severe or well defined
- May present with jaundice, if the gall-stone passes into and blocks the common bile duct, thus obstructing the flow of bile into the duodenum
- Transient obstruction of the gall bladder by a stone may cause episodes of severe pain that are called biliary colic caused by:
  - A sudden and complete obstruction of the cystic duct by a stone (Heitkemper *et al*, 2007)
  - There is severe pain, rising to a crescendo in a few minutes and continuing relentlessly
  - The pain may last several hours and may end spontaneously or may be relieved by pethidine analgesia
  - The patient may vomit
  - A history of similar attacks
  - No fever is present
- These may be accompanied with nausea and vomiting
- The obstruction may cause inflammation of the gall bladder which is called cholecystitis:
  - Is an acute inflammation of the gall bladder
  - The patient is unwell and often has a fever
  - The right upper outer quadrant of the abdomen is tender
  - The pain usually lasts for several days before subsiding
  - In its acute form this is a common cause of attendance to A&E
- If the infection persists an abscess may develop and is called an empyema of the gall bladder.

Investigations

- The pain must be differentiated from the pain caused by other disorder e.g. pancreatitis, MI and acute pyelonephritis of the right kidney (McCance *et al*, 2010)

- Ultrasound may show stones and a thickened gall bladder wall
- Gall bladder function can be demonstrated by an oral cholecystogram
- Endoscopic retrograde cholangiopancreatography (ERCP): small gall stones can be removed by slitting the sphincter at the lower end and using a balloon catheter or Dormia basket to retrieve them. This may make a potentially dangerous operation unnecessary
- Percutaneous cholangiography is used if ERCP is not available or is unsuccessful.

Treatment

- Pain control
- Replacement of fluid and electrolytes
- Antiemetic if required
- May require a period of fasting
- Cholecystectomy (removal of the gall bladder) may be required for complications
- A low-fat diet is prescribed.

Practice point

A patient should not be fasted for any longer than 12 hours, as by this time all glycogen stores are utilised and all body processes are utilising fats as a source of energy. The addition of stress will lead to the release of cortisol and the breakdown of protein, converted by the liver to enter the Krebs cycle, to form ATP.

CANCER OF THE LIVER

There are generally two types of liver tumours, primary and secondary.

Primary liver cancer

A primary tumour of the liver is usually hepatocellular carcinoma (HCC) which is the most common. A variant form of HCC is fibrolamellar carcinoma, which has a better prognosis as it can be removed:

- *Aetiology*
  - Infection with hepatitis B virus (HBV) even if it is a mild attack
  - Cirrhosis of the liver
  - Metabolic disorders

- *Pathology*
  - Primary liver cancer is a large single mass
  - It may be infiltrative or multifocal
  - It can spread through the portal vein and hepatic artery to the lung, brain or bone
- *Clinical features*
  - Hepatomegaly (enlargement of the liver)
  - Abdominal pain and discomfort
  - Ascites
  - Jaundice
- *Investigations*
  - The HCC cancer produces a marker called alpha (a)-fetoprotein (AFP) and is a useful blood test, as this is not normally found in the circulation after birth (Blows, 2005)
  - Liver function tests (LFTs) showing liver failure
  - Low blood albumin levels (hypoalbuminaemia)
  - Increased blood ammonia levels (hyperammonaemia).

Secondary liver cancer

The liver is the site for many metastases, as in the case of Joe, due to its vulnerable position, receiving blood from the systemic and portal circulation and as it is the largest organ in the body.

Case study 11.4

Joe is 70 years old and has renal pelvic cancer with metastatic liver disease. He complains of pain in his right shoulder. To relieve the pain oral morphine modified release (MST continues), 30 mg is prescribed b.d. He is also prescribed 4 mg dexamethasone orally o.d.

Practice point

In liver failure kidney function needs to be monitored. The liver converts ammonia (the waste product of cellular metabolism) into urea to be filtered by the kidney and excreted in urine. If the liver is unable to convert ammonia to urea, pure ammonia is filtered in the kidney damaging the renal tubule.

- *Aetiology*
  - The majority of liver cancers have spread from a primary elsewhere e.g. stomach, pancreas, gall bladder and bile ducts, large bowel, lung, breast, kidney (as in the case of Joe) or from a malignant melanoma
- *Pathology*
  - The tumours that arise from the metastases develop as nodules on the liver surface
  - Can occur deeper in the organ
- *Clinical features*
  - Weight loss
  - Pain over the liver
  - A palpable enlarged liver
  - Ascites
  - Jaundice
- *Investigations*
  - Serum level of alkaline phosphatase – an enzyme involved in phosphate metabolism, an early warning that liver metastasis is likely
- *Treatment*
  - Partial hepatectomy or laparoscopic liver resection – but can only be palliative
  - Chemotherapy
  - Poor prognosis – palliative care (required by Joe)
  - Survival can be a matter of months.

Pancreatitis

This is an acute inflammatory response resulting from premature activation of pancreatic enzymes (Hughes, 2004), and there are many pathophysiological hypotheses as to the reasons for the development of pancreatitis (Heitkemper *et al*, 2007). It can be acute or chronic and it is unclear whether acute and chronic pancreatitis are linked.

Case study 11.5

Jeffrey is a 34-year-old man who has a past medical history of pancreatitis. He is admitted with a sudden onset of central abdominal pain radiating to the back which is eased by sitting forward. He has vomited once in casualty and continues to feel sick.

On admission, Jeffrey is agitated and restless, which increases when his abdomen is touched or palpated. He has a temperature of 38.5°C and his BM stix is 20 mmol/L. His breathing is noisy and he has a slight wheeze.

Jeffrey has a distended abdomen and he is complaining that he has not had his bowels opened for 2 days. The extent of his distended abdomen is causing compression of the adjacent structures. There are indications of liver involvement.

Aetiology

- Alcohol, biliary and gastric disease, trauma, metabolic abnormalities
- Infection – mumps, viral hepatitis
- Drugs – thiazide diuretics, furosemide, oestrogens, tetracycline, salicylates, corticosteroids, immunosuppressive agents and methyldopa
- Activation of enzymes
- Metabolic disorders
  - Hyperlipidaemia
  - Hyperparathyroidism
  - Renal failure
  - Hypercalcaemia
- Trauma
- Tumours
- Pregnancy – third trimester
- Surgery
- Hereditary pancreatitis
- Scorpion venom.

Pathology

- Initiating process
  - Spontaneous, obstruction, bile, reflux, duodenal reflux
  - Oedema, vascular damage, rupture of pancreatic ducts
  - Activation of enzymes
  - Autodigestion
    - Trypsinogen activated into trypsin in contact with chyme leads to activation of all known pancreatic enzymes
    - Leads to oedema formation, haemorrhage, coagulation, necrosis, fat necrosis, vascular damage
- Obstruction blocks the outflow of pancreatic juices causing a back flow into the pancreas itself, leading to inflammation

- Duodenal reflux is when duodenal contents backflow into the pancreas, caused by a damaged Oddi's sphincter, which maintains a pressure gradient between the pancreatic duct lumen and the duodenum
- Bile reflux
- Chronic pancreatitis with chronic inflammation leading to permanent damage – diabetes is common, anorexia.

Clinical features

- Difficult due to differential diagnosis
- Pain which may radiate into the back due to the location of the pancreas
- Tenderness over the abdomen
- Reduced bowel sounds
- Abdominal distension
- Nausea/vomiting
- Pyrexia
- Hypotension
- Blue brown discolouration of limbs (Grey Turner's sign) is a late sign of pancreatitis.

Investigations

- Past medical history
- Serum amylase and lipase is raised
- Serum transferrin is raised if pancreatitis is due to alcohol
- Ultrasound and CT scan to evaluate involvement and seriousness of the condition
- Observe for abdominal compartment syndrome
- Differential diagnosis:
  - Duodenal ulcer
  - Acute cholecystitis
  - Small bowel obstruction
  - Kidney stones.

Treatment and drug therapy

Acute – there is no specific treatment, the major objective is to support the patient until the acute phase of the disease has subsided. This may require:

- Nasal gastric tube suctioning if severe vomiting
- Nil by mouth (NBM) – TPN may be required; for management of NBM see Whiteing and Hunter (2008)
- Analgesia – pethidine or buprenorphine

- IV infusion to maintain volume albumin, plasma, normal saline, whole blood
- Maintain electrolyte balance calcium, magnesium deficits
- May require critical care
- Stop alcohol consumption
- Pain control may require opioids, but simple analgesia paracetamol may also be required
- Control of diabetes – low doses of insulin if hyperglycaemia.

Pancreatic cancer

Pancreatic cancer is difficult to diagnose especially in the early stage (Blows, 2005). Palliative treatment is usually required, making prognosis very poor.

Aetiology

- Associated with genetic mutations – more common in non-ductal pancreatitis
- Smoking shown to have a strong link
- Viral infections.

Pathology

Pancreatic cancers are mostly:

- Adenocarcinoma derived from glandular epithelium
- Two forms are recognised:
  - Ductal
    - Most commonly seen in the elderly
    - More likely to arise in the head of the pancreas, which is the site where both the pancreatic and biliary duct enter the duodenum; the tumour here can obstruct either or both ducts (Blows, 2005)
    - Can be asymptomatic
    - A slow-growing tumour
  - Non-ductal associated with gene mutation
- Tumour spreads locally to involve the lymph nodes and the liver (Richards and Edwards, 2012).

Clinical features

- Biliary obstruction causes jaundice
- Pain is a feature in the later stage of the disease, usually too late for surgery
- Weight loss.

Investigations

- Ultrasound
- CT scan.

Treatment and drug therapy

- If diagnosed early then surgery may be a possibility, but often discovered too late for resection of the tumour or patient too elderly with co-mortalities to undergo a total pancreatectomy
- Survival rate measured at 5 years is very poor; only around 2% of patients are alive after 5 years (Blows, 2005)
- Jaundice is relieved by bypass under endoscopy and placement of a stent to aid drainage through the narrowed part of the common bile duct.

Overdose

Overdose can result from accidental ingestion or deliberate ingestion, overdose or poisoning from a variety of medications or environmental toxins. The clinical features, investigations and treatments are the same for both.

Accidental poisoning

Aetiology

In children accidental poisoning is commonest between the ages of 1 and 5 years when children like to explore the environment with their mouths as well as their eyes and fingers. In older children and adults accidental overdose is usually a result of a mishap at school or at work, e.g. inhalation of gases or fumes from organic solvents or ingestion while pipetting. In the older adult (as observed in the case study below) especially if a person is confused, they may forget they have taken a dose of their drug or make mistakes with doses.

Case study 11.6

Gordon is a 65-year-old man who goes to his GP feeling unwell, complaining of subcostal pain and tenderness. He has a past medical history (PMH) of chronic obstructive pulmonary disease (COPD) and arthritis. Gordon was at the GPs only 4 days ago with a flare-up of his arthritis. Through careful questioning of Gordon it arises that the last time Gordon attended the surgery his GP had prescribed him co-codamol tablets for his pain due to arthritis. Gordon found that these tablets were not controlling the pain, so he had taken paracetamol in between the prescribed medication given by the GP. At the same time Gordon had been feeling a 'cold' coming on, and fearing an exacerbation of his COPD his wife went to the chemist to get him some over-the-counter flu remedy, which he had been taking during the day as well. Gordon needed to be transferred to the hospital urgently.

Gordon was referred by his GP to A&E for investigation of an accidental overdose of paracetamol. He is admitted to your ward for observation. It is believed that in the period of 2–4 days Gordon had taken approximately 50 tablets. He seemed well on admission to the medical ward and his condition is stable.

Accidental overdose in the case of Gordon may be encountered at any age, but the causes differ:

- Neonatal poisoning – in utero from the parent
- Usually as a result of therapeutic doses of drugs or self-poisoning in the late stages of labour
- In elderly patients could be due to the miscalculation of doses.

Deliberate poisoning

Aetiology

This is the commonest form of poisoning in adults.

Case study 11.7

Hanna is a 15-year-old woman who is admitted to hospital following an overdose of paracetamol tablets; approximately 50 tablets have been taken. She is being nursed on a medical ward and her condition continues to deteriorate. She is semi-conscious but moves all limbs and is rousable to painful stimuli. An intravenous infusion of 5% dextrose and Parvolex has been commenced to maintain fluid intake.

Her past medical history is that Hanna has been depressed recently due to her boyfriend leaving her. This has caused her to feel periods of loneliness, insecurity and boredom. She does not get along very well with her parents, and is angry at them as she blames them for the split-up with her boyfriend. Due to this she has not been eating sufficiently, and could be potentially at risk from being undernourished or malnourished.

Deliberate poisoning counts for at least 95% of all poisoning admissions to hospital. The peak age is between 20 and 35 years but it is not uncommon below the age of 15.

Pathology

The pathology varies between the different drugs ingested, see clinical features below:

Clinical features

- Usually poisoned adults are able to inform healthcare staff what they have taken
- The presence of clinical features may help to see how severe the poisoning is
- Coma is the common clinical feature usually causes depression of the CNS, due to:
  - Hypnotics
  - Antidepressants
  - Anticonvulsants
  - Tranquillisers
  - Opioid analgesics
  - Alcohol
- Convulsions caused by CNS stimulation by:
  - Anticholinergics
  - Sympathomimetics
  - Tricyclic antidepressants
  - Monoamine oxidase inhibitors
- Respiratory features
  - Cough, wheeze and breathlessness often occur after inhalation of irritant gases such as ammonia, chlorine and smoke from fires
  - Cyanosis may be due to a combination of factors in the unconscious patient; can also be due to methaemoglobinaemia caused by poisons such as chlorates, nitrates, nitrites, phenol and urea herbicides
  - Hypoventilation is common with any CNS depressant
  - Usually respiration gets shallower rather than slower
  - Marked reduction in rate is likely to be due to opioids
  - Hyperventilation is most commonly due to salicylate poisoning and occasionally to CNS stimulant drugs and cyanide
  - Pulmonary oedema may follow inhaled poisons and paraquat poisoning (contained in some weed-killers)
- Cardiovascular features

    - Tachycardia may be due to anticholinergics, sympathomimetics and salicylates
    - Bradycardia may be caused by cardiac glycosides, e.g. digoxin and beta-blockers
    - Dysrhythmias may be caused by a variety of drugs and any antiarrhythmic drugs cause dysrhythmias if taken in excess
    - Hypotension may occur in any severe poisoning
    - CNS depressants may lower the systolic blood pressure to 70–80 mmHg. The BP falls lower as the coma gets deeper
    - Diuretics lower the blood pressure by depleting the blood volume
    - Hypertension is uncommon in overdosage
- Pupil changes
    - Very small and pinpoint pupils, especially if the respiratory rate is slowed, suggest opioid analgesics
    - Dilated pupils suggest tricyclic antidepressants or other anticholinergics or antihistamines
    - Tinnitus is a very common feature of salicylate poisoning.

Investigations

- The purpose of screening is to identify and quantify poisons amenable to treatment
- There is no point in doing an emergency screening if the result has no bearing on the treatment that will be given
- Paracetamol is the drug that is most likely to be screened for.

Treatment and drug therapies

- Naloxone (Narcan) is the antidote to all narcotic drugs. It may completely reverse a coma within 1–2 minutes and will increase the respiratory rate
- Flumenazil is the antidote for severe benzodiazepine poisoning but is not always used in less severe cases
- Acetylcysteine (Parvolex) is given in paracetamol poisoning and can prevent liver failure if given soon enough after the overdose
- About 90% of adults and children have minimal symptoms and require little medical care. Half the remainder are seriously ill and recovery depends upon good care. Management of coma is a vital part of this care
- Ensure the airway, breathing and blood pressure are adequate (ABC)
- Assess the level of consciousness using Glasgow coma scale (GCS) or alert, verbal, pain, unconscious (AVPU)

- Contact the poisons information services if there is any uncertainty about the toxicity of the substance or the management of the poison TOXBASE (www.spib.axl.co.uk)
- Consider whether an antidote is available or necessary
- Consider the need to prevent absorption of the poison
- Consider whether it is necessary to attempt to increase elimination of the poison
- Emptying the stomach:
  - There is an ongoing debate as to the usefulness of emptying the stomach
  - There are always dangers involved and sometimes it may lead to more rapid absorption of the drug
  - Gastric lavage is sometimes used
- Activated charcoal:
  - The charcoal is not absorbed but combines with some drugs in the stomach and intestine (adsorbs them) to prevent their absorption
  - Ten times as much charcoal is needed as the drug you wish it to combine with
  - The sooner it is given, the more effective it will be
  - It is best given within the first hour of ingestion but may be effective up to 2 hours after ingestion and longer if modified-release preparations are taken
  - It is a tasteless, black, gritty slurry and patients do not like to take it
  - It does not absorb all toxins but is good for:
    - Paracetamol
    - Benzodiazepines
    - Digoxin
    - Paraquat
    - Phenytoin
    - Salicylates
    - Quinine
  - It is useful for poisons that are toxic in small amounts such as tricyclic antidepressants. It can enhance the elimination of some drugs when they have been absorbed.

CONCLUSION

Nutrients are drawn from food for cellular functions, any undigested food is eliminated, and enzymes released from accessory organs facilitate these processes. Patients can suffer from disorders associated with the GIT system and be unable to tolerate food, and/or stress due to other illnesses or disease. Patients cannot replenish nutrients but utilise valuable nutrients required by the body, which can lead to a negative energy balance. The importance of feeding patients is imperative, as long periods of time without any nutrition can produce detrimental GIT responses and serious complications (see Best *et al*, 2004; Payne-James *et al*, 2001).

SELF-ASSESSMENT QUESTIONS

1. Provide an outline of the functions of the digestive system, organs of the alimentary canal and accessory organs.
2. Describe the major processes occurring during digestive system activity.
3. Identify the basic function of each accessory organ of the alimentary canal.
4. Define glycogenesis, glycogenolysis, and gluconeogenesis that takes place in the liver.
5. List the nutrients, essential nutrients and calories; the fat and water-soluble vitamins and minerals essential for health; dietary sources.
6. How are the events of the absorptive and post-absorptive state regulated?
7. Using the case studies provided in this chapter list several changes to the digestive system anatomy and physiology that may occur.

REFERENCES

Best, C., Wolstenholme, S., Kimble, J., Hitchings, H. and Gordon, H.M. (2004) How 'nil by mouth' instructions impacts on patient behaviour, *Nursing Times*, 100(39) 32–34.

Blows, W.T. (2005) *The Biological Basis of Nursing: Cancer*, London: Routledge.

Burkitt, H.G., Quick, C.R.G. and Gatt, D. (2002) *Essential Surgery: Problems, Diagnosis and Management*, 3rd edn, Edinburgh: Churchill Livingstone.

Edwards, S.L. (2000) Maintaining optimum nutrition (Chapter 27), in K. Manley and K.L. Bellman (eds) *Surgical Nursing: Advancing Practice*, Edinburgh: Churchill Livingstone.

Edwards, S. and Coyne I. (2012) *A Survival Guide to Children's Nursing*, Edinburgh: Elsevier.

Heitkemper, M., Croghan, A. and Cox-North, P. (2007) Liver, pancreas, and biliary tract problems, in S. Lewis, M. Heitkemper, S. Dirksen, P. O'Brian and L. Butcher (eds) *Medical-surgical Nursing Assessment and Management of Clinical Problems*, 7th edn, Mosby: St Louis, MO.

Hughes, E. (2004) Understanding the care of patients with acute pancreatitis, *Nursing Standard*, 18(18), 45–52.

Hughes, E. (2005) Caring for the patient with an intestinal obstruction, *Nursing Standard*, 19(47), 56–64.
Keshav, S. (2004) *The Gastrointestinal System at a Glance*, Oxford: Blackwell Science.
McCance K.L., Huether, S.E., Brashers, V.L., Rote, N.S. (2010) *Pathophysiology: The Biologic Basis for Disease in Adults and Children*, 6th edn, Edinburgh: Mosby Elsevier.
Malnutrition Advisory Group (MAG) (2003) *The MUST Report, Nutritional Screening of Adults: A Multidisciplinary Responsibility*, London: British Association for Parenteral and Enteral Nutrition.
NICE (National Institute for Health and Clinical Excellence) (2006) *Treatment for People Who are Overweight or Obese*, London: NICE.
Payne-James, J., Grimble, G. and Silk D. (eds) (2001) *Artificial Nutrition Support in Clinical Practice*, 2nd edn, London: Greenwich Medical Media.
Quigley, B.H., Palm, M.L., Bickley, L. (2012) *Bates' Nursing Guide to Physical Examination and History Taking*, Philadelphia: Wolters Kluwer Health/ Lippincott Williams & Wilkins.
Richards, A. and Edwards, S. (2012) *A Nurses' Survival Guide to the Ward*, 3rd edn, Edinburgh: Elsevier.
Whiteing, N. and Hunter, J. (2008) Nursing management of patients who are nil by mouth, *Nursing Standard*, 22(26), 40.

12 The musculoskeletal system

Sharon Edwards

FUNCTIONS OF THE MUSCULOSKELETAL SYSTEM

Bones and muscles work together to provide (Knight *et al*, 2005):

- Protection – e.g. the ribs give protection to the lungs and the kidneys
- Support, posture and body shape
- The manufacture of red blood cells, white blood cells and platelets in bone marrow
- Mineral homeostasis the release of calcium and phosphate when low levels detected in plasma
- Storage of calcium and phosphate in bone
- Leverage
- Venous return
- Limb movement, speech, non-verbal communication in the form of facial expression, hand movement, position
- Breathing for gas exchange
- Mobility and heat production.

BONES

There are 206 bones in the adult human body (Figure 12.1), divided into 2: the axial skeleton (trunk & head) and the appendicular skeleton (limbs). Bones are different shapes and sizes and are mainly made up of calcium, magnesium, phosphorus and collagen densely packed together resulting in the hard texture.

Bone cells

- Osteoblasts are bone-forming cells; their function is to lay down bone and once this is complete osteoblasts become osteocytes (McCance and Huether, 2010)

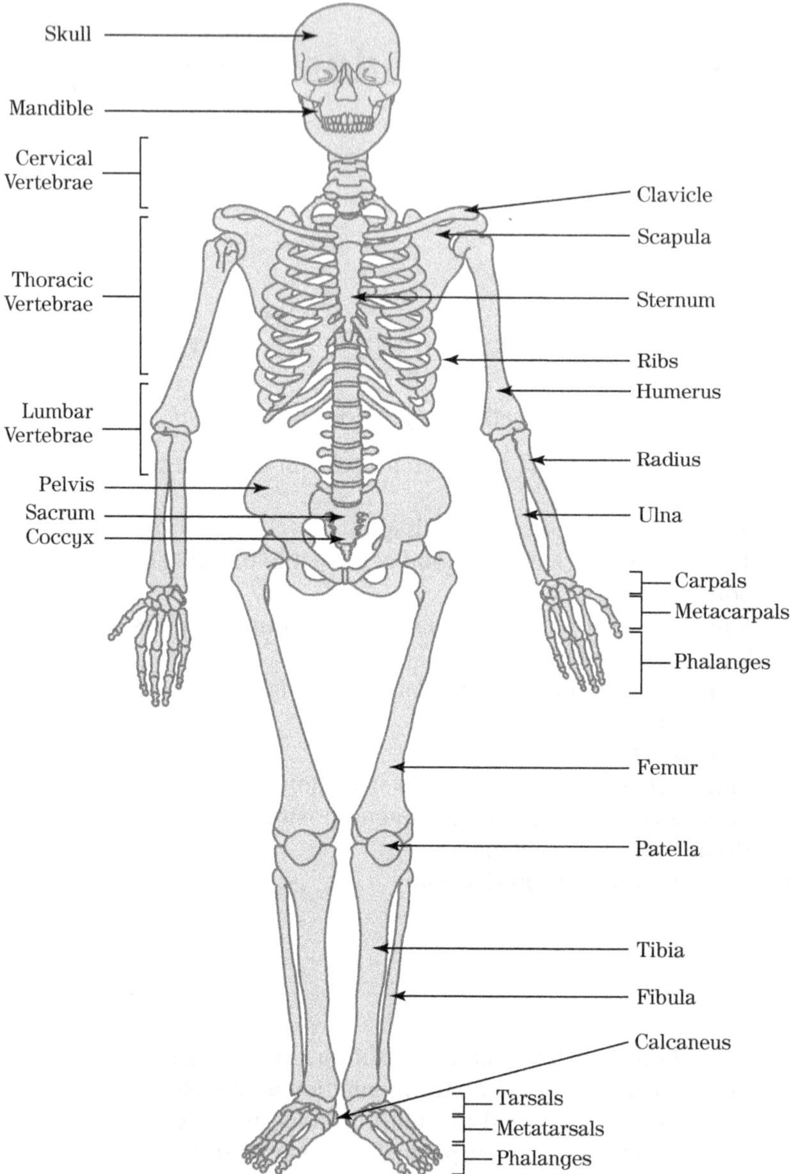

Figure 12.1 Bones of the body

- Osteocytes are the most plentiful cells in bone; which are embedded in the bone matrix
- Osteoclasts reabsorb bone; they contain lysosomes which digest old bone cells.

Bone matrix

- Organic components are collagen fibres
- Inorganic components are calcium and phosphorous
- Every bone has a texture:
  - Compact bone is the outer layer which gives bone its smooth and solid look and contains nerves, blood vessels and lymphatic vessels
  - Spongy or cancellous bone is the internal layer and helps the bone to resist stress.

Types of bones

There are 5 types of bones:

- Long bones:
  - Long and narrow shaft (diaphysis):
    - Contains yellow marrow, which produces red blood cells
    - Acts as lever for body movement in conjunction with contracting muscles (Judge, 2007), femur, tibia, humerus and radius
    - Merges into a broader neck (metaphysis); allows weight bearing to be distributed over a broad area
  - A broad end (epiphysis)
- Short (cuboidal) bones are found where only a limited range of movement is needed such as the carpal and tarsal bones
- Flat bones have a protective function and are thin to allow attachment of muscles such as the ribs or scapulae
- Irregular bones include vertebrae, hipbones and mandible
- Sesamoid bones are small, protective and found where a tendon passes over the joint of a long bone such as the patella.

JOINTS

- There are joints where 2 or more bones unite, providing the mechanism that allows them to bend and move
- Joints are classified as to the range of movement they can produce:
  - Diarthrosis – joints that allow free movement

- Synarthrosis – joints that are fixed
- Amphiarthrosis – joints that permit limited movement.

Classification of joints

- Occur when one bone meets another, classified as:
  - Synovial joints allow extensive movement (diarthrosis), are covered by articular cartilage and connected to ligaments, a space between them allows free movement and contains synovial fluids. There are a number of different types:
    - Pivot joints (radius, ulna)
    - Ball and socket joints (hip, shoulder)
    - Hinge joint (joints in the finger)
    - 'Plane' or gliding joint (vertebrae)
    - Condyloid joint (metacarpophalangeal joints e.g. the knuckle and radiocarpal e.g. wrist)
    - Saddle joint (thumb)
  - Cartilaginous – usually covered by a thin layer of hyaline or fibrous cartilage to allow slight movement such the pelvis or the vertebral bodies
  - Fibrous – are usually immovable, but some do allow minimal movement
- Cartilage is a cushion, which provides protection for joints when bones are exposed to forces during movement
- Ligaments help to provide joint strength
- Movement of a joint is achieved by the contraction of muscles that are attached to bones.

MUSCLES

There are more than 350 named muscles (Figure 12.2), which are nearly all in pairs. Muscles have the ability to contract and relax and are made up of contractile cells (Figure 12.3), which have the ability to shorten in length or contract (Judge, 2007).

Types of muscles

- There are 3 types of muscles:
  - Fusiform muscles, which are elongated and shaped like straps and run from one joint to another
  - Pennate muscles are broad and flat
  - Skeletal muscles

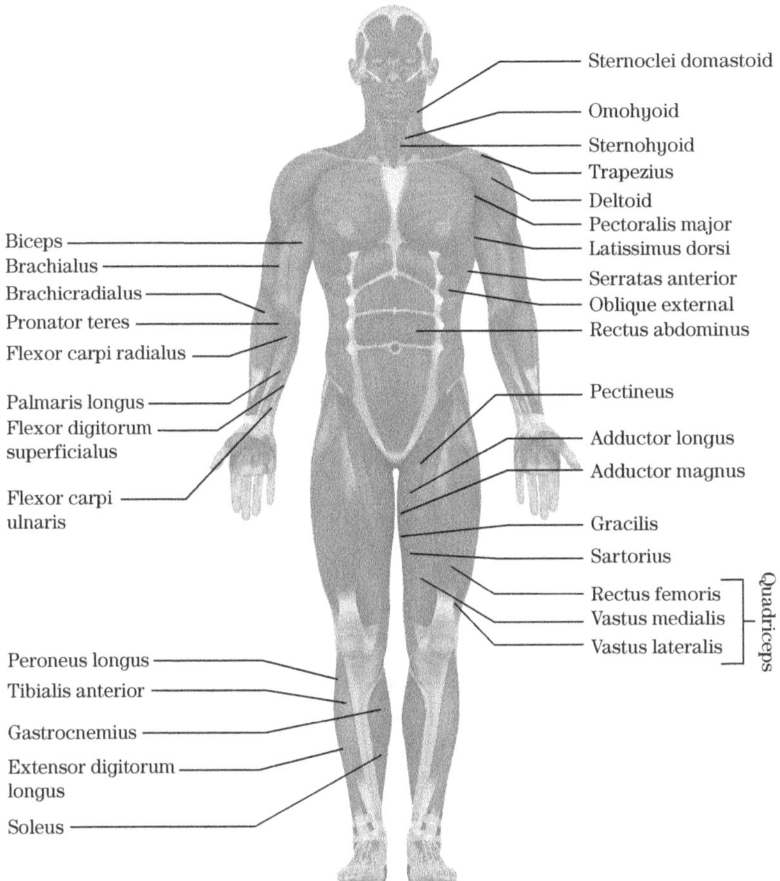

Figure 12.2 Muscles of the body

- Voluntary muscles are stimulated by the motor neurones of the somatic nervous system
- Striated muscles are contractile muscles, organised in units called sarcomeres
- Extrafusal muscles contains the sensory organs of the muscle

- Motor and sensory nerve fibres, which function together with muscles providing the electrical impulses required for movement.

Muscle contraction

- The function of muscles is to contract and undertake work observed as muscle movement

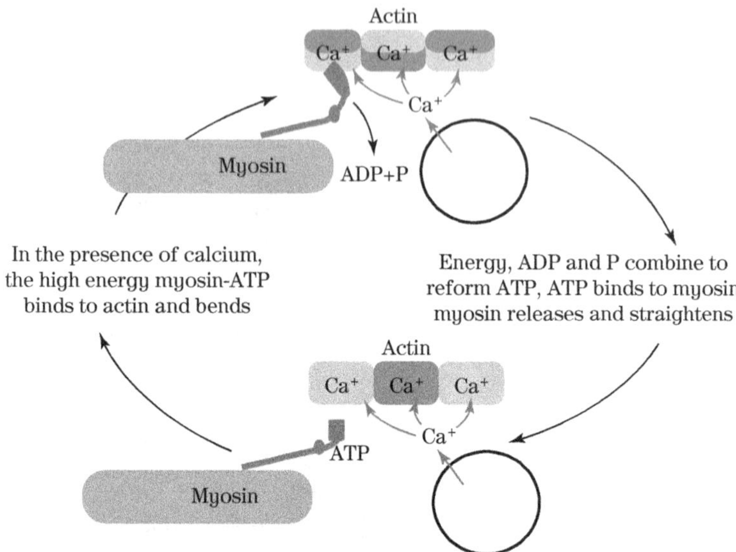

Figure 12.3 Muscle contraction

- To undertake work the muscle requires a source of energy, which depends on nutritional status (chapter 11):
  - A source of energy in the form of adenosine-triphosphate (ATP) obtained from glucose, glycogen or fats
  - A distribution of proteins (actin, myosin), which depend on inorganic compounds anions and cations to regulate protein synthesis and muscle contraction
  - Calcium, potassium and sodium for action potentials and depolarisation.
- Muscle contraction is a 4-stage process:
  - Excitation is when a nervous stimulus (action potential) reaches the neuro-muscular junction and causes rapid depolarisation of muscle fibres
  - Coupling is the electrical activity causes actin-containing filaments to shorten, and involves calcium and muscle
  - Contraction leads the muscle filaments to shorten using actin and myosin, adenosine-triphosphate (ATP) is released forming an actin-myosin complex and contraction occurs as the actin slides onto the myosin, causing the muscle to shorten
  - Relaxation is the removal of the actin-rich stimulus.

PATHOPHYSIOLOGY OF MUSCULAR SKELETAL SYSTEM

Muscular skeletal disorders can be directly related to the bone or muscle due to degeneration, reduction in hormones or vitamins, inflammation or infection, fracture or trauma to the bones. In addition, the nervous system can affect muscle and bone movement. Interventions and management for some of these conditions include long term support and medication to relieve symptoms, a loss of limb, limb movement, function and deformities. In other conditions early rehabilitation leading to full mobility and recovery can occur.

Osteoporosis

Osteoporosis is the most common metabolic bone disease – progressive decrease in bone mass with age, which decreases bone strength, predisposing women to an increased risk of fracture.

Aetiology

- 2 types of osteoporosis:
  - Type 1 or primary osteoporosis
    - Post-menopausal type occurs in middle age and older women and oestrogen levels fall too low to stimulate endometrial growth, bleeding stops
    - Senile type occurs after the age of 70
  - Type 2 or secondary osteoporosis
    - Caused by diseases or drugs
    - Can temporarily develop in patients receiving large doses of heparin
    - The 3rd trimester of pregnancy
- Changes in body oestrogen levels cause bone reabsorption in women after the menopause (McRee, 2006)
- Exercise throughout life helps to maintain bone mass
- Immobility for any reason may precipitate osteoporosis
- Direct causes can be found such as:
  - Cushing's syndrome
  - Diabetes
  - Thyrotoxicosis, hyperthyroidism
  - Chronic renal failure
  - Prolonged anorexia, low body mass index (BMI)
  - Smoking
  - Use of drugs such as glucocorticoids
  - Long-term heparin

- Alcohol abuse
- Immobility
- Coeliac disease.

Pathology

- Osteoporosis is not a disease of old age, as many older adults retain their bone density
- In osteoporosis the old bone is being reabsorbed faster than new bone is being made, causing compact and spongy bone to lose density (Allsworth, 2005)
- If this process continues the skeleton is no longer strong enough to give support and protection, bones can fracture spontaneously and become fragile leading to falls
- Reduced strength and the weakened bone fractures
- Damage to the femoral neck, the dorsal vertebrae and the distal radius are common
- With ageing bone reabsorption occurs
- Bone becomes more porous and thinner, making bones weaker and prone to fractures and curvatures
- Bone density can be used to define osteoporosis (McCance and Huether, 2010)
  - Normal bone is greater than 833 mg/cm^2
  - Osteopenia or decreased bone mass is 648–833 mg/cm^2
  - Osteoporosis is less than 648 mg/cm^2.

Clinical features

- Asymptomatic osteoporosis is common
- Backache is common
- Bone deformity
- The vertebrae may collapse due to typical crush fractures and there may be an exaggeration of the curvature of the thoracic spine
- Collapse of vertebrae may lead to loss of height
- Bone fractures may occur as the spongy bone becomes thin, sparse and the compact bone becomes porous:
  - Long bones femur or humerus, ribs
  - Fracture neck of femur.

Investigations

- X-ray will demonstrate decreased bone density and thinning of the cortex
- Specialist measures such as measurements of:

- Bone mineral density with a dual energy X-Ray absorptiometry (DXA) scan can asses the risk of osteoporosis
- Quantitative ultrasound (QUS) of heals can identify future risk of fracture, but is not recommended as a definitive diagnosis.
- Lumbar and thoracic vertebrae become biconcave in shape
- Blood levels of calcium, phosphate and alkaline phosphatase are normal
- Risk assessment using the WHO's fracture risk assessment (FRAX), a downloadable computer questionnaire (www.shef.ac.uk/FRAX).

Treatment and prevention

- Prophylaxis is preferred and will help:
  - A good diet with adequate amounts of calcium, magnesium and vitamin D
  - Additional calcium intake
  - Low alcohol intake
  - Moderate weight-bearing exercise
- Treatment can be unsatisfactory if the loss of bone mass has already occurred
- Attempts to prevent the progression by slowing down the rate of calcium and bone loss can be achieved with:
  - Bisphosphonates reduce risk of vertebral fracture
  - Short-term HRT as there are side effects of long-term use (BNF, 2014)
  - Selective oestrogen receptor modulators (SERMs) e.g. raloxifene
  - Fractures caused by osteoporosis should be treated as appropriate e.g. total hip replacement for a fractured neck of femur (Temple, 2004).

Osteomyelitis

This is infection in the bone, which is difficult to treat and can lead to physical disability. The infection can be blood borne or occur from direct spread of micro-organisms.

Aetiology

- Often caused by bacteria, a mixture of aerobic and anaerobic organisms, which is either:
  - Exogenous osteomyelitis enters the body from the outside and spreads from soft tissues into adjacent bone, through:
    - Open fractures
    - Penetrating wounds

    - Surgical procedures e.g. replacement joints
    - Human bites or fist blows to the mouth
- Endogenous osteomyelitis is caused by bacteria transmitted in the blood from infection sites elsewhere in the body (McCance and Huether, 2010):
    - Skin sepsis or ulcer
    - Intravenous drug abuse
    - Chronic urinary tract infection
    - Sickle cell disease
    - Chronic diverticulitis.

Pathology

- Once infection has gained access to bones and bypassed the body's natural defences the bone becomes vulnerable to damage and destruction by the bacterial toxins
- Bone cells have limited capacity to replace bone damaged by infection (Davies *et al*, 2006)
- The bacteria lead to stimulation of the inflammatory response
- Increased swelling can deprive underlying bone of a blood supply, leading to necrosis and death of bone
- This can lead to amputation.

Clinical features

- There is fever, pain, swelling and tenderness over the affected bone
- Chronic osteomyelitis from untreated or undertreated acute osteomyelitis can lead to:
    - Bone erosion
    - Areas of degeneration
    - May be intermittent flare-ups of the infection over a period of years with fever, local pain and sinus formation.

Investigations

- Blood culture or bone biopsy can be undertaken to determine diagnosis
- Diagnosis is possible from the clinical picture alone
- Increased white blood cell count
- CT scan, MRI.

Treatment and drug therapy

- Antibiotics
- Drainage of inflammatory exudates and debridement

- Evaluation is by bone scanning and MRI
- Chronic osteomyelitis may require a combination of surgery and antibiotic therapy
- Hyperbaric oxygen is sometimes used.

BONE TUMOURS

Osteosarcomas

Aetiology

- These are the most common form of malignant bone cancer (Blows, 2005)
- Sometimes there is a coincidental history of trauma
- Sometimes may present with a fracture of unknown cause
- Can develop as a complication of Paget's disease (Blows, 2005).

Pathology

- A malignant bone-forming tumour
- It is aggressive as it destroys the cortex of the bone and extends outward into surrounding soft tissues and inwards into the bone canal
- Found in bone marrow
- The diagnosis is made on the basis of the production of osteoid produced by the malignant cells
- There are 3 types of osteosarcomas depending on how much osteoid is present in the tumour:
  - Osteoblastic
  - Chondroblastic
  - Fibroblastic.

Clinical features

- The commonest sites are the knee, lower femur and upper tibia
- Inflammation leading to swelling and pain which is:
  - Slight and intermittent at first
  - Becomes more intense and of longer duration
  - Often becomes worse at night
  - Analgesia becomes necessary.

Investigations

- The earlier the tumour is identified the better the prognosis

- Many could be diagnosed earlier but often the signs are ignored and the individual does not seek medical attention
- Radiologic studies include:
  - Plain X-ray
  - CT scan
  - MRI to enable:
    - Diagnosis
    - Staging of the cancer
    - The progress of the tumour with treatment.

Treatment and drug therapy

- Chemotherapy and surgery
- Chemotherapy is usually given both pre- and postoperatively using combinations of drugs
- There is the possibility of limb salvage by the removal of the tumour.

Chondrosarcoma

Aetiology

- The causes of the tumour are not fully understood.

Pathology

- A cartilage or cartilage like forming tumour
- Usually occurs in middle age and older adults.

Clinical features

- Most common complaint is pain and swelling leading an individual to seek treatment.

Investigations

- Bone scan
- Biopsy
- Chest X-ray and chest CT to detect metastasis.

Treatment and drug therapy

- Surgery
- Amputation may be necessary.

JOINT DISORDERS

Rheumatoid arthritis

Rheumatoid arthritis (RA) is a classic autoimmune disorder with self-perpetuating inflammation in the joints.

Aetiology

- The trigger factor is unknown and various agents have been suggested
- Genetic susceptibility to the disease seem to be vitally important, with genetic markers such as the human leucocyte antigens identified as playing a role (Martin, 2004).
- Hormonal factors may have an influence
- Normally the immune system does not attack 'self', in autoimmune disorders the body starts to make antibodies to body proteins
- Rheumatoid factor present in serum can lead to changes in the synovial fluid, such as:
  - Increase in volume occurs
  - Increase in turbidity occurs and the joint fluid looses its transparency and becomes cloudy
  - Mucin decreases
  - The numbers of white cells are increased.

Pathology

- Early in the disease the synovial membrane tissue that lines the joint cavity and joints become, warm, swollen and tender
- As the condition progresses there is joint cartilage, capsule and deformity
- May lead to the progressive destruction of articular cartilage
- Usually affects more than one joint at the same time, more commonly small joints of the hands and feet (Dandy and Edwards, 2004).

Clinical features

- Pain and swelling in symmetrical small joints (e.g. fingers and toes)
  - Morning stiffness in affected joints
- May be tired, irritable, with acute fever, weight loss and excessive fatigue
- Gradually the disease spreads, joints take on a deformed appearance, difficulties occur

- The patient can become depressed and anxious
- Periods of exacerbation and remission
- Other changes throughout the body
  - Subcutaneous nodules in 25% of cases
  - Vasculitis – involves arterioles, venules and capillaries and leads to localised purpura
  - Fibrinous pleurisy and fibrosis of the lungs
  - Cardiac involvement – pericarditis
  - Neuropathy – decreased touch sensation in the feet
  - Carpal tunnel syndrome
  - Eye changes: Keratoconjunctivitis (dry eyes) pain, photophobia and impairment of vision
  - Splenomegaly
  - Anaemia
  - Fatigue, malaise and depression.

See case study 12.1.

Case study 12.1

Mary, a 49-year-old receptionist, was admitted to the Day Surgical Unit for the removal of a fatty lump from her left axilla. She has been given an afternoon appointment because she suffers from rheumatoid arthritis and has a problem getting going in the morning. Mary has suffered from rheumatoid arthritis for 15 years. She accepts that her rheumatoid arthritis is a way of life and she has a very positive attitude towards her condition. Prior to her admission to the Day Surgical Unit Mary was seen in the Pre-Assessment clinic where she had many tests to assess how active her rheumatoid arthritis was. The disease is most dominant in her wrists and fingers of both hands. Although Mary has the disease in other joints she feels the wrists and fingers are the most debilitating. With this in mind Mary chooses to wear her splints at night otherwise she feels her hands take longer to get going in the mornings. It is now 3 years since Mary has been able to drive her car.

Investigations

- X-rays can appear normal, but later erosions can give diagnostic information
- The metatarsals of the feet and the metacarpophalangeal joints in the hands are used to help monitor the progression of the disease (Martin, 2004).

- Blood tests:
  - Rheumatoid factor (RhF) may be positive
  - Erythrocyte sedimentation rate (ESR) raised due to inflammation, not specific to RA, but can aid diagnosis
  - C-reactive protein (CRP) a non-specific inflammatory marker, but only significantly raised in server uncontrolled RA
  - Haemoglobin (Hb) can be depressed in patients with RA (normochromic normocytic anaemia).

Treatment and nursing management

- Reduce pain, enable patient to lead a normal life, reduction in symptoms:
  - Application of heat:
  - Wax, heating pads
  - Whirlpool-type baths
- Physiotherapy with exercises maintains joint movement and strengthens weak muscles
- Occupational therapists provide splints, as well as aids and appliances
- Drug treatment
  - NSAIDs – decrease pain, GIT side effects, no effect on the underlying disease process
  - Corticosteroids in low doses can, in combination with other agents, can reduce the rate of progression of joint damage
  - Immunosuppressive drugs
  - Disease-modifying antirheumatic drugs (DMARDs), which must be monitored regularly for safety and efficiency (Martin, 2004).

Osteoarthritis

Aetiology

- Contributing factors include:
  - Obesity
  - Postural defect
  - Malformed joint
  - Long-term occupational or athletic stress on a joint.

Pathology

- A common degenerative disease, where there is a progressive breakdown of the joint surface resulting in a loss of articular cartilage and exposure to underlying bone (Judge, 2007)

- In osteoarthritis inflammation of the joints is an important feature (McCance and Huether, 2010)
- It commonly affects the weight-bearing joints:
  - The knees
  - Inter-phalangeal joints of the hands
  - Common in the hip joint
- It may be:
  - Primary – a degenerative disease and the result of wear and tear on the joint
  - Secondary – attributable to other causes, e.g. joint injury in athletics or trauma.

Clinical features

- Joint aches and stiffness, increase with activity and decrease with rest
- No systemic signs or symptoms
- Pain becomes more persistent and stiffness increases and degeneration progresses
- Limitation of movement in the affected joint
- Loss of mobility is from hip and knee involvement.

Investigations

- Diagnosis is confirmed by X-ray or imaging.

Treatment and drug therapy

- No prevention or arrest of the process
- Analgesia is helpful, NSAIDs
- Physiotherapy and the use of activities that reduce strain can help
- Joint replacement often becomes necessary, as in the case of Sheree in case study 12.2.

Case study 12.2

Sheree is a 75-year-old retired nursery school assistant. She lives in a one-bedroom flat within a sheltered accommodation unit. She has two sons who live nearby with their families. Sheree has severe osteoarthritis of both hips, the left being worse than the right. She is overweight, but otherwise is generally healthy. She was admitted to the ward for an elective left total hip replacement. It was recognised that she is at risk of the usual range of potential post-operative complications; however this type of surgery in particular contributes a significant risk factor for the development of a deep vein thrombosis (DVT). On return to the ward Sheree is provided with controlled analgesia (PCA) with morphine for pain relief, an intravenous infusion to ensure fluid and electrolyte balance, and a wound drain in situ.

Practice point

Long-term therapy using NSAIDS is not recommended and patients on these drugs need to be aware of the complications. They should consult their doctor if they experience bleeding gums or excessive vaginal bleeding. NSAIDs are not recommended for patients with renal impairment or asthma.

Fractures

A fracture is a complete break, incomplete break or crack in the continuity of bone.

Classification of fractures

- Classifications/terminology used (Judge, 2007):
  - Complete – the bone is broken all the way through
  - Incomplete/partial – the bone is damaged but still in one piece
  - Open fracture – the bone is protruding through the surface of the skin
  - Closed – the fracture has not penetrated the skin
  - Comminuted – the bone is broken into more than 2 fragments
  - Linear – the fracture runs the parallel to the axis of the bone
  - Oblique – fractured at a 45° angle to the long bone axis
  - Spiral – fracture twists around and encircles the bone
  - Transverse – fracture occurs straight across the bone
  - Impacted – one part of a bone is forcefully driven into another.

Aetiology

- Usually due to trauma e.g. falls, road traffic accidents (RTA)
- Pathological fractures can be:
  - A break at a pre-existing site or abnormality
  - Disease of the bone such as:

    - Tumours
    - Osteoporosis
    - Infection
    - Metabolic bone disorders
- Stress fracture often seen in athletes. There are 2 types:
  - Fatigue fractures caused by abnormal stress and can recover
  - Insufficiency fractures occur in bone that is lacking the normal ability to reform and recover
- Transchondral fracture when a fragment of cartilage fragments and separates causing friction and pain; common in the distal femur, ankle, kneecap, elbow and wrist (McCance and Huether, 2010).

Pathology

- Pain starts as soon as the bone is broken, several stages until the break is healed:
  - Haematoma formation around the fracture
  - Cellular proliferation by the osteoblasts
  - Laying down of calcium to form callus
  - Consolidation into mature bone
- Restoration of function
  - Rehabilitation is always necessary and should begin as soon as the fracture is treated; if ignored and immobile the muscles will waste and the joints will stiffen
  - There may be permanent impairment of function.

Clinical features

- Soft tissue injury – swelling, haematoma, oedema
- Blood vessels and nerves may be damaged, impaired sensation and numbness
- Painful and there is loss of function – muscle spasm and is worse on movement
- Deformity (unnatural alignment), shortening of the limb and rotational deformities
- Tenderness
- Crepitus may occur – abnormal movement at the fracture site, bone ends grind against each other.

Investigations

- X-ray of the whole length of the bone, including the adjacent joints, should be done

    - Range of movement (ROM), which assesses the amount of deviation away from the neutral position in both passive (the patient moves the joint) and active (the examiner provides the movement) (Judge, 2007).

Treatment and drug therapy

- Fundamentals of treatment:
    - Reduction – realignment of the bone fragments
    - Manipulative reduction – under general anaesthesia skin is not opened and the bones are moved back into place
    - Mechanical traction – draws the bone fragments back to their normal length
    - Operative reduction – fragments will be fixed internally to ensure maintenance of their position
    - Immobilisation – rigid splinting to maintain their position:
        - Prevent displacement of the bone fragments
        - Prevent movement that may interfere with union
        - Relieve pain
- Methods of immobilisation include:
    - Micro-fibre plaster or other external splint
    - Continuous traction
    - External fixation
    - Internal fixation
- In open fractures there is a high risk of infection
    - Antibiotics are always administered e.g. broad spectrum such as cephalosporin
    - Tetanus prophylaxis must be given if not up to date
    - The patient should be closely observed for signs of infection, especially a sustained rise in temperature
    - The wound should be kept covered with a sterile dressing and not disturbed until the patient can urgently go to theatre:
        - The wound can be cleaned
        - Dead tissue removed
        - Wounds immediately sutured
- Monitoring of any complications of fractures
    - Accompanying damage to neighbouring structures:
        - Nerves
        - Blood vessels
        - Tendons
    - Depressed fracture – segment of bone is depressed below the level of the bone – common in skull fractures
    - Displacement – bone ends have moved from each other

  - Dislocation – loss of congruity between the articular surfaces of a joint e.g. a Pott's fracture is dislocation of the ankle joint with fracture of the tibia or fibula
  - Compartment syndrome (Edwards, 2004)
- May only be a small part of the damage:
  - Multiple injuries
  - Other trauma is more important
  - Maintaining the airway is always the first priority
  - There may be spinal injuries or head injuries also
- The prevention and identification of complications from the fracture:
  - Infection
  - Delayed union, non-union, mal-union
  - Shortening
  - Avascular necrosis – death of bone due to interference with its blood supply
  - Blood vessel injuries – observation of the peripheral circulation, numbness of the digits and pain due to ischaemia
  - Compartment syndrome
  - Injury to nerves
  - Injury to viscera – lung complications following fractured ribs and bladder injury following a fractured pelvis
  - Tendon injuries
  - Injuries to joints
  - Fat embolism – globules of fat enter the venous circulation pass through lungs.

Compartment syndrome

Acute compartment syndrome is a common but potentially life-threatening condition. It occurs in limbs and the abdomen, and requires prompt recognition and intervention (Edwards, 2004).

Aetiology

- Stimulation of the inflammatory response due to soft tissue injury:
  - Traumatic
  - Haemorrhage
  - Surgical
  - Vascular
  - Complication of another injury
- Tight fitting casts, compression bandage.

Pathology

- There are 4 compartments in the legs and in compartment syndrome following trauma or haemorrhage severe swelling occurs within one or more of the enclosed muscle compartments
- The swelling leads to fluid moving into compartments increasing perfusion pressure, which can lead to a reduction in blood flow to muscle from which it never recovers (Edwards, 2004)
- More commonly found in the lower limbs.

Clinical features

- Myoglobinuria is the excretion of globulins (proteins present in muscle tissue) in urine, appear as a dark reddish brown colour
- Increase in the serum enzyme creatine kinase (CK), which can be 100 times greater than normal
- An increase in myoglobinurea (rhabdomyolysis) indicates a severe life-threatening muscle trauma.

Investigations

- Urinalysis
- Pain that is disproportionate to the apparent injury, difficult if the patient is receiving regular analgesia
- Paraesthesia not expected to occur
- Sensory deficit
- Can only be identified in fully conscious patients
- Measure of intercompartmental pressure (ICP) should be between 10–30 mmHg.

> **Practice point**
>
> The pain experienced by a patient with compartment syndrome is inconsistent with the injury obtained and should be investigated immediately.

Treatment

- Removal or relief from tight bandage or cast
- Elevation of limb
- Fasciotomy is an incision through fascia (layer of tissue that envelopes the body beneath the skin):

- Used to release swelling which could compromise blood flow
- Indicated to decompress the compartment and allow reperfusion of the muscle.

Nervous disorders

Nervous disorders affect both muscle and bones:

- Multiple sclerosis is demyelination at many sites in the brain and the spinal cord
- Motor neurone disease is a progressive degenerative disease but cognitive level is spared
- Disease of voluntary muscles:
  - Myasthenia gravis is an autoimmune disease where antibodies destroy acetylcholine receptors
  - Muscular dystrophy – some are inflammatory, associated with drugs, toxins and endocrine weakness
  - Potassium deficiency (hypokalaemia) may cause a generalised flaccid weakness if severe
- Epilepsy – bursts of excessive electrical activity
- Parkinson's disease – loss of nerves in the substantia nigra which regulates motor function:
  - Muscle cells require neurotransmitter dopamine
  - Symptoms of Parkinson's disease are due to a decline in dopamine and a relative excess of acetylcholine.

For more information see chapter 10.

CONCLUSION

The skeleton, muscles and joints allow the body to move and much of what the body does is related to mobility. Therefore, immobility can lead to dangerous consequences, which come about through disabling conditions such as arthritis and osteoporosis. The outcomes of these and other muscular skeletal conditions are variable from the possibility of regaining full mobility and recovery (fracture), the risks of surgical procedures, the loss of limb (compartment syndrome), long-term drug therapies (pain killers), disability or deformity (arthritis), depression or mental health problems due to the long-term nature of some of these conditions. The healthcare professional plays an active role in minimising the risks and returning the patient to optimum mobility.

Self-assessment questions

1. Provide an outline of the functions of the musculoskeletal system.
2. Describe the structure of bones and muscle identifying the different types.
3. Identify the role the nervous system plays in movement and posture.
4. Using the case studies provided in this chapter list several changes to the musculoskeletal anatomy and physiology that may occur.

REFERENCES

Allsworth, A. (2005) Osteoporosis nursing implications, in J. Keale and P. Davis (eds) *Orthopaedic and Trauma Nursing,* 2nd edn, Edinburgh: Churchill Livingstone.

Blows, W.T. (2005) *The Biological Basis of Nursing: Cancer*, London: Routledge.

BNF (British National Formulary) (2014) *BNF 66: The Authority on the Selection and Use of Medicines*, London: The British Medical Society, The Royal Pharmaceutical Society.

Dandy, D.J., Edwards, D.J. (2004) *Essential Orthopaedics and Trauma,* 4th edn, Edinburgh: Churchill Livingstone.

Davies, R., Everitt, H. and Simon, C. (2006) *Musculoskeletal Problems*, Oxford: Oxford University Press.

Edwards, S. (2004) Acute compartment syndrome, *Emergency Nurse*, 12(3), 32–38.

Judge, N.L. (2007) Assessing and managing patients with musculoskeletal conditions, *Nursing Standard*, 22(1), 51–57.

Knight, C., Mathew, A. and Muir, J. (2005) The locomotor system, in J. Kneale and P. Davis (eds) *Orthopaedic and Trauma Nursing*, 2nd edn, Edinburgh: Churchill Livingstone.

McCance, K.L. and Huether, S.E. (2010) *Pathophysiology: The Biologic Basis for disease in Adults and Children,* 6th edn, Missouri: Mosby Elsevier.

McRee, R. (2006) *Pocketbook of Orthopaedics and Fractures*, 2nd edn, Edinburgh: Churchill Livingstone.

Martin, L. (2004) Rheumatoid arthritis: symptoms, diagnosis and management, *Nursing Times*, 100(24), 40–44.

Temple, J. (2004) Total hip replacement, *Nursing Standard,* 19(3), 44–51.

13 The endocrine system and associated disorders

Ann Richards

THE ENDOCRINE SYSTEM

- The endocrine system along with the nervous system is important in communication within the body
- The two systems together control the internal functioning of our body and regulate metabolic activity
- Endocrine glands are ductless glands and secrete chemical messengers called hormones directly into the bloodstream
- These messenger molecules are transported all over the body but the system is precise because only target cells respond to a hormone
- The target cell has receptors (binding sites) that a specific hormone will fit into, rather like a key fitting a lock. After acting on the specific receptor, the hormone is metabolised or inactivated and excreted
- Hormones released by endocrine glands control metabolic processes and help to regulate our blood pressure, water and electrolyte balance and blood glucose levels. Hormones are also important in reproductive functioning, growth and development.

Most hormone release is controlled by a negative feedback mechanism.

- An example is the hormone insulin which is released by the pancreas in response to a rise in blood glucose levels. When the blood glucose levels fall, the release of insulin is decreased
- Some hormones are released at reasonably constant levels e.g. thyroxin from the thyroid gland
- Others are released in cycles e.g. oestrogen from the ovaries
- Others are released intermittently, as needed, such as the insulin described earlier.

The major endocrine glands are scattered all over the body and are shown in Figure 13.1.

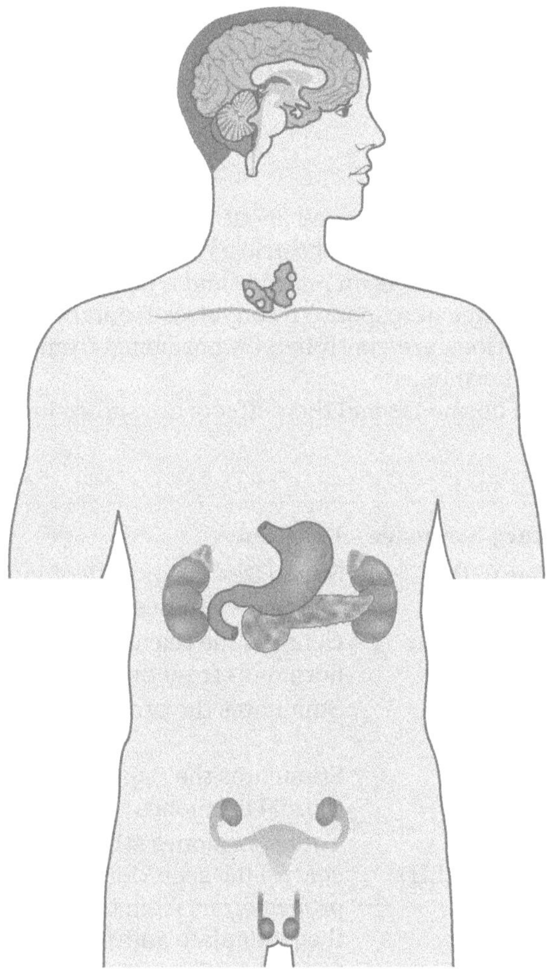

Figure 13.1 The major endocrine glands

Endocrine disorders are usually due to either excessive amounts of the hormone or a deficit of the hormone. Sometimes it may be the target cell that is resistant to the hormone and so does not respond to its secretion. This may be seen in type 2 diabetes mellitus for example (Insulin resistance).

Treatment depends on the problem – for example a hormone deficit can be treated by replacement therapy. One example is the administration of insulin in type 1 diabetes mellitus. Sometimes surgery is needed, especially if there is a tumour (an adenoma). Tumours of the pituitary can compress brain tissue and press on the optic chiasma causing blindness.

We will now look at each endocrine gland in turn describing its physiology and pathophysiology. The most common disorders will be the ones described in the most detail.

The pituitary gland

Situated at the base of the brain and about 1 cm in diameter, this small gland is known as 'the leader of the orchestra' as it secrets hormones that control other endocrine glands. It has an anterior and a posterior lobe. The posterior lobe releases hormones in response to impulses from the hypothalamus. The anterior lobe secretions are controlled by hormones from the hypothalamus known as 'release hormones'.

Pituitary gland hormones and their effects are shown in Table 13.1 below.

Anterior pituitary hormones	**Function**
Growth hormone (GH)	Stimulates the growth of long bones Increases synthesis of proteins
Adrenocorticoid hormone (ACTH)	Controls the release of corticosteroid hormones from the adrenal cortex
Melanocyte stimulating hormone (MSH)	Stimulates the production of melanin
Thyroid stimulating hormone (TSH)	Stimulates the thyroid gland to produce thyroid hormones
Gonadotrophins Luteinising hormone (LH) Follicle stimulating hormone (FSH)	These hormones stimulate ovulation and control the secretion of oestrogen and progesterone from the ovaries. In males they stimulate androgen synthesis and the formation of sperm in the testes
Prolactin	Stimulates milk production after childbirth
Posterior pituitary hormones	
Antidiuretic hormone (ADH) or vasopressin	Prevents water loss from the body by reducing urine output Constricts the blood vessels
Oxytocin	In labour, stimulates contraction of the uterus Increases the flow of milk from the breast

Table 13.1 Pituitary gland hormones and their effects

Hypopituitarism

This is likely to cause a deficiency of several hormones and may be due to pressure from a pituitary adenoma.

- May present as amenorrhoea in women due to reduction in gonadotrophins or erectile dysfunction in men with loss of libido
- There may be an underactive thyroid and also adrenals which may result in hypotension, nausea and collapse
- Pituitary adenomas make up about 10% of intracranial tumours and are often found at autopsy having given no symptoms during life
- Larger tumours may cause headaches or visual symptoms if they press on the optic chiasma.

Growth hormone

Secretion is regulated by two hormones from the hypothalamus. Growth hormone release factor stimulates secretion and somatostatin inhibits release.

Acromegaly

Excessive secretion of growth hormone in adult life. The most common cause is a pituitary adenoma. The patients has very large hands and feet with a widening of the nose and a large jaw. Internal organs such as the heart may enlarge and there may be hypertension. Cardiovascular complications may lead to early death if the disorder is not treated.

Gigantism

This occurs when there is an excess of growth hormone secreted before the epiphyses of long bones have fused.

Hypersecretion of other pituitary hormones

- Examples are hypersecretion of thyroid-stimulating hormone which is a rare cause of hyperthyroidism
- Hyperprolactinaemia may cause amenorrhoea and infertility if occurring before the menopause
- Over-secretion of ACTH leads to Cushing's syndrome described below.

Posterior pituitary

Diabetes insipidus

- This is caused by a decreased release of ADH resulting in the passage of large quantities of dilute urine, often over 10 litres in 24 hours
- This results in thirst and polydipsia (drinking large quantities of water)

- It is treated by replacement of the hormone in the form of a more powerful alternative, desmopressin, which may be taken by nasal spray or tablet.

The thyroid gland

The thyroid gland is situated in the neck, just below the larynx and either side of the trachea. The two lobes are joined together by a broad bridge, the isthmus. The gland is very vascular and is able to extract iodine from the blood. The iodine is needed to produce the two thyroid hormones. These are thyroxine (T4) and triiodothyronine (T3), containing 4 and 3 atoms of iodine respectively.

- The hormones are involved in regulating metabolism and increase the rate of energy release form carbohydrates, increase protein synthesis and fat breakdown
- They control our basal metabolic rate (BMR) which is the amount of energy (calories) the body uses while at rest
- Thyroid hormones are also needed for normal growth and the development of the nervous system
- The level of thyroid hormones is controlled by TSH from the anterior pituitary gland
- Thyroxine is the less potent hormone but makes up at least 95% of the thyroid hormones circulating in the bloodstream.

The thyroid gland also produces calcitonin which is synthesised by different cells within the gland. This hormone plays a part in the control of calcium and phosphate levels in the blood.

- Calcitonin decreases the level of calcium and phosphate ions in the blood by decreasing their release from bone
- It increases the rate calcium and phosphate ions are deposited in bone
- Also increases the removal of calcium and phosphate ions by the renal system
- Its release is stimulated by high blood calcium levels in the blood
- Reduces bone resorption during pregnancy and breast feeding when calcium is needed for the baby.

Disorders of the thyroid gland

Goitre

This is an enlargement of the thyroid gland and may be seen in the neck.

- A large goitre can compress the trachea, causing difficulty with breathing or may compress the oesophagus causing difficulty swallowing. It may cause concern to the patient because it can be seen
- It may be caused by both under-secretion and over-secretion of the thyroid gland
- Used to be common in areas where there was a low level of iodine in the soil but iodine is now added to table salt
- Toxic goitre is due to hyperactivity of the thyroid gland often due to increased secretion of TSH.

Hyperthyroidism (thyrotoxicosis)

Usually (about 80% of cases) due to Graves disease which is an autoimmune disease of the thyroid that occurs more frequently in women.

- The patient shows signs of a generally increased metabolism
- Heat intolerance
- Excessive activity (hyperkinetic)
- Excessive sweating
- Weight loss although eating well
- Anxiety and emotional lability
- Tachycardia and palpitations
- May develop atrial fibrillation and heart failure if older
- There is sometimes exophthalmos where the eyeballs protrude.

Other causes of hyperthyroidism include toxic nodular goitre and a thyroid adenoma.

Treatments include surgical removal of the thyroid gland, treatment with radioactive iodine or antithyroid drugs.

Hypothyroidism

This is an interactivity of the thyroid and is often linked to autoimmune disease.

In Hashimoto's thyroiditis there is a painless goitre. This is 20 times commoner in women than men and may be linked to other autoimmune disorders.

Primary myxoedema occurs when the thyroid atrophies, and, again, is commoner in elderly women than men and is linked to autoimmune disease.

- Hypothyroidism leads to a slowing of metabolism and the patient may present with hypothermia
- Other symptoms include weight gain but decreased appetite
- Bradycardia
- Tiredness and lethargy with slow thought processes
- Cold intolerance.

Treatment is replacement therapy with thyroxine in tablet form.

The adrenal glands

These are situated above each kidney. The gland has an outer cortex and an inner medulla. The medulla secretes the hormones adrenaline and noradrenaline. The cortex secretes steroid hormones – glucocorticoids, mineral corticoids and sex hormones (mainly androgens).

The adrenal medulla

A rare benign tumour of the adrenal medulla is a phaeochromocytoma.

- This secretes adrenaline and noradrenaline and the patient presents with intermittent hypertension related to this excess
- Palpitations, sweating and sometimes collapse may occur
- There is a raised blood sugar and glycosuria due to adrenaline raising blood glucose levels
- Treatment is removal of the tumour.

The adrenal cortex

Consists of 3 zones. The zona glomerulosa secretes aldosterone, a mineralocortidoid that controls the sodium and potassium balance in the blood and fluid volume. Its secretion is regulated by the renin-angiotensin system in the kidney.

The other 2 zones produce glucocorticoids, the main hormone being cortisol.

Cortisol has many effects on metabolism and is important in dealing with long-term stress.

- It increases blood sugar by stimulating glucose breakdown and inhibiting protein synthesis
- Has anti-inflammatory and immunosuppressive effects. Synthetic steroids are used in the treatment of some skin conditions and other inflammatory disorders such as asthma
- Excess steroids affect bone metabolism and can cause osteoporosis.

The gland does secrete small amounts of sex steroids too.

Cushing's syndrome

This is an over-secretion of cortisol by the adrenal cortex that occurs most commonly in women.

- There is fat deposition around the trunk, around the face giving a typical 'moon face' and on the back giving a 'buffalo hump'

- Increased protein breakdown leads to thin arms and legs
- Stretch marks (striae) occur on the abdomen due to collagen breakdown
- Hypertension is present
- Osteoporosis may lead to a collapse of the vertebrae
- Hyperglycaemia may be present
- Swinging moods with depression and sometimes psychosis
- Androgen release may be increased causing hirsuitism (facial hair growth in women) and amenorrhoea.

Causes of Cushing's syndrome

- Excessive release of ACTH from the pituitary
- Tumour of the adrenal cortex
- Iatrogenic due to the administration of steroids.

Conn's syndrome

Due to hypersecretion of aldosterone and thus sodium retention, potassium loss and fluid retention. Usually caused by an adrenal adenoma.

- Hypertension
- Muscle weakness, muscle cramps and tetany
- Polyuria
- Hypokalaemia.

Adrenocorticoid hypofunction

May be acute or chronic. About 90% of the adrenal cortex has to be destroyed before there are symptoms.

Addison's disease

Chronic insufficiency that can become acute.

- Usually due to autoimmune disease and often associated with other autoimmune diseases such as pernicious anaemia
- General lethargy, muscle weakness and anorexia are present
- There is pigmentation of the skin and other membranes
- Hypotension is present.

Acute insufficiency

- Presents with vomiting, hypotension, dehydration and hypoglycaemia
- Acute insufficiency may occur in meningococcal septicaemia
- Acute failure may occur when there is already chronic failure in Addison's disease

- May occur when synthetic steroids are suddenly withdrawn if treatment has been long term
- Treatment is by the administration of steroids.

Parathyroid glands

There are 4 parathyroid glands situated one at each pole of the thyroid gland. They secrete parathyroid hormone which is responsible for regulating calcium levels and exerts its effects on blood bone and the gut. Secretion is controlled by the level of calcium in the blood.

Over-secretion is hyperparathyroidism and may be due to an adenoma of the gland which can be removed.

- The patient presents with tiredness and muscle weakness
- Due to excess calcium, renal calculi may form and bone disease may develop.

Under-secretion of parathyroid hormone leads to a low blood calcium.

- This results in increased muscle tone and tetany if severe
- It is usually due to removal of the glands in a thyroidectomy. It can be difficult to distinguish the parathyroids.

The pancreas and diabetes mellitus

Diabetes mellitus is a syndrome characterised by a persistently raised blood glucose level. Diabetes is associated with either an absence of insulin (type 1 diabetes) or a resistance to insulin action (type 2 diabetes).

The normal range for blood glucose levels in health is 3.5–8.0 mmol/litre.

- A random blood glucose of above 11.1 mmol/L is diagnostic of diabetes mellitus if symptoms are present. Without symptoms, two raised blood glucose measurements must be measured. These measurements should be taken in the laboratory. A fingerprick glucose measurement cannot be used for a diagnosis
- Glucose levels over a period of months can be measured by taking blood for a HbA1c measurement. This measure how much of the haemoglobin in the red cells is carrying glucose i.e. glycosylated. If the HbA1c is above 48 mmol/L (6.5%) this can be used as a diagnosis of diabetes in some cases.

Insulin and glucagon are hormones produced by the islets of Langerhans in the pancreas. They control the level of glucose in the blood. Insulin lowers blood glucose and glucagon raises blood glucose. The two hormones have a much greater impact on overall metabolism than this though.

- There is a low level of insulin release all day (basal level) but this level increases dramatically when our blood glucose rises following a meal
- Insulin secretion is dependent on the blood glucose levels and rises rapidly after a meal
- Insulin is an anabolic (building up) hormone and its release leads to the utilisation of glucose and its removal from the bloodstream to be stored as glycogen in the liver or as fat in adipose cells
- Insulin also increases protein synthesis and inhibits protein breakdown; it inhibits lipolysis (fat breakdown)
- Although insulin is needed to transport glucose into our body cells, it is not needed for glucose to enter brain cells. This is because neurones have a constant requirement for glucose in order to function Exercising muscle can also utilise glucose with very little insulin
- If there is not enough insulin available, the body cannot utilise glucose effectively and the glucose will build up in the bloodstream. It will also be eliminated in the urine when the blood glucose rises above the renal threshold (usually about 10 mmol/L).

Diabetes mellitus

Type 1 diabetes is due to destruction of the islets of Langerhans usually by an autoimmune process. The patient eventually cannot secrete insulin and must receive insulin by injection at regular intervals.

Type 2 diabetes is a different disease and is due to insulin resistance. The pancreas still produces insulin but the cells do not respond to it.

- Type 2 diabetes is associated with obesity and lack of exercise. It is increasing in incidence in developed countries and is much more common than type 1 diabetes
- Type 1 diabetes is always treated with insulin replacement. Type 2 diabetes may be controlled by diet alone, tablets or sometimes insulin by injection
- Type 1 diabetes has a peak incidence around puberty. Type 2 diabetes occurs more frequently in older people although it is now seen in younger patients as inactivity and obesity increase
- Both types of diabetes are extremely dangerous to health is not controlled
- Acute complications are more likely to occur in type 1 diabetes but chronic complications occur in both types of diabetes.

Type 1 diabetes

As insulin production decreases and blood glucose rises, there are symptoms.

- The high blood glucose level in the blood causes an increase in urine production called polyuria

- As the patients passes more urine, they become thirsty and drink large amounts of water – polydipsia
- This leads to frequency in passing urine and may lead to a child wetting the bed at night. Adults will have to get up in the night to pass urine (nocturia)
- Although the glucose is high in the blood, it cannot be utilised by the cells for energy without insulin and so the patient feels tired and lethargic
- Body fat is broken down to produce energy and the waste products of this fat breakdown (ketones) cannot be eliminated via the normal route without glucose being available
- Ketones accumulate in the blood and as they are volatile, they may be smelt as acetone (pear drops) on the breath
- Excess ketones cause the blood to become more acid (acidosis) and the patient now feels sick. They have diabetic ketoacidosis (DKA)
- Drinking is reduced due to nausea and vomiting and dehydration occur
- Eventually the patient will lose consciousness if not treated. This is a diabetic coma (ketoacidotic coma) and can be lethal
- Treatment is by fluid replacement and insulin
- The patient with type 1 diabetes will require insulin throughout their life.

DKA can occur in someone who is already diagnosed with diabetes. When we are ill and have an infection e.g. a urinary tract infection, our bodies require more insulin.

Practice point

The person with diabetes may lose their appetite if unwell and omit their insulin. They must never do this unless advised to by a medical professional.

If they omit their insulin they can develop a high blood glucose and ketoacidosis.

Hypoglycaemia

This is a low blood glucose below 4 mmol/L.

- It occurs in patients with type 1 diabetes when they have too much insulin or do not eat sufficiently after injecting insulin
- It can also occur following exercise as the muscles utilise glucose from the bloodstream

- It can occur when alcohol is consumed
- In type 1 diabetes the patient regularly checks their blood glucose so that they can prevent hypoglycaemia as well as hyperglycaemia
- Symptoms of hypoglycaemia include hunger, aggressiveness (due to lack of glucose in the brain), sweating and tremor (due to increased adrenaline release) and loss of consciousness
- The treatment is administration of glucose by mouth if the patient is conscious or intravenously if they are unable to swallow.

Type 2 diabetes

This is an increasingly common disorder and nearly 1 in 20 people in the UK may develop diabetes in their lifetime.

- The islets are not destroyed by antibodies in type 2. The patient develops a resistance to insulin and at first the pancreas responds by hypersecretion. This controls the blood glucose for some time
- The symptoms are slow to develop and many patients are diagnosed in routine medicals when their blood glucose is found to be high. They can have had the condition for years and not known
- There is a hereditary factor involved in insulin resistance
- Type 2 diabetes may be delayed by eating a healthy diet and keeping a normal weight. Exercise is also important in its prevention as this enables greater utilisation of insulin
- Treatment other than diet may not be necessary if weight is lost and exercise increased
- Many patients take oral medication to control their blood glucose. Some may need insulin eventually.

Case study 13.1

Martha is a 47-year-old woman who works at a desk all day and has little time for any physical activity. She finds meals are rather rushed and so healthy eating has been replaced by snacking on high calorie meals. Over the past year she has put weight on and her BMI (body mass index) is now 35 (obesity is defined as a BMI over 30).

On a recent visit to the doctor because she was feeling tired, her blood glucose was raised and following more blood tests at the hospital, she has now been diagnosed as having type 2 diabetes mellitus. Martha is determined to reduce her weight, eat healthily and do more exercise as the doctor has told her that this may be sufficient to control the diabetes and prevent any complications occurring.

Chronic complications of diabetes mellitus

These occur in both types of diabetes. Some affect small blood vessels (microvascular) and others affect large blood vessels (macrovascular).

Small blood vessels are affected by the raised glucose levels in the blood.

- This leads to damage that has an impact especially on the retina causing retinopathy. This is treated by laser therapy but may lead to loss of vision eventually
- Vessels in the kidneys can be affected causing nephropathy. This can be treated by antihypertensive drugs but may lead to chronic renal failure eventually
- Peripheral neuropathy is the impact of glucose on the nerves. This can lead to loss of sensation in the fingers and toes and may also be painful.

Large blood vessels are affected by the laying down of fatty tissue (atheroma) which occurs more readily in diabetes.

- This may lead to cardiovascular disease, angina and a myocardial infarction. About 70% of people with diabetes die from cardiovascular disease
- It may also lead to peripheral vascular disease where the arteries in the legs are affected leading to pain on walking any distance
- A combination of poor circulation and loss of feeling means that many patients with diabetes may develop ulcers and gangrene leading to amputation of toes or the lower limb.

The person with diabetes needs to be educated in the control of their blood glucose and those with type 1 diabetes can regulate their insulin doses according to their needs. Most complications can be greatly reduced if both type 1 and type 2 diabetes are treated effectively, a healthy diet is eaten and blood glucose levels controlled.

CONCLUSION

This chapter has looked at the major endocrine organs in the body, their functions and some of the disorders that may affect them. Each gland has been considered in turn but the commonest disorder described is type 2 diabetes. The patient may be admitted with another diagnosis such as kidney failure but it may be that diabetes is the causal factor. It is important that the healthcare worker understands this increasingly common, but largely preventable, disorder.

SELF-ASSESSMENT QUESTIONS

1. List the major endocrine glands in the body and the hormones they produce
2. Describe how negative feedback is involved in the control of hormone release.
3. Describe the function of the thyroid gland.
4. List the signs and symptoms of hypothyroidism.
5. Explain the effects of oversecretion of cortisol from the adrenal cortex.
6. Compare and contrast the aetiology of type 1 and type 2 diabetes.
7. Explain what is meant by 'diabetic ketoacidosis'.
8. List the chronic complications of diabetes mellitus.

FURTHER READING

Holt I.G. and Hanley N.A. (2012) *Essential Endocrinology and Diabetes*, 6th edn. Wiley-Blackwell.

Kumar P. and Clark M.L. (2012) *Clinical Medicine* 8th edn. Edinburgh: Saunders.

Whettem, E. (2012) *Diabetes Survival Guide*. Harlow: Pearson.

14 The renal system

Sharon Edwards

The renal system has a prime role in maintaining normal, healthy life and many early changes that occur in the body may be reflected in the urine well before they become clinically obvious.

ANATOMY OF THE RENAL TRACT (FIGURE 14.1)

There are:

- Two kidneys
  - Situated either side of the midline in the upper part of the abdominal cavity at the back, well protected by the abdominal contents in front and the lower ribs and lumbar muscles behind
  - Nephrons are the structural and functioning unit of the kidney:
    - The inner layer, the medulla, contains rows of tubules arranged next to each other (Figure 14.1)
    - The outer layer, the cortex, contains the glomeruli and convoluted tubules (Figure 14.2).
    - Urine is formed in the nephrons and drains through the tubules into collecting ducts, the calyces combine within the renal pelvis of the kidney, and flows into the ureters
- There are two ureters, which run down the posterior wall of the abdominal cavity to the floor of the pelvis where they enter the bladder
- The bladder then acts as a distensible reservoir, storing the urine until it is convenient to void it through the urethra.

The functions of the kidney

- To regulate:
  - Body fluid volume
  - The composition of urine
  - Electrolyte balance – calcium, sodium and potassium levels
- To maintain acid base balance

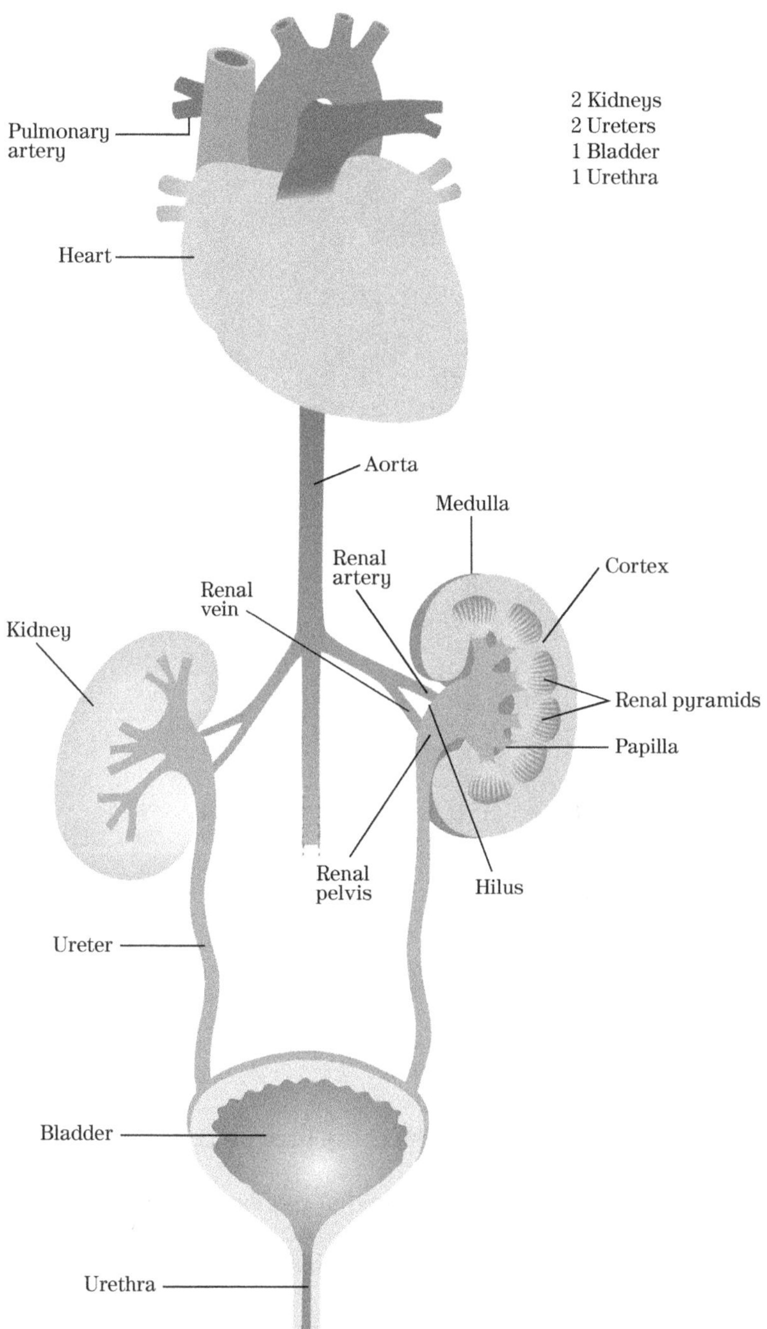

Figure 14.1 The renal system and kidney anatomy

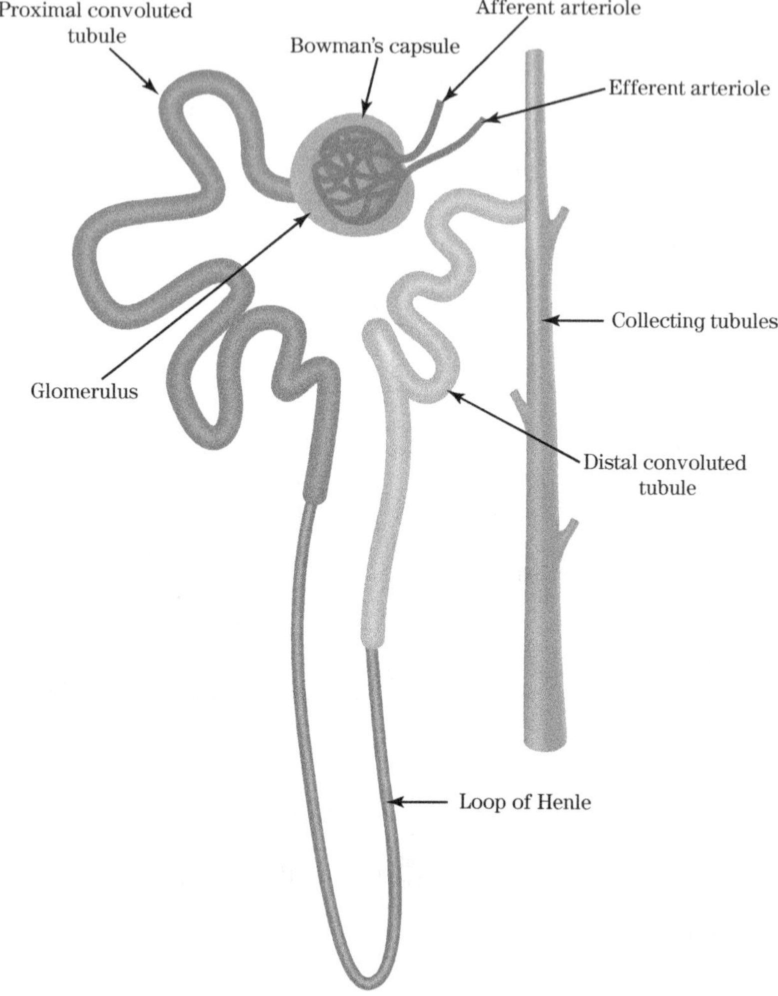

Figure 14.2 The convoluted tubes of the nephron

- Metabolism of vitamin D
- To excrete other waste products e.g. urea and creatinine
- To produce and secrete:
  - The hormone erythropoietin that regulates red blood cell (RBC) production
  - Renin that maintains blood pressure and glomerular filtration rate (GFR)
  - Prostaglandins – involved in the inflammatory immune system and maintains GFR.

KIDNEY PHYSIOLOGY

Mechanisms of urine formation

- The kidneys filter the entire plasma volume more than 60 times/day
- The kidneys account for about 1% of body weight, but consume 20–25% of all oxygen used by the body
- The kidneys process 180 L of blood derived fluid daily; only 1% of this amount (1.5 L) leaves the body as urine
- Urine formation and the adjustment of blood composition involves three major processes (Figure 14.3):
    - Glomerular filtration (GF) contains everything in the blood except proteins, thrombocytes, erythrocytes, and leukocytes; by the time it reaches the collecting ducts it has lost most of its water, nutrients and ions
    - Tubular re-absorption is the movement of fluid and solutes from the renal tubules to the capillary plasma
    - Tubular secretion is the transfer of substances from the capillary plasma to the renal tubules.

Tubular re-absorption and secretion are both carried out by the renal tubules.

Urine production

The glomerulus acts as a high-pressure filter, extracting water, dissolved salts and other compounds and molecules, which are small enough to pass through the membrane. Far more water is filtered at the glomerulus than ultimately appears in the urine, since a considerable amount is re-absorbed before urine reaches the bladder. During this process the concentration of the electrolytes and other constituents of the filtrate are finely adjusted as it passes along the tubules.

The formation of urine is complex but it is possible to divide the process into a series of stages according to what happens at various parts of the nephron, as each part of the tubule has different functions.

Glomerular filtration (GF)

GF occurs across the membranes of the glomerulus and Bowman's capsule, and is determined by:

- Net filtration pressure (NFP) determined by blood pressure in the renal artery between the range of 65–180 mmHg
- Glomerular filtration rate (GFR):
    - Total surface area available for filtration
    - Filtration membrane permeability
    - Net filtration pressure

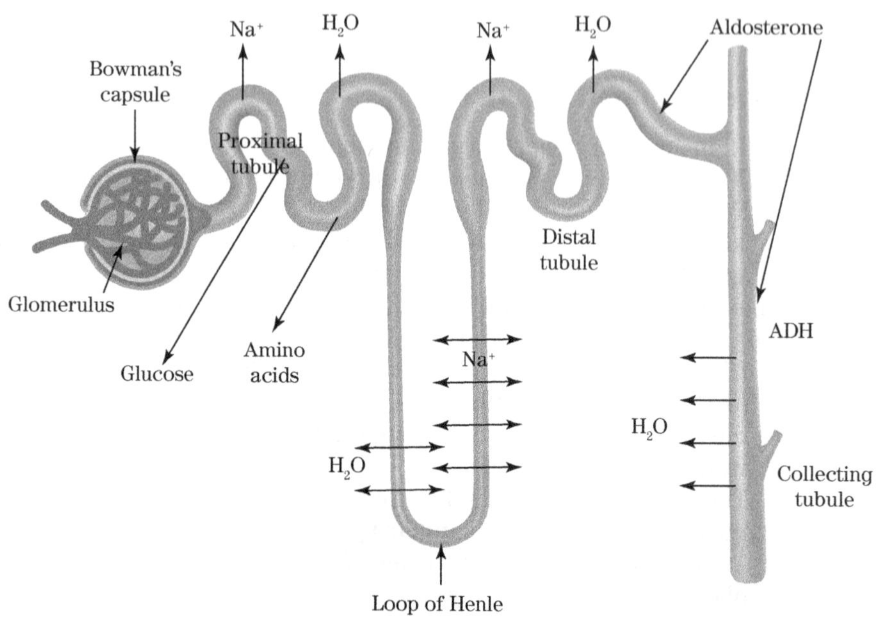

Structure of glomerulus	**Proximal tubule**	**Loop of Henle**	**Distale tubule**	**Collecting tubule**
Function is filtration	Reabsorption of: NaCl (majority), Glucose K^+ Amino acids HCO_3^- PO_4^- Protein Urea H_2O (ADH not required) Secretion of: H^+, Foreign substances, organic anions, organic cations	Concentration of urine (a counter-current mechanism) Descending loop water reabsorption NaCl diffuses in Ascending loop Na^+ reabsorbed (active transport) water stays in Urea secretion	Reabsorption of: NaCl H_2O (ADH required) HCO_3^- Secretion of: K^+ Urea H^+ NH_3^+ Some drugs	Reabsorption of: H_2O (ADH required) Reabsorption or secretion of: Na^+ K^+ H^+ NH_3^+ Urea secretion in medulla
Tonicity of fluid within ducts	Isotonic	Isotonic Hypertonic Hypotonic	Isotonic or hypotonic	Final concentration

Figure 14.3 Glomerular filtration, tubular secretion and tubular reabsorption

- The filtrate consists of water and salts, no protein or other large molecules/cells
- 1.3 L/min of blood passes through the kidney, 127 ml/min of fluid plus salts pass through the pores = GFR
- In 24 hours 170–200 L of filtrate formed, but only 1.5–2 L of urine passed
- 99% of filtrate is reabsorbed
- Regulation of GFR if threatened is maintained by increasing systemic blood pressure using the following mechanisms:
  - Renin-angiotensin-aldosterone (RAA) mechanism (see below)
  - Stress response via the sympathetic nervous system (SNS).

Tubular re-absorption

Tubular re-absorption takes place in:

- The proximal (first) convoluted tubule
  - Most of the tubule contents are quickly reclaimed and returned to the blood, water and many other ions are continuously regulated in response to hormonal signals:
    - All nutrients glucose, amino acids, vitamins; and bicarbonate and chloride are reabsorbed here
    - Sodium and potassium blood levels maintained by the RAA mechanism
    - Calcium is regulated by two hormones:
      - Parathyroid hormone (PTH) stimulated when there is a reduction in serum calcium levels
      - Calcitonin is released when there is a high serum calcium
    - Urea, creatinine and uric acid
- The distal (second) convoluted tubule further absorption of:
  - Water influenced by ADH
  - Sodium influenced by aldosterone
  - Chloride.

Tubular secretion

Tubular secretion is effectively re-absorption in reverse composed of both filtered and secreted substances, mostly hydrogen ions:

- The proximal (first) convoluted tubule
  - Disposes of substances not already in the filtrate, such as certain drugs (penicillin and phenobarbital)
  - Eliminating undesirable substances that have been reabsorbed by passive processes e.g. urea and uric acid
- The distal (second) convoluted tubule further absorption of:
  - Potassium influenced by aldosterone

  - Hydrogen and ammonium ions in exchange for sodium, which is then available for reabsorption:
    - Acidification of the urine
    - Conservation of body sodium.

Urine output (UO)

- The kidney receives about 25% of the cardiac output and determines GFR, which is dependent on an adequate renal perfusion
- The process of passing urine or emptying the bladder is called micturition also known as voiding or urination
- Occurs generally when about 200 ml of urine has collected in the bladder activating stretch receptors
- When tissue perfusion is adequate the production of urine will exceed 0.5 ml/kg per hour or around 1.5 to 2 L/day. The minimum urine output is equal or less than 30 ml/hour, some practitioners prefer 50–70 ml/hour (Edwards and Sabato, 2009). When tissue perfusion is adequate urine production will exceed 0.5 ml/kg per hour – 30–70 ml or more/hr
- When blood flow to the kidneys is reduced vasoconstriction occurs – GFR decreases, reducing UO
- If there are concerns about the patient's kidney function, overall fluid and electrolyte balance, quality of urine and circulatory status, then urinary output should be measured at regular intervals and accurately recorded.

Monitoring of urine output

- The significance of fluid balance charts and measuring a patient's urine:
  - Fluid intake (IV, oral, or enteral feeding)
  - Fluid output (urine, wound/chest drains, vomiting, diarrhoea, insensible loss)
  - A balance between the two can either be negative or positive over a 24-hour period and has implications for the patient's condition:
    - Positive fluid overload, heart failure
    - Negative can indicate dehydration, hypovolaemia, bleeding, third space fluid shift
- UO reduces during:
  - Stress to increase BP
  - Loss of circulating volume
  - Renal failure, hypoxic injury to the kidney e.g. acute tubular necrosis (ATN), retention

    - Heart failure following on from conditions such as left ventricular failure (LVF), acute coronary syndromes (ACS), and myocardial infarction (MI)
- UO increases:
    - In diabetes insipidus inability of the pituitary gland to excrete adequate anti-diuretic hormone (ADH)
    - Diuretic phase of renal failure
    - Following the administration of diuretics
    - In hypothermia (massive diuresis, due to extreme cold)
- A catheter monitors kidney function, if UO falls below 30 ml per hour, fluid administration may be necessary
- When there is an increase in fluid administration causing hypervolaemia (fluid overload), cardiac failure and pulmonary oedema may occur – kidney function may also become impaired, due to:
    - Reduction in the pumping action of the heart
    - Reduced cardiac output
    - Reduced blood flow to the kidneys
- In dehydrated or hypovolaemic states the kidneys restore extracellular fluid volume and increase BP
- UO should be measured, either at hourly intervals via a catheter or from a bedpan or bottle, and recorded
- Interpretation of UO should also consider overall fluid balance (positive or negative over a 24-hour period), the quality and colour of urine
- This elaborate set of interlinked processes involves the renin-angiotensin-alderosterone system, osmoreceptors and baroreceptors.

Homeostatic control by the kidneys

Homeostatic control by the kidney is fluid and electrolyte balance, and can conceal the signs of dehydration, hypo- or hypervolaemia (fluid overload) and prevent renal failure. The re-absorption of fluid and electrolytes is adjusted to meet the needs of the body by the action of hormones. The major hormones involved in this process are antidiuretic hormone (ADH), released by the posterior pituitary and aldosterone, secreted by the adrenal cortex.

Anti-diuretic hormone (ADH)

The release of anti-diuretic hormone (ADH) by the posterior pituitary is regulated by the osmoreceptors in the hypothalamus. These receptors are stimulated by:

- An increase in the osmolarity of the blood (determined by an increase in sodium in relation to water), as in dehydration

- A decrease in osmolarity (determined by a reduction in sodium in relation water), as in the administration of too much intravenous crystalloid fluid.

The ADH released in response to dehydration and promotes the re-absorption of water from the renal tubules, resulting in:

- The retention of water
- Dilution of the blood sodium
- A decrease in the osmolarity of the blood back to the normal level
- The excretion of a small volume of highly concentrated (hypertonic) urine (e.g. with a high specific gravity).

Aldosterone

The secretion of aldosterone by the adrenal cortex may be stimulated by:

- An increase in blood potassium (e.g. over-infusion of potassium chloride)
- A decrease in blood sodium (reduced blood osmolarity), blood volume or BP (e.g. haemorrhage)
- An increase in blood potassium directly stimulates the adrenal cortex to secrete aldosterone.

A decrease in blood sodium, blood volume and BP indirectly affects aldosterone secretion by stimulating the kidneys to secrete the enzyme renin into the blood (Figure 4.2):

- Renin released by the juxtaglomerulus apparatus in the kidney is immediately:
  - Catalysed by angiotensinogens that leads to a the formation of angiotensin I
  - Angiotensin I is converted into angiotensin II by the angiotensin converting enzyme (ACE)
  - Stimulating the release of aldosterone from the adrenal cortex
- Aldosterone promotes:
  - The reabsorption of sodium from the glomerular filtrate into the blood, in exchange for potassium, which is secreted from the blood back into the renal tubules
  - When sodium ions are reabsorbed, water follows passively owing to the osmotic gradient that is created
- Angiotensin II has two other major effects:
  - Enhances the release of noradrenaline, thus stimulating vasoconstriction and thereby increasing the blood pressure further
  - Stimulates the release of ADH from the pituitary gland.

The net effect

- When kidney blood supply or blood pressure is threatened:
  - There is an increase in vasoconstriction, causing the circulating blood flow to the kidneys to be reduced
  - The blood pressure and GFR decreases, reducing urinary output
  - Stimulating both the osmoreceptors and the release of renin to prevent further loss of water and electrolytes from the circulation
- Administration of IV fluid challenge can, prevent damage to kidney function there will be:
  - Reduced nervous stimulation to the osmoreceptors and a decrease in the production of renin, to increase the GFR, urine production and thus urine output.
  - An over administration of IV fluids can lead to fluid overload, LVF, pulmonary oedema, heart failure, stimulating the release of renin worsening fluid overload.

Normal urine constituents

A normal sample of urine has a pH of 4.5–8 with no detectable glucose, protein or blood. The concentration of sodium, potassium or other ions depends on dietary intake. The kidney has a role in maintaining a balanced internal environment, and therefore, will adjust the amount of constituents in the urine according to their concentration in the body. Excess of any one substance will result in an increased amount appearing in the urine to maintain equilibrium in the body, thus an examination of the constituents of the urine will give an indication of the general state of health (see below).

THE PATHOPHYSIOLOGY OF RENAL FAILURE

Renal function can be affected by a variety of disorders; the most common is an infection. The urinary tract can be obstructed by kidney stones or by a tumour from inside or outside the renal system. Renal function can also be impaired by disorders of the kidney itself or by many other systemic diseases. Because the kidney filters the blood, it is directly linked to every other organ system including the heart. Therefore, conditions that lead to renal failure can be life threatening. A simple urine test can be an early indicator of disease, as changes in the urine may occur before other symptoms develop.

Urine testing for disease

Urine examination can yield important information about the early signs of disease, as many life-threatening conditions of insidious onset such as diabetes, cancer of the bladder or renal disease may be revealed by the analysis of the constituents of the urine. Taking notice of some of the areas measured in routine urine test helps to provide valuable clues to the patient's condition or the effectiveness of treatment. Some clues suggesting a preliminary urine test may be required can be viewed in Table 14.1.

> **Practice point**
>
> The significance of urine testing can be found in the specific gravity, pH or whether blood, protein, bilirubin and urobilinogen, nitrates, glucose and ketones are present (Table 14.2).

Appearance

The appearance of the urine should be noted for colour and clarity (Table 14.3):

- Colour changes may be due to endogenous pigments such as haemoglobin (red or red/brown colour), bilirubin (yellow) or intact red cells (smoky red)
- Exogenous pigments may also cause colour changes: red-coloured urine may be due to eating beetroot or to contamination with menstrual blood
- Orange discolouration may be due to the pigments found in some laxatives and a blue/green colour may be caused by ethylene blue in some proprietary medicines.

Symptom or sign	Possible diagnosis	Tests to consider
Weight loss, perhaps with an increase in thirst	? Diabetes	Look for glucose and ketones
Frequency of micturition	? Infection	Test for bacteria (i.e. indicated by the presence of nitrites) or protein
	? Renal disease	Test for specific gravity and protein
Yellow tinge to skin	? Jaundice	Test for urobilinogen and urine bilirubin

Table 14.1 Clues suggesting preliminary urine tests are required

Urine test	Significance	Measure	Condition
Specific gravity (SG) to determine hydration and the amount of waste products to be excreted	To determine if hydration is adequate.	SG varies between 1,005 and 1,035	Low SG – diabetes insipidus (dilute urine) Increase SG dehydration (concentrated urine)
The pH reflects acid-base balance of the body	Excess hydrogen or bicarbonate ions are excreted by the tubules to maintain the normal blood pH.	Urine has a pH of around 6 (range from about 5–8.5).	Metabolic acidosis Renal calculi prevented by adjusting pH UTI proteinurea + alkaline pH – bacterial infection
Blood	The presence of blood is serious rapid investigation	Should not appear in the urine The blood will disappear with resolution of the infection, or stone	Earliest sign of cancer of the bladder Trauma, infection or stones, glomerulonephritis, polycystic disease or warfarin excess
Protein early renal disease, glomerulus and tubules may leak small amounts of protein into the urine	As renal disease progresses, detectable levels of protein will be found in the urine	Proteinuria an early sign of disease Monitoring the progress of disease or response to therapy	Renal disease, UTI, hypertension, pre-eclampsia heart failure, diabetes with nephropathy, nephrotic syndrome, systemic lupus erythematosis (SLE), and myeloma
Bilirubin and urobilinogen	Red blood cells are broken down after about 28 days; waste products excreted 98% as bilirubin in bile via the bile duct	Bilirubin is not found in the urine	Liver disease e.g. bilirubin or its metabolites can be found in the urine

Table 14.2 Urine testing

Urine test	Significance	Measure	Condition
	The other 2% excreted in the urine as urobilinogen (is normally present in urine)	Urobilinogen should appear in the urine	Elevated levels can indicate liver abnormalities or excessive destruction of red blood cells, such as in haemolytic anaemia
Nitrates	Urine normally contains nitrates from dietary metabolites, and some of the common bacteria responsible for urinary infections will convert these nitrates to nitrites	Nitrates are not normally present in urine Visible sign is the specimen clear or cloudy? If clear and blood, protein, leukocytes and nitrates are not present, you can be sure there is not a UTI	Nitrates are produced in increasing numbers when gram negative bacteria such as E. coli convert dietary nitrates (found in the preservatives n meat products and cheese and smoked food) to nitrites
Glucose	Valuable in monitoring diabetes and complications secondary to prolonged hyperglycaemia	Not normally found in urine	It can be associated with many medical conditions such as diabetes mellitus, stress, sepsis, Cushing's syndrome, renal tubular disease, corticosteroids, and acute pancreatitis
Ketones	When the body metabolises fat waste, the breakdown products are the ketone bodies, which are excreted in the urine	Quantities are detectable in urine Ketones are acidic substances and when present in excess can lead to metabolic acidosis	Usually ketones found in people who are fasting, and with uncontrolled diabetes

Table 14.2 Continued

Colour	Cause
Yellow-orange to brownish green	Bilirubin from obstructive jaundice
Red to red-brown	Haemoglobinuria
Smoky red	Unhaemolysed RBCs from urinary tract
Dark wine colour	Haemolytic jaundice
Brown-black	Melanin pigment from melanoma
Dark brown	Liver infections, pernicious anaemia, malaria
Green	Bacterial infection (*Pseudomonas aeruginosa*)

Table 14.3 Appearance of urine and cause

Odour

The odour of a urine specimen should be noted:

- Normal, freshly voided urine has very little smell, but develops an ammonia-like smell when left standing exposed to air
- Infected urine smells foul and may have a characteristic fishy smell on voiding and the smell worsens on standing
- Substances such as acetone excreted by diabetics with ketoacidosis, or in patients who have been starving or suffering from anorexia, gives urine a characteristic smell. Eating fish, curry or other strongly flavoured foodstuffs can also make the urine smell.

The urinary system plays an important role in transporting, storing and eliminating waste products as urine from the body. Other organs e.g. the heart and liver contribute in many ways. Therefore, any changes in urine can be a good indication of developing disease not only in the kidney but in other organs as well, long before other symptoms occur. It is imperative that HCPs view urinalysis and urine output as a valuable contribution to the overall knowledge and assessment of their patients' condition.

Generalised causes of renal failure

Inflammation (see Figure 2.3)

- Infection usually bacterial
- Obstruction from kidney stones
- Tumours.

Reduced blood supply to the kidneys (see Figure 2.2)

- Hypoxic damage
- Acute tubular necrosis (ATN)
- Hypovolaemia.

Urinary tract infection (UTI)

An infection of the urinary tract, highlighted in the case of Carole:

> **Case study 14.1**
>
> Carole is a 55-year-old woman who enjoys eating and has a body mass index >30 kg/m^2. Recently passing urine has become very painful. Her GP diagnoses a urinary tract infection (UTI). To treat the pain and inflammation she is prescribed a non-steroidal anti-inflammatory drug (NSAID). The GP also sends a midstream urine sample for culture and sensitivity. Depending upon the result of this test she may be prescribed antibiotics.

Aetiology

- Inflammation of the urinary epithelium
- Usually caused by bacteria from gut flora from retrograde movement into urethra and bladder.

Pathology

- Inflammation of the bladder is the most common site
- More common in women
- Common organisms
  - *Escherichia coli* 80–90%
  - *Klebsiella, proteus and enterobacter cloacae* 5%
  - *Pseudomonas*
  - *Staphylococcus saprohphticus* – remaining 10–5%
- The different types of UTI need to be identified to determine appropriate treatments (Naish and Hallam, 2007)
  - Asymptomatic bacteria – the absence of symptoms, the evidence of infection is provided by urinalysis, common in pregnant women, patients with diabetes and older adults, can lead to symptomatic invasive disease
  - Symptomatic bacteria – gives symptoms of UTI
  - Uncomplicated UTI – infection of the bladder (cystitis) or kidney (glomerulonephritis, pyelonephritis) without structural or

functional abnormality of the urinary tract, can occur in healthy individuals

- Complicated UTI – is an infection in the presence of one or more of the conditions of acute kidney injury (AKI) detailed below.

Clinical features

- Dysuria
- Frequency of micturition
- Urgency of micturition
- Loin pain
- Blood in the urine
- Pyrexia
- Abdominal pain
- Offensive smelling urine
- Cloudy urine.

Investigation

- Diagnosed by microscopy, culture and sensitivity (mc & s) of specific organisms
  - Counts of 100,000 bacteria/ml of freshly voided urine
- Can occur anywhere along the urinary tract
- Urinalysis – pH indicate the presence of calculi, specific gravity the presence of dehydration.

Treatment and drug therapy

- If asymptomatic no treatment may be required
- If symptomatic treatment with micro-organism specific antibiotics.

> **Practice point**
>
> Patients with UTIs should be encouraged to drink fluids; an increase in urine output will serve to excrete the bacteria from the system.

Acute kidney injury (AKI)

The term 'acute kidney injury' was previously known as 'acute renal failure' (Murphy and Byrne, 2010). It stipulates that an increase in serum urea and creatinine does not mean failure of the kidneys, but a dysfunction that may or may not lead to failure (Vijayan, 2008).

Classification system for AKI

This is known as the RIFLE system using grades of severity risk, injury, failure, loss and end stage kidney failure (Bagshaw *et al*, 2008):

- **R**isk – increased serum creatinine (SGr) x 1.5 baseline or GFR decreases ≥25%, urinary output <0.5 ml/kg/hr for 6 hours
- **I**njury – increased SGr x 2 baseline or GFR decreases ≥50%, urinary output <0.5 ml/kg/hr for 12 hours
- **F**ailure – increased SGr x 3 baseline or GFR decreases ≥75% or SGr ≥354 μmol/L with an acute rise of at least 44 micro mol/L, urine output <0.3 ml/kg/hr for 24 hours or anuria for 12 hours
- **L**oss – persistent acute renal failure – complete loss of kidney function >4 weeks
- **E**nd stage kidney disease (ESKD) – >3 months.

Pre-renal failure

Pre-renal failure is a reaction to renal hypoperfusion:

- Failure of blood supply to kidneys, which effects the arteriolar blood volume and the kidneys are deprived of blood flow (hypovolaemia):
  - Reduced effective circulating volume (ascites, oedema, inflammation, heart failure)
  - Altered vascular capacity (sepsis, shunting, vasodilation)
- Decrease in cardiac output (CO)
  - Myocardial infarction (MI)
  - Pulmonary embolism (PE)
  - Heart failure (HF)
- Hypotension
  - Gastrointestinal loss (vomiting, diarrhoea)
  - Haemorrhage
  - Fluid loss (diuretics, laxatives)
  - Skin loss (excessive sweating, burns).

A decline in perfusion can lead to intrinsic or intrarenal failure (Blackeley, 2008).

Intrarenal (intrinsic) renal failure

Intrarenal failure occurs as a result in injury to the kidney itself or nearby vasculature:

- Tubular necrosis occurs due to extreme pre-renal failure e.g. sepsis, pancreatitis, haemorrhagic shock

Referred to as an acute tubular necrosis (ATN) caused by:

- Ischaemic – due to prolonged pre-renal failure

- Nephrotoxic changes – due to:
    - Nephrotoxic drugs like aminoglycoside antibiotics, radio contrast dye, ethylene glycol (antifreeze) and anaesthetics
    - Endogenous toxins such as incompatible blood transfusions
- Glomerular such as glomerulonephritis an inflammation of the glomerulus, which can be acute, rapidly progressive or chronic, caused by:
    - Immune responses
    - Toxins or drugs
    - Vascular disorders
    - Systemic diseases e.g. systemic lupus erythematosis (SLE)
    - Can lead to nephrotic syndrome
        - Excretion of at least 3.5 g protein in urine per day
        - Hypoproteinaemia, hyperlipidaemia and oedema
        - Caused by loss of plasma proteins across the injured glomerular filtration membrane
        - Reduced protein leads to oedema
        - Treatment involves normal-protein, low-fat diet, salt restriction, diuretics, steroids, occasionally albumin replacement
    - Interstitial due to autoimmune, toxic, infectious, sometimes referred to as acute interstitial nephritis (AIN) and can be drug induced inflammation (antibiotics, diuretics, NSAIDs, anticonvulsants, allopurinol) (Faubel *et al*, 2008)
    - Vascular when large or small vessels may be involved.

Post-renal failure

Post-renal failure is due to an obstruction that can occur anywhere along the renal tract due to structural abnormalities to the kidneys such as blockage of the urinary outflow. Can last up to 6 weeks. The structral abnormalities can be intrinsic or extrinsic:

- Intrinsic
    - Renal stones – formed from calcium loading in the urethra. This can lead to an obstruction anywhere in the urinary tract and renal colic, in Edward's case:

Case study 14.2

Edward is a 35-year-old man who has presented with severe left loin pain. This is unrelieved by support and positioning. A urinalysis is performed which reveals haematuria and proteinuria. Renal colic is diagnosed.

- Tumours
  - Neural lesions interrupt innervations of the bladder
  - Renal cell carcinoma is a common neoplasm, transitional cell carcinoma of the renal pelvis and ureter, and carcinoma of the bladder
  - Bladder tumours have a high rate of recurrence
  - Clinical features
    - Frank haematuria
    - Loin pain
    - Loin mass
    - Weight loss, hypertension, anaemia, fatigue and peripheral oedema
  - Investigations
    - CT renal scan
    - Intravenous urogram (IVU)
    - Blood pressure
  - Treatment
    - Surgery – radical nephrectomy
    - Radiotherapy and/or chemotherapy
    - Metastases to the liver, lung, bone.

- Extrinsic
  - Surrounding or infiltrating tumour
  - Large inflammatory abdominal aortic aneurysm.

The obstruction resulting from intrinsic and extrinsic post-renal failure leads to a collection of urine behind the obstruction, affecting surrounding organs leading to inflammation and ischaemic atrophy. The severity of the obstruction is dependent on:

- Location with the urinary tract
- Unilateral or bilateral
- Partial or complete – GFR reduced or zero
- Acute or chronic duration – chronic partial obstruction causes compression of kidney structures reducing renal ability
- The underlying cause.

The relief of a renal obstruction is followed by a variable period of diuresis, with losses of large amounts of urine:

- Lasts for a few days
- Usually without symptoms of volume depletion
- Check for fluid and electrolyte imbalances if there is a rapid post obstructive diuresis.

Clinical features of AKI

- Asymptomatic
- Oliguria
- Increasing blood urea and creatinine
- Hyperkalaemia – K^+ levels >6.5 mmol/L (less if showing EGG changes)
- Nausea and vomiting
- Confusion
- Loss of appetite
- Metabolic acidosis.

Investigations of AKI

- Urinalysis – protein, pH, specific gravity
- Bloods for:
  - Biochemistry
  - Haematology
  - Immunology – antibodies
  - Virology – Hep B and C, HIV
- Radiology
- Renal biopsy.

Treatments of AKI

- Correct the primary disorder
- Remove the obstruction
- Correction of fluid and electrolyte disorders
- Prevention of infection
- Maintain optimal nutrition
- Systemic effects of uraemia
- Correct metabolic acidosis
- Education and support to the patient and family
- Renal replacement therapy initiated if other treatments are ineffective (see below for more information).

Chronic kidney disease (CKD)

Chronic kidney disease is a permanent loss of kidney function (Redmond and McCelland, 2006). It cannot be cured, but interventions can be instigated that slow its progress and improve symptoms.

Aetiology

- Any of the causes from pre-, intra- and post-renal causes
- Other conditions include:

- Diabetes mellitus
- Chronic pyelonephritis – an infection of the renal pelvis, acute or chronic (persistent or recurrent)
  - Cause is usually bacterial, but can be due to fungi or viruses
  - Generally spread by ascending organism along the ureters, but may occur via the bloodstream
  - Responds well to 2 weeks of organism-specific antibiotics
- Polycystic kidneys
- Hypertension.

Pathology

There are a number of stages that patients with progressive renal failure follow before reaching the need for renal replacement therapy (Redmond and McCelland, 2006):

- Stage 1 – chronic kidney disease with normal GFR >90 ml/min/1.73 m^2
- Stage 2 – mild chronic kidney disease with decrease in GFR 60–90 ml/min/1.73 m^2
- Stage 3 – moderate chronic kidney disease 30–59 ml/min/1.73 m^2
- Stage 4 – severe chronic kidney disease 15–29 ml/min/1.73 m^2
- Stage 5 – established renal failure <15 or on dialysis.

Patients at stages 1–3 chronic kidney disease can be asymptomatic and few will require dialysis. Those patients in stages 4–5 are at a greater risk of hypertension, cardiovascular disease and premature death.

Treatment and drug therapies

- Control cause such as diabetes, ischaemic heart disease, hypertension, alcohol consumption
- Maintain nutrition levels, regular weight and body mass index (BMI), nutritional assessment
- Blood and urine analysis
  - Check haemoglobin for anaemia
  - Electrolytes e.g. sodium, potassium and calcium
  - Creatinine and urea
  - Urine testing for protein
  - Arterial blood gases for pH balance
- Fluid and electrolyte balance
  - Potassium – ECG changes
  - Sodium
  - Mainly through diet
  - Phosphate and calcium balance

    - Fluid and diet intake is strictly controlled
    - Fluid input and output
    - Acidosis
        - Metabolic acidosis begins to develop when GFR decreases by 30–40%
        - Maintained by respiratory system removal of carbon dioxide
- Renal replacement therapy
    - Haemofiltration
        - Usually continuous
        - Less traumatic to the circulation
    - Renal dialysis
        - Intermittent
        - Traumatic to the circulation and reduces BP
        - Home dialysis is available so may opt to self-manage
    - Peritoneal dialysis
        - Intermittent generally at home at night, but may involve at least 3 more during the day
        - Managed by the patient
    - Transplantation has varied success, improvements have been shown using live donors.

There are a number of broader issues to consider in relation to caring for a patient with AKI e.g when to stop dialysis and instigate end of life care

End stage kidney disease (ESKD)

This is terminal renal failure as in Jenny's case:

Case study 14.3

Jenny is a 65-year-old woman who has had chronic renal failure for over 10 years and has been using overnight peritoneal dialysis at home. She has been on the renal transplant waiting list since she was 55 years old and it is unlikely that at her age she is going to get a satisfactory match.

For Jenny this is a difficult time and careful planning and palliative care issues may need to be considered.

However, renal failure accounts for a small group of patients' deaths:

- Death can sometimes be easy to predict because dialysis has been discontinued
- They can suffer from pain during the last days and this underscores the necessity for medical and nursing staff to be skilled providers of modern palliative care

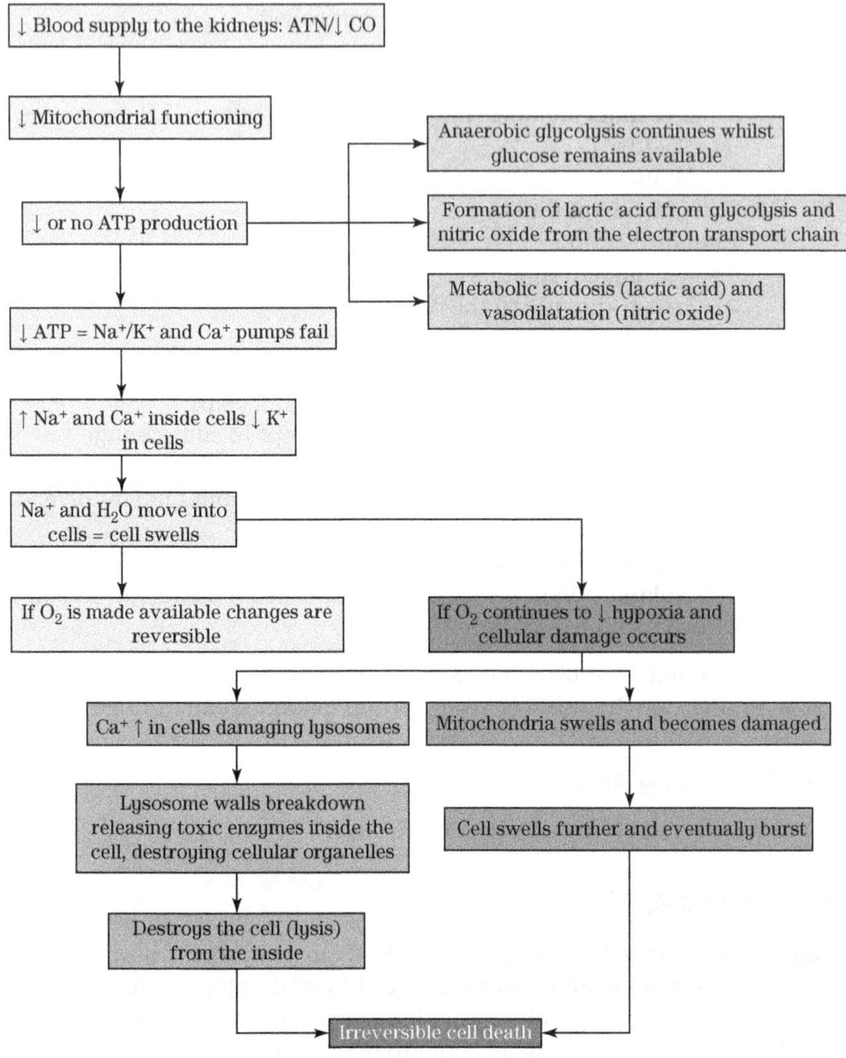

Figure 14.4 Hypoxic death of the kidney

- If the symptoms of ESRF are poorly managed this leads to misery at the end of life
- Knowledge of palliative care in these instances is essential.

Inflammation and reduced blood supply can cause damage to renal function, e.g MI as outlined in the case below:

Case study 14.4

George is a 65-year-old man with a past medical history of unstable angina and a heart condition. He was admitted after being found wandering in the local shopping centre in a confused state, holding his chest and groaning as if in severe pain. George had suffered an inferior myocardial infarction (MI) with changes on his 12 lead ECG in leads II, III and AVF. During the acute episode of his MI, George's blood pressure dropped for a short period to below 60/40.

CONCLUSION

The kidneys and internal structures transport, store and eliminate waste from the body as urine. Other organ systems contribute to healthy function of the kidneys such as the heart (providing adequate pressure for GF) and the lungs (as together they maintain acid base balance). Without kidney function, excessive fluids, wastes and electrolytes accumulate in the blood, which harm cells and affect body processes. The processes stimulated are the IIR and reduction in blood supply leading to hypoxia and cellular death (Figure 14.4). These occur in a number of conditions such as a urinary obstruction, urinary tract infections, glomerular disorders, drug overdose or other disorders. The diagnosis of renal failure is a life-changing event and HCP need to offer support, as the end result can be fatal.

SELF-ASSESSMENT QUESTIONS

1. Provide an outline of the renal system from the two kidneys, the ureters, bladder and into the urethra.
2. Describe the anatomy of the kidney and nephron.
3. Identify the different parts of the nephron responsible for filtration, re-absorption and secretion.
4. Track the blood supply from the heart through to the kidney.
5. Compare the male urethra with the female urethra.
6. List the functions of the kidney.
7. List several abnormal urine components, and name the condition when each is present in detectable amounts.
8. List several changes that may occur to the urinary system anatomy and physiology.

REFERENCES

Bagshaw, S.M., George, C. and Bellomo, R. (ANZICS database management committee) (2008) A comparison of the RIFLE and AKIN criteria for acute kidney injury in critically ill patients, *Nephrology, Dialysis and Transplant*, 23(5), 1569–1574.

Blackeley, S. (ed) (2008) *Renal Failure and Replacement Therapies*, London: Springer.

Edwards, S. and Sabato, M. (2009) *A Nurse's Survival Guide to Critical Care*, Edinburgh: Churchill Livingstone Elsevier.

Faubel, S., Cronin, R.E. and Edelstein, C.L. (2008) The patient with acute renal failure, in R.W. Schrier (ed) *Manual of Nephrology*, 7th edn, Philadelphia: Lippincott Williams & Wilkins.

Murphy, F. and Byrne, G. (2010) The role of the nurse in the management of acute kidney injury, *British Journal of Nursing*, 19(3), 146–152.

Naish, W. and Hallam, M. (2007) Urinary tract infection: diagnosis and management for nurses, *Nursing Standard*, 21(23), 50–57.

Redmond, A. and McCelland, H. (2006) Chronic kidney disease: risk factors, assessment and nursing care, *Nursing Standard*, 20(10), 48–55.

Smith, G. (2012) *ALERT: A Multi-professional Course in Care of the Acutely In Patient*, 3rd edn, Portsmouth: Portsmouth Hospital NHS Trust.

Vijayan, A. (2008) Overview of the management of acute kidney injury and acute tubular necrosis, in D. Windus, (ed) *The Washington Manual Subspecialty Consult Series, Nephrology Subspecialty Consult*, Philadelphia: Williams and Wilkins.

15 The reproductive system

Sharon Edwards

THE ANATOMY OF THE REPRODUCTIVE SYSTEM

Male reproductive system

The organs of the male reproductive system are the testes and its ducts, the prostate gland and penis. The urethra is important as it acts as a duct for both urine and sperm (Figure 15.1).

Penis

- The urethra leaves the prostate and extends into the penis and opens at the tip of the glans penis, which is covered with a fold of skin
- The penis is muscular and consists of erectile tissue used for sexual intercourse.

Testes

- There are two bilateral testes, which lie outside the body in the fold of skin known as the scrotum. Their function is to produce:
  - Sperm (spermatogenesis) necessary for reproduction
  - The hormone testosterone, which stimulates the production of sperm
- The testes are divided into lobules each containing seminiferous tubules, where spermatogenesis takes place
- The seminiferous tubules unite into an opening into the head of the epididymis where the sperm is stored
- Spermatogenesis – is the production of sperm, which is produced in the seminiferous tubules from germ cells called spermatogonia (Blows, 2005)
  - In a healthy male, sperm are produced at a rate of 200–400 million per day
  - Sperm production requires a supply of testosterone and two specialised cells in the testes:

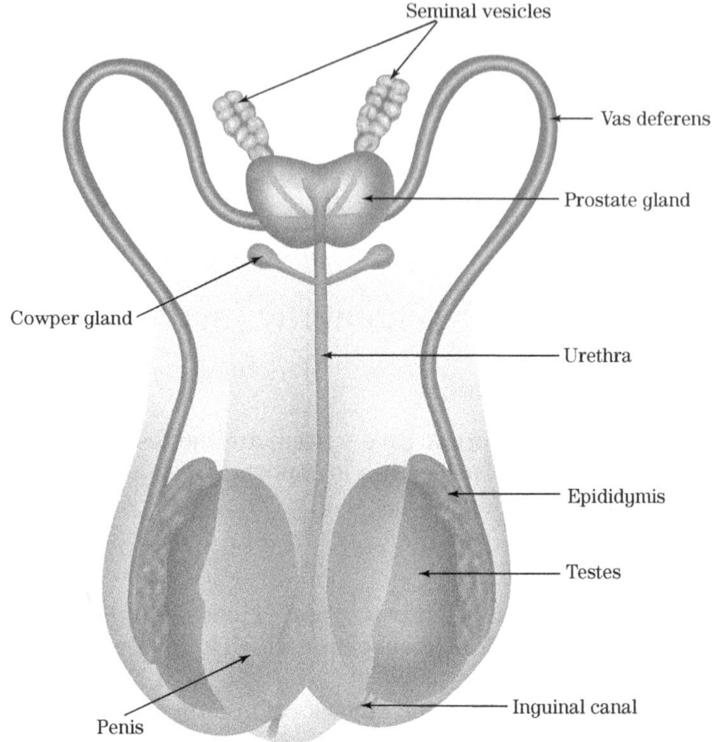

Figure 15.1 The male reproductive organs

- Leydig cells, which produce testosterone and are under the control of the (Intestinal cell-stimulating hormone ICSH released from the anterior pituitary gland)
- Sertoli cells, found in the lining of the seminiferous tubules are under control of the follicle-stimulating hormone (FSH) controlled by the anterior pituitary gland. Sertoli cells also:
  - Form the blood-testes barrier between the outer surface of the tubule (the basal compartment) and the inner lumen of the seminiferous tubule (the adluminal compartment). The fluid in each compartment is different; the inner tubule fluid contains the correct constituents needed for developing sperm, and the blood-testes barrier is needed to maintain the difference
  - Produce the hormone inhibin, which provides a negative feedback mechanism regulating the release of FSH, and ensures the correct concentration of testosterone needed for sperm production

- The ductus deferens are two ducts one from each testes, which extend into the abdomen, over the urinary bladder to join the duct from the seminal vesicles on each side (Figure 15.1):
  - Seminal vesicles – produce fluid, (60% of the component of semen) substance in which sperm is carried. Semen is an alkaline fluid containing sugar and vitamin C for nutrition for the sperm
  - Ejaculatory duct – the ductus deferens join to form a single duct from each side, which extend into the prostate gland on both sides and join with the urethra inside the prostate
- Male hormones are known as androgens and are produced by the adrenal gland, but the main source in males is the testes. Androgens have masculinisation effects e.g. building of muscles and bone (can be misused by athletes) of which there are 3:
  - Testosterone the most potent
  - Dehydroepiandrosterone (DHEA)
  - Androstenedione.

The prostate gland

- The prostate gland lies at the base of the urinary bladder and consists of 3 lobes or zones:
  - The central zone
  - The transitional zone
  - The peripheral zone
- The zones of the prostate gland circle the urethra with the bladder and seminal vesicles, vas deferens and ureters lying behind and above
- The gland consists of minute tubes, which contain prostatic fluid squeezed out by contraction of the muscles during ejaculation
- The gland secretion:
  - Provides liquid that acts as a transport medium and facilitates movement
  - Is a fructose-based nutrient to provide the sperm with energy to continue on their journey
  - Acts as a lubricant
  - Contains chemicals to protect and activate the sperm.

Female reproductive system

The female reproductive system is made up internal and external genital organs. The system has a 28–32 day cycle known as the menstrual cycle, beginning with ovulation and the release of an ovum or egg, which flows down the fallopian tube where if it meets a sperm can become fertilised. If the fertilised egg embeds in thickened lining of the uterus it will form an embryo and later the foetus (McCance and Huether, 2010). If fertilisation does not occur the egg will travel to the uterus and menstruation will occur. There are two breasts made up of glandular tissue, used to produce milk following the delivery of a baby.

The external genitalia (Figure 15.2)

- This consists of the vulva which is divided into the:
  - Mons pubis or veneris is the skin covering the symphysis pubis and is covered in pubic hair
  - Labia majora is the covering of skin over the vestibule
  - Labia minor is the inside part of the labia majora, which encloses the vestibule
  - Clitoris is an erectile organ, which is positioned where the two labia minora meet

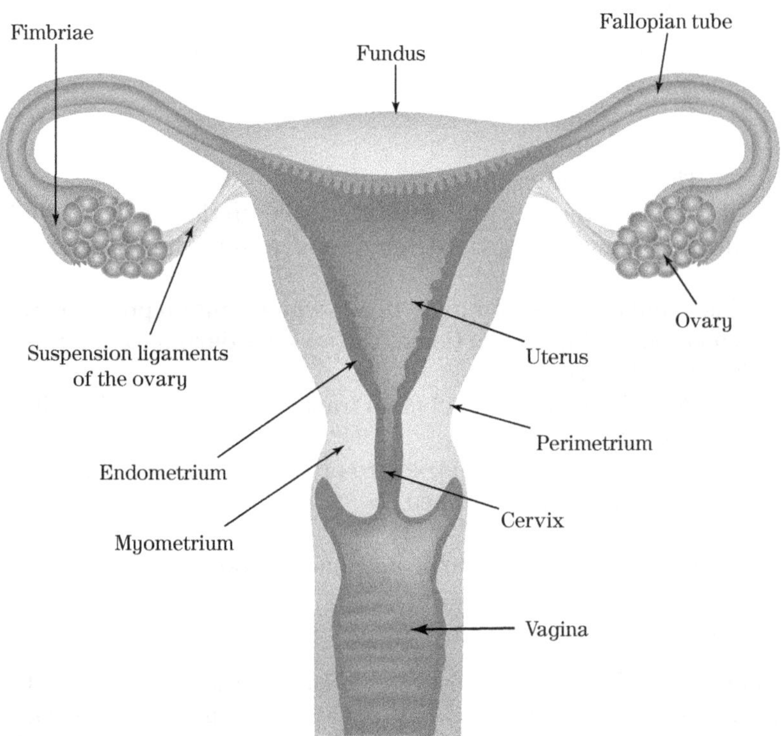

Figure 15.2 The female reproductive organs

  - The vestibule contains the:
    - Urethral opening – for the passage of urine
    - Vaginal opening – positioned posterior to the urethral opening
- Bartholin's and Skene's glands produce lubricating fluid and mucus in response to sexual stimulation and both facilitate and prepare the area for coitus.

The internal genitalia

- Ovaries
  - These are the primary female reproductive organs, which have two main functions:
    - Secretion of female sex hormones
    - Development and release of female ova
  - Each month one mature follicle in the ovary releases a mature ovum, an event referred to as ovulation. After ovulation, the follicle develops into the corpus luteum, whose fate depends on whether it becomes fertilised or not:
    - If fertilisation does not occur, the corpus luteum secretes progesterone and some oestrogen for approximately 10 days and then degenerates, triggering the maturation of another ovum.
    - If fertilised the corpus luteum enlarges and continues to secrete hormones that supports pregnancy for the first 3 months until the placenta takes over
  - The pituitary and thyroid glands regulate ovarian functions and disruption of these can affect fertility and lead to ovarian dysfunction
    - Oestrogen is the most potent female hormone and is principally produced by the ovaries; it is derived from cholesterol obtained in the diet
    - Progesterone is stimulated by luteinising hormone (LH) and released by the corpus luteum; LH is reliant on levels of oestrogen and maintains pregnancy
    - Androgens are primarily male hormones, but a small amount are produced in the ovary and adrenal cortex, and contribute to the changes that occur during puberty
- Fallopian tubes:
  - Link the ovaries to the uterus, one on each side
  - These pass the ova from the follicle of the ovary to the uterine body.
  - Once the ovum has entered the fallopian tubes, cilia and peristalsis move it toward the uterus
  - If fertilisation of the ova by sperm takes place (in the fallopian tube) then the developing cells travel to the uterus and attach themselves to the endometrium and become implanted

  - If fertilisation of the ova does not take place, it continues to travel to the uterus, where it breaks down and is released as part of the normal menstrual cycle
- Uterus
  - The uterus is sometimes referred to as the womb, which is a hollow pear-shaped organ with three layers:
    - Perimetrium – the serous (peritoneal) coat of the uterus
    - Myometrium – the smooth muscle wall
    - Endometrium – the inner lining of glandular cells, which has a rich blood supply and is shed regularly as part of the menstrual cycle
  - The function of the uterus is to:
    - Protect and secure a fertilised ovum
    - Provide an optimal environment while the ovum grows
    - Facilitate the delivery of the foetus at birth
- Cervix
  - The lower part of the uterus is the cervix, which is very small, preventing bacteria and other organisms from entering the vagina
- Vagina
  - The cervix opens into the vagina, which lies between the urethra and part of the bladder and the rectum. The vagina:
    - Allows menstrual fluids to pass out of the body
    - Widens to allow babies to be delivered
    - Receives the penis during sexual intercourse
    - Can defend itself from infections by:
      - Producing an acid which prevents the growth and replication of most bacteria
      - Has a thick epithelial lining
- Breasts
  - The breasts are mainly fatty in youth and glandular in adults; breast cancer is commonly associated with glandular tissue
  - Each breast consists of between 15–20 sections or lobes, which contain smaller sections called lobules composing of glandular cells which, following childbirth, secrete milk
  - The glandular cells each have small drainage ducts that join at the nipple.

Physiological changes in pregnancy

The changes that occur during pregnancy are normal to allow survival of the foetus. However, these changes can lead to serious complications that can be life threatening e.g. adult respiratory distress syndrome (ARDS), myocardial infarction, deep vein thrombosis (DVT) and pulmonary embolism (PE) (Edwards, 1998).

Respiratory changes during pregnancy

- These respiratory alterations during pregnancy occur gradually, beginning in early pregnancy and continuing throughout gestation (Edwards, 1998):
  - The change in tidal volume, the volume of gas that is exchanged with each breath, progressively increases and begins in the first trimester
  - The diaphragm elevates about 4 cm, causing a decrease in the length of the lungs
  - The minute ventilation increases by 50% by term because of the increase in respiratory rate of 15% and tidal volume by 30–40%, thus decreasing the arterial carbon dioxide tension ($PaCO_2$)
  - This results in an increase in ventilation and decrease in arterial partial pressure of carbon dioxide to about 27 to 32 mm Hg (3–5 kPa)
  - The pH is not altered from the non-pregnant level of about 7.35 to 7.45
  - Oxygen demand and consumption are greater resulting in a reduction in arterial partial pressure of oxygen (PaO_2)
  - The functional residual capacity and residual volume of the lung are decreased in pregnancy, reducing the ability of the pregnant patient to compensate for any respiratory compromise.

Cardiovascular changes during pregnancy

- Maternal blood volume increases markedly
  - The elevation of oestrogens and progesterone during pregnancy increases plasma renin and aldosterone levels to promote sodium and water retention
  - The increase in total volume for a single pregnancy is between 1000 and 1500 ml; in multiple gestation the increase is greater and the heart increases in size
  - Cardiac output (CO) increases secondary to increased blood volume, but may decrease in the supine position
  - This hypovolaemia of pregnancy ensures adequate perfusion of foetal and maternal needs and is a protective mechanism for blood loss that occurs with delivery
  - The increase in progesterone level decreases systemic vascular resistance (SVR) and produces vasodilation of peripheral vessels
  - Heart rate increases by 10 to 15 beats per minute by the fourteenth week of pregnancy, but mean arterial blood pressure is altered very little

- These haemodynamic alterations are intended to protect the mother and foetus, but consequently impose a 40% increase in maternal cardiac workload. Generally, healthy expectant mothers adjust readily to the cardiovascular changes.

Haematological changes during pregnancy

- Haematological changes are reflected in increases in plasma volume at a proportionately greater rate than erythrocyte volume, resulting in a physiological anaemia of pregnancy, most apparent from the seventh month
- There is an increase in clotting factors and fibrinogen may result in hypercoagulation and thrombus formation in women with decreased mobility, as such both haemoglobin and haematocrit values are lower during pregnancy
- The production of red blood cells (RBC) increase, to deliver more oxygen to cope with the increasing demand required by the organs of the body and developing foetus, but the overall erythrocyte count will decrease because of physiologic haemodilution
- These changes are thought to enhance homeostasis at the time of delivery, but this particular adaptation predisposes the mother to an increased risk of clot formation.

THE PATHOPHYSIOLOGY OF THE REPRODUCTIVE SYSTEM

Male reproductive system conditions

Testicular cancer

The male has 2 testes, which are the site of sperm manufacture. Testicular cancer is malignant changes in the testes tissue and is fatal if left untreated.

Aetiology

There are a number of factors that might lead to testicular cancer:

- Undescended testicle – if a male child's testicles are not in the scrotal sac at birth, they can have a higher risk of testicular cancer
- Family/genetic
- Inguinal hernia/hydrocele
- Trauma – testicular tumours are known to occur following traumatic injury
- Can be metastatic spread from prostatic cancer
- Human immune-virus disease (HIV).

Pathology

- Testicular cancer arises from the germ cells within the lining of the seminiferous tubules (Blows, 2005)
- Testicular cancer falls into 4 main categories:
  - Germ cell tumours, spread can be via the lymph nodes or into the blood to the liver, bone and lung. There are 2 types of germ cell tumours:
    - Seminomas
    - Teratomas
  - Spermatic cord stromal tumours
  - Mixed germ cell tumours
  - Others:
    - Leydig cell tumours
    - Malignant lymphoma
    - Adenomatoid tumours
- There are 4 stages of testicular tumours, used for all types:
  - Stage 1 is when the tumour is confined to the testes
  - Stage 2 is lymph node involvement below the diaphragm
  - Stage 3 is lymph node involvement above the diaphragm
  - Stage 4 indicates the tumour has spread to lungs and liver.

Clinical features

- A painless lump or swelling in 1 of the testes
- Enlargement of one or both of the testes
- Groin or abdominal heaviness
- A dull ache in the scrotum
- Acute pain
- Metastases includes:
  - Back pain may indicate spinal metastases
  - Breathlessness, coughing up blood-stained sputum may suggest metastatic involvement of the lungs
- Differential diagnosis can delay the diagnosis and treatment of testicular cancer:
  - Benign epididymitis
  - Acute orchitis
  - Seminal granuloma which can follow vasectomy.

Investigations

- Testicular self-examination (TSE)
- Ultrasound scan
- Blood test markers:

  - The enzyme placental alkaline phosphatase (PLAP) secreted by gonadocytes
  - The hormone human chorionic gonadotrophin (HCG) secreted by trophoblastic cells
  - Alpha-fetoprotein (AFP) secreted by yolk-sac cells
- Surgical exploration of the testes under a general anaesthetic
- Computerised axial tomography (CT scan) will determine any lymph node involvement and any spread.

Treatment/drug therapy

The type of treatment will depend on the stage and type of the testicular cancer:

- Germ cell tumours:
  - Surgical removal of the tumour
  - Cisplatin has improved the prognosis of germ cell tumours and a cure is possible in most cases
- Other tumours:
  - Surgical removal of the testis (orchidectomy)
  - Chemotherapy as follow up treatment
- Psychological and sociological support
  - Body image, virility and sexuality
  - Infertility issues, relationships
  - The treatment of surgery, radiotherapy and chemotherapy can be disturbing
  - Ongoing care post-operatively and following treatment.

Prostate cancer

Aetiology

- Family/genes
- Chances of prostate cancer increases after the age of 50, but usually occurs after the age of 65
- Dietary factors e.g. high in animal fat and dairy products, low in fruit and vegetables increases the risk.

Pathology

- Prostate cancer is rare in young men, but more common in older men, as it is associated with the ageing process
- Prostate cancer is usually the result of adenocarcinomas derived from glandular tissue

- The cancer is a chaotic mass of rapidly dividing cells
- Benign hypertrophy is common in middle-aged and older men, usually arises in the inner lobe, but malignant changes usually occur in the outer lobe (Johnson, 2004a)
- The grading of prostate cancers uses the tumour node metastasis (TNM) system; an example can be found in Figure 6.1.

Clinical features

- Difficulty and pain on passing urine
- Poor urinary flow with hesitancy
- Involuntary stopping and starting of urination
- Dribbling at the end of micturition
- Feeling that the bladder is not completely empty following voiding
- Frequency and urgency due to bladder instability
- Increasing nocturia
- Haematuria
- If spread there may be pain in the back and pelvis.

Investigations

- Often found by chance in patients who have been offered a transurethral prostatectomy for benign hypertrophy of the prostate
- Blood screening for markers (Blows, 2005):
  - The prostate specific antigen (PSA) a glycoprotein found in the endoplasmic reticulum of prostatic cells, large amounts of which is released into the blood when the gland is diseased. The normal is 4 ng/ml
  - The prostate specific acid phosphatase found in the lysosomes of prostate cells and released into the blood in disease of the gland
- Digital rectal examination (DRE) – a gloved finger is inserted into the rectum, from which an enlarged (benign prostate hyperplasia) or hard and lumpy prostate (tumour) can be felt (Ahmed *et al*, 2007)
- Transrectal ultra sound and prostatic biopsy
- CT scan, magnetic resonance imaging and bone scans may be used to determine the extent of the disease (Johnson, 2004a).

Treatment/drug therapy

- Regular monitoring as if localised the disease rarely progresses significantly over a decade
- Radiotherapy and chemotherapy are considered depending on the individual

Infection *(Pathogen)*	Aetiology	Pathology	Clinical features	Investigations	Treatment and drug therapy
Genital herpes *(Herpes simplex* virus) Most genital herpes is caused by HSV-1	Vaginal or anal sex with infected partner who is shedding the virus Oral sex if partner has cold sores Any skin-to-skin contact, although the virus passes more easily through the moist skin that lines the genitals, mouth and anus	Secondary infections to open lesions In older people, herpes infection can be severe as they already have suppressed immune systems	Following incubation period of 2–20 days: fever, headaches, fatigue, aching muscles, pain, localised itching, sweats, dysuria, urethral discharge, swollen lymph glands Men – lesions of external genitalia Women – lesions on the cervix and urethra Both genders – lesions on anus, mouth, lips, eyes, side of finger nails (whitlow)	Swab from blister to undergo molecular studies *OR* Blood test if symptoms have subsided (ineffective for 3 months after exposure)	Antiviral drugs speed recovery from primary outbreak Virus becomes resident in nervous system and reactivation with clinical symptoms is unpredictable
Genital warts (Human papilloma virus)	Unprotected vaginal, anal or oral sex Skin-to-skin contact, particularly with the thinner skin on the vulva, vagina, cervix or scrotum	Increased rate of cervical and penile cancer	Some HPV infections may be asymptomatic as virus has long incubation period	Examination of warts	Most disappear without treatment, but topical chemical solution, cyrotherapy or diathermy is available for wart removal

Table 15.1 Additional sexually transmitted diseases

Adapted From: McCance and Huether (2010), Marieb (2012)

	Pregnant mothers can pass the virus to their baby during delivery, causing throat ulcers	Urinary retention caused by pain as urine passes over lesions	Warts developing on or around penis, vagina or anus In severe cases, warts appear as large cauliflower-like masses on or around the genital area		
Trichomoniasis *(Trichomonas vaginalis)*	Unprotected vaginal sex or vulva-to-vulva contact Sharing sex toys which have not been cleaned in between Rarely, can be passed on by sharing towels, clothes or hot baths Women can pass infection to baby during vaginal delivery	If left untreated, individuals may be more at risk of becoming infected with HIV	After an incubation period of 1–3 weeks: Women – 5% are asymptomatic Change in vaginal discharge, inflammation and itching in and around the vagina, dysuria, cystitis, discomfort or pain during sex Men – 15–50% are asymptomatic Discharge from urethra, dysuria, itching, burning after urination or ejaculation	Women – pelvic examination and high vaginal swab/smear test Men – urethral swab *OR* First-pass urine sample for culture	Course of antibiotics, usually metronidazole

Table 15.1 Continued

- Prostatectomy may be offered early in the disease, but a radical prostatectomy can lead to impotence and/or urinary incontinence in some men, but can increase survival rate up to 15 years in a high percentage of men (Kirby, 2011)
- Bilateral sub-capsular orchidectomy
- In later disease e.g. when the prostate cancer has advanced:
  - Therapy may be palliative
  - Treatment is designed to contain, shrink and reduce symptoms rather than cure the disease
  - Many of these patients may already have undetectable metastasis
- Hormone therapy can be used with widespread disease, suppressing testosterone secretion or androgen depletion:
  - Cyproterone acetate which reduces prostatic cell growth, but it is hepatotoxic
  - Gosereline antagonises luteinising hormone release and can be prescribed with cyproterone acetate
- Safeguard the individual patient's interests, considering their psychological and sociological needs, taking into consideration:
  - Sexual dysfunction following surgery
  - The slow-growing nature of the cancer
  - Follow-up investigations.

Female reproductive system conditions

Menopause

Aetiology

- Age:
  - Occurs in women aged 45–56 years.
  - From around the age of 35 years the natural cycle becomes less predictable and bleeding may be irregular
  - Can occur at an early age in some women, even as early as 20, described as premature menopause
- Surgery
  - Bilateral oophorectomy
  - Hysterectomy
- Genetic factors
- Autoimmune disease
- Radiotherapy and/or chemotherapy
- Infection.

Pathology

- Oestrogen levels fall, in an attempt to try to stimulate ovarian function and ovum releases more follicle-stimulating hormone (FSH)
- When oestrogen levels fall too low, bleeding will stop altogether (RCN, 2003).

Clinical features

- Hot flushes and night sweats
- Psychological upset e.g. crying at what seems unimportant
- Poor memory and concentration
- Tiredness, mood swings
- Vaginal itching, dryness
- Painful intercourse (dyspareunia)
- Frequency of micturition, urgency, mild stress incontinence.

Investigations

- It is diagnosed by the last menstrual bleed, but the symptoms go on for before and after
- History of mental, urinary and vaginal changes
- Blood tests for oestrogen and FSH.

Treatment

- There is no treatment required, but after the menopause women are more prone to some diseases e.g. osteoporosis and as such need to be monitored
- Hormone replacement therapy:
    - Can help in the short term with hot flushes, sweats and vaginal dryness
    - But there are risks of complications:
        - Heart disease, stroke, DVT
        - Endometrial cancer
        - Breast cancer.

Sexually transmitted diseases

Aetiology

- Gonorrhoea:
    - Caused by a bacterium called gonococcus
    - Transmission is by:
        - Sexual, oral or anal intercourse, finger contact between genitals
        - Rimming (tongue is used to stimulate the anus)

    - Sharing of sex toys that have not been washed or covered with a new condom
  - Mother can pass the infection to her baby at birth, causing conjunctivitis
- Syphilis:
  - Caused by an anaerobic bacteria *Treponema pallidum*
  - Transmitted through:
    - Sexual contact with infected lesions
    - Non-sexual direct contact with syphilitic ulcer
- Chlamydia:
  - Is the most commonly diagnosed STI in genito-urinary medicine (GUM) clinics in the UK (McIntosh, 2008)
  - Transmitted by unprotected vaginal or oral sex
  - Genital contact with infected partner
  - Pregnant mothers can pass infection to baby during delivery
- Human immunodeficiency virus/acquired immunodeficiency syndrome (HIV/AIDS):
  - Unprotected vaginal, anal or oral sex
  - Sharing of sex toys which have come into contact with blood or semen
  - Blood transfusion (particularly before 1985 when blood products were not tested for HIV)
  - Sharing contaminated needles
  - Mother can pass virus to baby during pregnancy, labour and when breastfeeding.

Pathology

- Gonorrhoea:
  - An aerobic gram-negative micro-organism *gonococcus*
  - Can be transported from the cervix into the uterus and fallopian tubes by sperm
  - Can lead to pelvic inflammatory disease
  - Syphilis becomes a systemic disease shortly after infection
  - Progression consists of 4 stages:
    - Primary syphilis is the site of the infection, micro-organisms drain into the lymph and stimulate a specific immune response
    - Secondary is systemic and infection spreads to all major organs, the immune system is able to suppress the infection
    - Latent stage whereby no clinical manifestations are shown, transmission to others is still possible
    - Tertiary syphilis is the severe stage

- Chlamydia:
  - A sexual infection, which is caused by the bacterium *Chlamydia trachomatis*
  - Gram-negative bacteria, which can only reproduce within host cells (similar to a virus)
  - Requires epithelial tissue but does not invade deeper tissues or organs
- HIV lives in the T-helper cells of cell-mediated immunity (see chapter 5) and it can lay dormant for many years.

Clinical features

- Gonorrhoea is asymptomatic, but following an incubation period of 2–5 days:
  - In men a thick purulent discharge is noticed from top of penis, urethral infection and dysuria, urethral itching, inflammation of the testicles and tender scrotum
  - In women acute dysuria, vaginal discharge, dysmenorrhoea or dyspareunia, bleeding between periods
  - Both genders – sore throat or eyes, discharge from the anus, anal itching, bleeding or painful bowel movements
- Syphilis:
  - Primary stage – a sore or ulcer appears on the penis, vagina, cervix or rectum, with enlarged lymph nodes, usually disappears within 2–8 weeks
  - Secondary stage – variable systemic symptoms, fever, malaise, sore throat, all-over body rash, lesions around the vulva such as warts are highly contagious, pruritus and alopecia are common
  - Usually treatment is instigated prior to features occurring in the latent and tertiary stages
- Chlamydia is usually asymptomatic, but following an incubation period of 1–3 weeks:
  - In men – urethritis, discharge from tip of penis similar to gonorrhoea, burning sensation on urination
  - In women – change in vaginal discharge, bleeding between periods or after sex, lower abdominal pain, cystitis, can lead to tubal infertility
  - Both genders – rectal pain, bleeding, conjunctivitis, throat irritation
- HIV may have no symptoms for a number of years:
  - Short periods of illness such as sore throat, fever, rash, pyrexia, aches and pains, nausea, vomiting, diarrhoea
  - If virus is allowed to take hold the immune system becomes weakened and cannot protect the body against invading organisms leading to AIDS.

Investigations

- Gonorrhoea:
  - In men microscopic examination of swab from discharge
  - In women a cervical swab is required
  - Patients can also have chlamydia infection, accompanying gonorrhoea
- Syphilis:
  - Blood tests (may give false negative results up to 3 months after infection)
  - Microscopy of a specimen from a lesion
  - Urine sample
  - Internal examination in women
- Chlamydia:
  - Screening in asymptomatic women in GUM clinics using tissue culture techniques
  - Microbiological culture with cervical, urethral or penile swab
  - Urine sample (nucleic acid amplification test)
- HIV/AIDS:
  - Blood test to show positive reaction for antibodies approximately 3 months after infection.

Treatment and drug therapy

- Gonorrhoea:
  - Penicillin or tetracycline (some resistant strains)
  - Cephalosporins are now recommended (McCance and Huether, 2010)
- Syphilis treatment for all stages is benzathine penicillin G (other antibiotics can be used for those allergic to penicillin)
- Chlamydia responds well to antibiotics (azithromycin, erythromycin, ofloxicin) for the infected individual and contacts
- HIV/AIDS early treatment with anti-retroviral drug therapy can delay development of AIDS.

For additional STDs see Table 15.1.

Ovarian cancer

Aetiology

- The cause of ovarian cancer is unknown (McCance and Huether, 2010)
- Is associated with early menstruation, late menopause.

Pathology

- The ovaries are composed of 3 kinds of tissue (West, 2005):
  - Germ cells, which produce the eggs (ova) formed on the inside of the ovary
  - Stromal cells, which produce most of the female hormones, oestrogen and progesterone
  - Epithelial cells, which cover the ovary and most ovarian cancers start in this epithelial covering
- The histological hallmark of malignant ovarian cancer is usually the invasion of the stromal cells
- Ovarian tumours of low malignant potential or borderline tumours and there are several types (Chen *et al*, 2003).

Clinical features

- Usually asymptomatic
- Vague symptoms of abdominal discomfort
- Abnormal vaginal bleeding
- Gastrointestinal problems:
  - Dyspepsia
  - Bloating
  - Vomiting
  - Change in bowel habits
- Pelvic discomfort
- Backache
- Increase in abdominal size
- Enlarged ovaries.

Investigations

- Ultrasound – fails to differentiate between benign and malignant lesions
- Diagnosis is confirmed by biopsy
- The extend of the disease is determined by computerised tomography (CT scan)
- Increased serum levels of the marker antigen CA125, which is present in both borderline and invasive malignant tumours
- Increase in the tumour marker carcino-embryonic antigen (CEA) can also indicate ovarian cancer (West, 2005)
- Diagnosis is confirmed by biopsy.

Treatment

- Due to the lack of symptoms in the early stages, the disease is usually advanced by the time treatment is instigated

- Surgical intervention is the preferred option
  - Unilateral salpingo-oophorectomy – removal of 1 ovary and one fallopian, usually recommended if there is potential for childbearing
  - Bilateral salpingo-oophorectomy – removal of both ovaries and both fallopian tubes
  - Total hysterectomy and bilateral salpingo-oophorectomy – removal of the uterus, cervix, and both ovaries and fallopian tubes. If removed vaginally, the operation is called a vaginal hysterectomy
  - Partial oophorectomy – removal of 1 ovary or part of both ovaries
  - Omentectomy – removal of the omentum (tissues lining the abdominal wall).

Cervical cancer

The majority of cervical cancers are squamous cell; adenocarcinoma of the cervix is rare. This is highlighted in the case study below:

Case study 15.1

Honeysuckle is a 47-year-old female patient, with a history of excessive menstrual bleeding and lower abdominal pain. Honeysuckle went to her GP complaining of these symptoms. The GP informed Honeysuckle that her symptoms could be due to fibroids or to something more serious. She was sent for a pelvic examination, cervical smear and colposcopy, which confirmed the diagnosis of cervical cancer. Removal through the vagina was impossible for Honeysuckle as the cancer was large and complications would be more likely using this method. Therefore, Honeysuckle was seen by a gynaecologist and booked in for a routine abdominal hysterectomy.

Aetiology

- There is a link between squamous cell carcinoma and the number of sexual relationships and the age a woman started sexual intercourse, as exposure to the risk factors are increased
- Smoking and poor diet increase the risk of cervical cancer
- Can be caused by cervical human papillomavirus (HPV) infection acquired by adolescents and young women within 3 years of initiation of sexual intercourse. The majority of infections are

generally cleared by the immune system and do not go on to develop invasive cervical cancer.

Pathology

- The cervix is the inferior narrower part of the uterus, which is subject to friction during intercourse
- Cancer is more likely to develop in the transformation zone, as in this zone columnar epithelium are constantly being replaced by squamous epithelium in a process known as metaplasia, which is effected by hormonal levels.

Clinical features

- Early features can be asymptomatic, but may experience:
  - Vaginal discharge, which is:
    - Watery
    - Blood stained
    - May have a foul odour
  - Inter-menstrual bleeding that is painless (metrorrhagia)
  - Heavy lengthy menstrual bleeding (menorrhagia), which is interrupting the patient's physical, social and emotional wellbeing, leading them to seek medical attention, as in the case of Honeysuckle
  - Bleeding can lead to anaemia
  - Ulceration of the vulva or pelvic area
  - Bleeding following intercourse
- Late features
  - Pelvic or epigastric pain can be experienced
  - Back or leg pain
  - Ankle oedema
  - Urinary or rectal symptoms
  - Vaginal haemorrhage.

Investigations

- Cervical smear and cytology
- Differential diagnosis e.g. fibroids
- Blood tests e.g. haemoglobin levels to determine anaemia
- Regular HPV screening
- Colposcopy to examine the cervix
- Cervical biopsy is the removal of a small section of tissue for microscopy or histological examination for any changes.

Treatment/drug therapy

- Hysterectomy
- Cryotherapy is when freezing is used to destroy the cancerous tissue, but is usually reserved for smaller lesions and does not compromise fertility. It does not require an anaesthetic
- Diathermy is considered to be more effective than freezing, but requires a local anaesthetic. It can destroy cancerous tissue, but can lead to vaginal discharge and scarring of the cervix
- Laser (light amplification by stimulated emission of radiation) therapy is direct heat to the cancerous tissue, offering precision and control of destruction of normal healthy tissue
- Radiotherapy can be used for larger cervical tumours to reduce pelvic metastasis
- Chemotherapy can be used to reduce the size of the tumour prior to surgery to improve access to the malignant lesion
- Good psychological and sociological care prior to, during and after treatment:
  - Allow time to voice anxieties
  - For those women undergoing hysterectomy it will remove fertility
  - The side effects of surgery include continence problems and sexual difficulties
  - Under- or over-estimation of the seriousness of malignancy
  - Depression.

Breast cancer

Defined as malignant changes in any of the breast tissues, it may occur at any time of life and if not treated can lead to serious illness and death (Johnson, 2004b). Breast cancer can occur in men, but with a much lower incidence (Ahmed *et al*, 2007).

Aetiology

A number of factors increase the risk of a women developing breast cancer:

- Family history, genetic – 10% of breast cancer is genetically predisposed, and a family history potentiates all risk factors (Johnson, 2004b), the 2 genes are:
  - BRCAI on chromosome 17
  - BRCA2 identified on chromosome 13
- Previous history of a benign tumour
- Exposure to oestrogen – e.g. early menstruation, late menopause
- Age – likelihood increases with age

- Nationality – a woman living in Western countries is 5 times more likely to develop the disease than a women living in far Eastern countries (Johnson, 2004b)
- Lifestyle includes diet, alcohol and smoking
- Prolonged use of hormone replacement therapy (HRT).

Pathology

- The most common type of breast cancer is infiltrating intra-ductal carcinoma
- There are two stages of breast cancer (Ahmed *et al*, 2007):
  - Non-invasive – the cancer is contained within the ducts and at this stage is almost completely curable
  - Invasive, which is sub-divided into 4 stages:
    - Stage 1 – the tumour measures less than 2 cm in diameter, and there is no spread into the lymph nodes
    - Stage 2 – measures between 2–5 cm and/or there are affected lymph nodes
    - Stage 3 – tumour measures larger than 5 cm diameter and may be attached to a muscle or skin, the lymph nodes at this stage are usually affected
    - Stage 4 – describes a tumour of any size; the lymph nodes are generally affected and the cancer has spread
- Microscopic examination shows the cancer cells' appearance, this is graded 1–3:
  - The lower the grade the cells are closer to normal in the appearance
  - The higher the grade indicates the tumour cells have an abnormal appearance and characteristics of a fast-growing and aggressive tumour.

Clinical feature

- A small, painless lump that is irregular in shape felt in breast, and is not cyclical with menstruation
- Usually there may be no other symptoms
- Veins in the breast become more visible
- Changes in the colour and texture of breast skin
- Dimpling over the breast or nipple
- Discharge or bleeding from the nipple.

Investigations

- Breast self-examination – lumps can often be felt when the breast is examined

- Mammogram – tumours can be detected at an early stage (Crouch, 2003)
  - A 2 view mammography is now recommended and all women screened for breast cancer should be offered these scans of their breasts
  - One taken from above and 1 taken diagonally from the armpit (Crouch, 2003)
- Ultrasound can detect small lumps that cannot be felt
- Fine needle aspiration
- Core biopsy of breast lump to determine malignancy or benign tumour
- Immuno-histo-chemical examination is undertaken in the UK on all women with early stage breast cancer, to detect expression the over-expression of human epidermal growth factor receptor-2 (HER2) proteins on the surface of the cancer. The presence of these molecules indicates that cell division is increased by naturally occurring oestrogens and hormone therapy may be indicated
- Histological frozen section may be undertaken to:
  - Confirm diagnosis of malignancy prior to surgery
  - Assess excision margins after mastectomy to ensure complete removal of malignant breast tumour
  - Assess the involvement of axillary lymph nodes in the cancerous disease, to identify dissection limits.

Treatment/drug therapy

- Mastectomy – removal of the breast tissue and nipple
- Radical mastectomy – removal of the breast, lymph nodes removed as well
- Axillary clearance – is when lymph nodes are cleared under the arm
- Complications of a mastectomy
  - Bruising and swelling
  - Stiffness especially in the shoulder
  - Pain and tightness
  - Oedema and lymphoedema
  - Phantom pain
- Breast can be reconstructed following removal
- Alternatives to mastectomy:
  - Lumpectomy – the cancer only is removed, the breast is left intact
  - Chemotherapy – cytotoxic chemicals are used to destroy cancerous cells, unpleasant side effects, can be used with radiotherapy in advanced cancer when the cancer has infiltrated surrounding cells

    - Radiotherapy – deep X-ray to kill cells, can be followed by chemotherapy, targeted to specific area localised to the tumour, has side effects
    - Drug treatment
        - HER2 positive tumours can be treated with Herceptin, recommended in the treatment for early breast cancer and as combination therapy with paclitaxel or docetaxel for metastatic breast cancer (BNF, 2014)
        - Selective oestrogen receptor drugs used to suppress the growth of the cancer e.g. Fareston, tamoxifen
        - Anti-oestrogen drugs – slow growth of cancer and reproduction of cells, reduce chances by 50%, have side effects such as hot flushes, irregular periods, bleeding
- Chemotherapy and/or radiotherapy can be used in combination with surgery
- Need to consider sociological/psychological aspects of treatment:
    - Patients with cancer living on the poverty line, not being able to afford transport to attend clinics/treatment sessions or diet, access financial help or support
    - Encourage to talk about it, reduced sexuality, loss of hair, relationships afterwards, not feeling a woman any more
    - Consideration as to how the patient may be feeling, counselling may be needed, disfigurement and the personal impact of this considered
    - Involve the family
    - Depression is common, coping
    - Consider supportive services e.g. Macmillan, other charities.

Practice point

Women with conditions such as described above can require emotional support regarding fertility and self-esteem.

CONDITIONS DURING PREGNANCY

Trauma during pregnancy

Aetiology

Anatomic and physiological changes during the gestational period predispose pregnant women to accidental injury. The most common causes of trauma during pregnancy are:

- Motor vehicle accidents
- Falls
- Industrial accidents
- Burns
- Firearm injuries
- Direct assault to the abdomen caused by violence.

Pathology

- As the pregnancy progresses, alterations in balance and gait increase the likelihood of falls
- The enlarged abdomen becomes more susceptible to injury from blunt and penetrating trauma (Edwards, 1998).

Clinical features

Factors that influence the effect of trauma on pregnancy include:

- Length of gestation
- Type and severity of the trauma
- Degree of disruption of uterine and foetal physiology.

Severe pre-eclampsia

Pre-eclampsia is known as pregnancy-induced hypertension (PIH).

Aetiology

The cause of PIH has never been identified, but thought:

- Calcium
- Antithrombotic agents
- Angiotensin II
- Prostaglandins
- Hereditary factors.

Clinical features

- Hypertension
- Proteinurea
- Oedema from vascular endothelial damage, which leads to:
  - Plasma leakage from blood vessels
  - Colloid osmotic pressure, normally decreased during pregnancy, further decreases as protein enters the extra-vascular space via the damaged endothelium with risks of:
    - Hypovolaemia
    - Alterations in tissue perfusion and oxygenation.

Treatment/drug therapies

- Induced labour and delivery of the baby
- If the baby is not viable, to save the mother the child may have to be aborted
- Severe pre-eclampsia can lead to haemolysis, elevated liver enzyme, low platelet count (HELLP syndrome), and is associated with significant perinatal mortality and morbidity. Liver enzymes become elevated as hepatic endothelial damage eventually leads to ischaemia and decreased liver function.

Rupture of the mother's (gravid) uterus

This is an uncommon but serious obstetric emergency that presents a lethal threat to both foetus and mother. Such rupture usually involves dehiscence of a previous uterine scar from Caesarean section or myomectomy, but occasionally occurs spontaneously or following blunt trauma.

> **Practice point**
>
> It is important for healthcare practitioners to remember and have insight into the pleasure that is associated with reproduction, which is important to individuals on a number of different levels.

CONCLUSION

The reproductive system is responsible for ensuring optimal conditions for producing, maintaining and delivering of a baby. The pathological changes to the mother during pregnancy can lead to conditions requiring emergency interventions. The hormones produced by the male and female genitals influence other body organs, which can lead to abnormal conditions unrelated to the reproductive system. Like any other organs this system is prone to infections and cancer, some of which have been discussed in this chapter.

SELF-ASSESSMENT QUESTIONS

1. Provide an outline of the male and female reproductive systems.
2. Identify the different parts of the male and female genitalia responsible for reproduction.
3. List the functions of the male and female reproductive organs.

4. List several abnormal conditions of the male and female reproductive organs.
5. List several changes to the male and female anatomy and physiology that may occur in diseased states.

REFERENCES

Ahmed, N., Dawson, M., Smith, C. and Wood, E. (2007) *Biology of Disease*, London: Taylor & Francis Group.
Blows, W.T. (2005) *The Biological Basis of Nursing: Cancer*, London: Routledge.
BNF (British National Formulary) (2014) *BNF 66: The Authority on the Selection and Use of Medicines*, London: British Medical Society, The Royal Pharmaceutical Society.
Chen, V. W, et al. (2003) Pathology and classification of ovarian tumours, *Cancer*, 97(10), 2631–2642.
Crouch, D. (2003) Does screening save lives? *Nursing Times*, 99(19), 22–25.
Edwards, S. (1998) Haemodynamic monitoring of the pregnant woman in intensive care, *Nursing in Critical Care*, 3(3), 112–121.
Kirby, R.S. (2011) *The Prostate, Small Gland, Big Problem: A Guide to the Prostate, Prostate Disorders and Their Treatments*, London: Prostate Research Campaign, UK.
Johnson, S. (2004a) Men's cancers, in N. Whittaker, *Disorders and Interventions*, London: Palgrave Macmillan.
Johnson, S. (2004b) Women's cancers, in N. Whittaker, *Disorders and Interventions*, London: Palgrave Macmillan.
Marieb, E. (2012) *Essentials of Human Anatomy and Physiology*, 9th edn, San Francisco, CA: Benjamin Cummings.
McCance, K.L. and Huether, S.E. (2010) *Pathophysiology: The Biologic Basis for Disease in Adults and Children*, 6th edn, Missouri: Mosby Elsevier.
McIntosh, M. (2008) *The Bigger Picture: The National Chlamydia Screening Programme*, London: NHS report, chlamydiascreening.nhs.uk.
RCN (Royal College of Nursing) (2003) *Health and Menopause*, London: RCN.
West, V.A. (2005) Ovarian tumours of low malignant potential, *Cancer Nursing Practice*, 4(7), 35–39.

16 The skin

Sharon Edwards

THE ANATOMY OF THE SKIN

The skin is surprisingly versatile: it invisibly repairs small cuts, grazes and burns, and epithelial cells are constantly lost and replaced. It is the largest organ of the body, and together with its derivatives (sweat and oil glands, hairs and nails) makes up a very complex set of organs that serves several functions, mainly protective. Together, these organs form the integumentary system.

The skin is made up of 3 distinct regions: the epidermis, dermis and hypodermis. The underlying dermis is composed of connective tissue, is tough, makes up the bulk of the skin and contains the blood vessels and nerve endings (Figure 16.1). The hypodermis is the deep tissue, consists mainly of adipose tissue or fat store, and anchors the skin to the underlying muscles. This layer thickens when gaining weight.

Epidermis

The epidermis is composed of epithelial cells and is the outermost protective cover of the body. The epidermis is continuously shedding the superficial layer of stratum corneum primarily made up of keratinocytes and melanocytes. This layer contains no blood vessels or nerve endings. Nutrients reach the epidermis by diffusion through the tissue fluid from blood vessels in the dermis. The epidermis is formed of squamous epithelial tissue and this is usually made up of 5 layers of cell types (Figure 16.1). It is therefore a stratified epithelium, with cells being produced in the basal layer and moving through the other layers over a period of approximately 35 days, that regenerates the epidermis.

The cells of the epidermis

- Keratinocytes produced from keratin, a substance that makes the epidermis tough as a barrier, an insoluble fibrous protein molecule made up of 18 amino acids, gives the epidermis its protective properties:

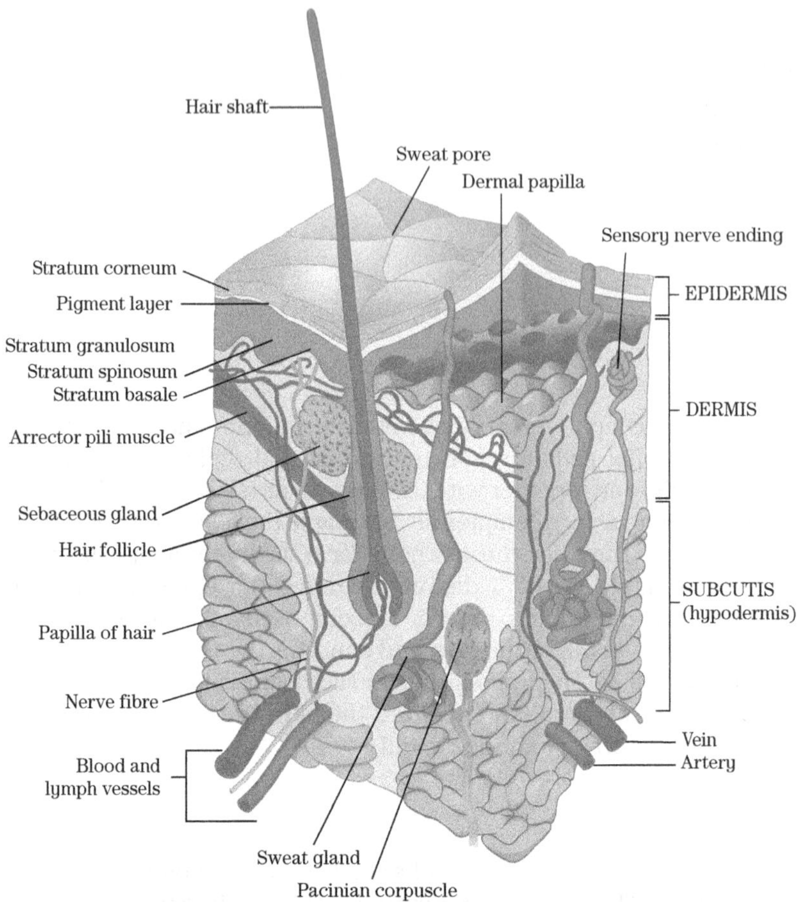

Figure 16.1 The skin

   - Arises in the deepest part of the epidermis from a layer of basal cells (stratum basale), which undergo continuous mitosis
   - The keratinocytes are pushed towards the surface by the production of new cells beneath them by the time the keratinocytes reach the surface of the skin they are dead
   - Millions of the dead cells rub off the skin surface every day, giving a new epidermis every 25–45 days
- Melanocytes synthesise the pigment melanin and are found in the deepest layer of the epidermis:
   - Form a pigment shield that protects the keratinocyte nucleus from the damaging effects of ultraviolet (UV) radiation in sunlight

    - The differences in skin colouring are due to the variation in melanocyte activity or the speed of melanin breakdown within the keratinocytes (Marieb, 2012)
- Langerhans cells arise from bone marrow and migrate to the epidermis and help to activate the immune system
- Merkel cells are relatively small in number and act as a sensory receptor for touch.

The layers of the epidermis

- Basal layer (stratum basale) is the single layer nearest to the dermis, where cell division occurs:
    - The cells dip down into the dermis to surround sweat glands and hair follicles
    - As long as that part of the dermis is retained which contains the hair roots or sweat glands, then some epidermal regeneration can occur from the remaining basal cells
- Spinous layer (stratum spinosum) – is several layers thick and is attached to desmosomes, which prevent cell separation (something which could otherwise occur as a result of surface stresses). In order to facilitate the protein synthesis the cells are rich in ribonucleic acid (RNA)
- Granular layer (stratum granulosum) – the cells contain a waterproofing glycolipid that is in the extracellular space and slows water loss across the epidermis
- Clear layer (stratum lucidum) – only present in thick skin such as that on the palms of the hands and soles of the feet
- Horny layer (stratum corneum) – forms the surface layer of cells, all of which are dead:
    - Constantly shed from the body's surface with movement
    - Provides a durable layer for the body, protecting deeper cells from a hostile environment and from water loss
    - Renders the body relatively insensitive to biological, chemical and physical assaults.

The normal flora of the skin epidermis

- On each square centimetre of skin there may be up to 3 million micro-organisms, most of which are commensals. The bacteria commonly presenting as commensals on the skin are *Corynebacterium and Staphylococcus epidermis*
- Individuals live in harmony with commensals as long as the skin remains an intact barrier

- If these micro-organisms are given the opportunity to invade the dermis or body cavities, for example the bladder, these normally harmless bacteria turn against us and may then act as opportunistic pathogens.

Dermis

The dermis is a fibrous elastic bed, supporting and providing nourishment for the epidermis and its appendages (the hairs, sweat glands, blood vessels, lymphatic vessels and nerve endings (Figure 16.1). The dermis ranges in thickness from about 0.5 mm thick in the eyelid, penis and scrotum to over 4 mm thick on the soles of the feet and the palms of the hands. It gives mechanical strength to the skin.

Layers of the dermis

The dermis is formed of two distinct layers:

1. The papillary layer lies next to the basal layer of the epidermis and forms a series of undulations called dermal papillae, which alternate with epidermal or rete pegs
2. The reticular layer is deeper and contains fewer blood vessels and is less reactive.

The 2 layers slot into one another and a polysaccharide gel serves to bind the 2 layers together. This cellular arrangement prevents the epidermis shearing off the dermis when shearing forces are applied to the skin.

Ground substance, fibres and cells of the dermis

The dermis is formed of a ground substance or matrix, fibres and cells:

- Ground substance supports fibres and cells and fills the spaces between them. Substances in solution travelling between blood vessels and cells must cross through this matrix
- There are 3 main fibres, all produced by mesodermal fibroblasts:
  - Collagen – a fibrous protein with the tensile strength of steel wire of the same diameter and has a protective function:
    - It binds to water avidly and the dermis contains 18–40% of the total body water. This water can be mobilised in dehydration or haemorrhage. The water-binding properties of collagen decrease with age, and the wrinkled appearance of the skin in elderly people is due to the decreased water-holding power of the collagen
    - Ascorbic acid is necessary for collagen formation and hence an adequate intake is essential for efficient wound healing

    - The bundles of collagen fibres run in diverse directions, in certain areas they lie in the same direction. Surgeons make their incision in the direction in which the fibres lie. This results in a fine scar, which tends to heal faster and gape less than one made across the line of cleavage
  - Reticular fibres form a loose framework in the dermis and envelop the collagen. They help to disperse mechanical forces applied to the dermis
  - Elastin fibres are yellow fibres, which are elastic but may rupture when stretched by pregnancy, obesity or prolonged ascites. When this occurs, silvery linear scars appear, called striae or stretch marks
- Cells may either be resident (synthesising ground substance or fibres) or blood-borne and thus transient:
  - Fibroblasts are resident and lie between the bundles of collagen and are concerned with collagen and elastin synthesis. Their numbers increase considerably during wound healing
  - Tissue macrophages or histiocytes are wandering phagocytic cells (derived from the monocytes in blood), which engulf particulate matter and are protective in function
  - Tissue mast cells (analogous to the basophils in the bloodstream) produce both histamine and heparin, and play a role in hypersensitivity reactions in the skin (McCance and Huether, 2010)
  - Transient cells include neutrophils, lymphocytes and monocytes. They move constantly between the blood vessels of the dermis, moving out of the blood in large numbers as part of the inflammatory reaction, which occurs in response to trauma. Normally, the dermis is free from bacteria.

Skin colour

The 3 pigments which contribute to skin colour are melanin, carotene and haemoglobin. These are pigment-producing cells, which are present over the entire skin:

- Melanin:
  - Colours hair and there is a biochemical difference in the melanin produced by blondes, brunettes and redheads which results in different tones of hair pigment colour
  - Colours the iris of the eye and differs structurally between individuals
  - Production is influenced by sunlight. After exposure of skin to sunlight, new melanin is not formed immediately. Erythema

    (reddening of the skin) due to inflammation occurs initially, and this lasts approximately 2 days. Then melanin production is evident as the skin colour changes from pink to brown
    - Melanin production is under genetic control, and is regulated by melanocyte-stimulating hormone (MSH) secreted from the anterior lobe of the pituitary. Melanocytes are found in the epidermis and dermis
- Carotene is a yellow to orange pigment found in certain products such as carrots. It accumulates in the stratum corneum and in fatty tissue in the hypodermis
- Haemoglobin gives the pinkish hue of fair skin and reflects the crimson colour of oxygenated haemoglobin in the red blood cells circulating through the dermal capillaries. White skin only contains small amounts of melanin; the epidermis is nearly transparent and allows haemoglobin colour to show through.

Blood vessels

The cutaneous blood vessels lie entirely within the dermis and have an essential role in transporting nutrients to, and waste substances from, the dermal tissues. Cutaneous blood vessels have a rich sympathetic nerve supply. Under normal conditions, there is always a certain amount of background vasoconstrictor tone. Circulating adrenaline and noradrenaline enhance the vasoconstrictor effect of the sympathetic nerves. They are also of major importance in the regulation of body temperature:

- The number of vessels is much greater than would be necessary for purely nutritional purposes, and so the skin is capable of accommodating varying amounts of blood
- In some exposed areas, for example the hands, feet, ears or nose, large numbers of arterio-venous anastomoses exist (Figure 16.1). At normal body temperatures, these anastomoses are kept almost closed by sympathetic vasoconstrictor nerves
    - When body temperature rises, the sympathetic vasoconstrictor tone is reduced and the anastomoses open, allowing blood to short-circuit the deeper capillary beds, so that a large volume of warm blood enters the superficial vessels, promoting heat loss
    - When the environmental temperature drops, the sympathetic nerves are stimulated and so vasoconstriction occurs; vasodilation results from sympathetic inhibition in warm conditions.

Lymphatic vessels

- Lymphatic vessels are found throughout the dermis and they have a major role in draining excess tissue fluid and any plasma proteins that may have leaked into the tissues. The leaked fluid must be carried back to the blood to ensure sufficient blood volume (Marieb, 2012)

- This explains why patients who have had surgical removal of their lymph glands, following carcinoma of the breast, frequently have arm oedema. The lymphatics are therefore important in maintaining interstitial fluid volume and composition.

Nerve supply

- The skin is the largest sensory organ in the body. Its dermis contains free nerve endings (pain receptors) and touch receptors (Meissner's corpuscles). Sensory receptors are specialised so they each respond to a different form of energy – chemical, mechanical or thermal – thus the modalities of touch-pressure, cold, warmth and pain can be consciously appreciated
- The receptors act as transducers, and convert the energy into action potentials
- The skin contains 3 main types of sensory nerve endings (Figure 16.1):
  - Naked nerve endings
  - Encapsulated endings (Pacinian corpuscles, Meissner's corpuscles and Krause's end-bulbs)
  - Expanded endings (Ruffini's organs). These are in addition to the petrichial sensory endings supplying hair follicles.

Hypodermis

Sometimes called the superficial fascia (Figure 16.1) and not always considered as part of the skin, but it shares the skin's protective functions. It contains most of the body's stores of fat up to 60%.

Subcutaneous fat

Adipose tissue, or fat, forms a valuable store of triglycerides for the body, and this is a potential source of energy:

- 60% of the total body fat stores are subcutaneous, and this fat insulates the body and prevents heat loss from the core
- Fat also protects from trauma, in that it acts as a shock absorber. Blows to the body surface cause lateral displacement of the skin due to the presence of subcutaneous fat, and hence the full force of the blow is not transmitted to the deeper structures
- Fat distribution, under the skin, differs between the sexes; this difference becomes evident at puberty:

    - Females have greater deposits on the upper limbs, breasts and buttocks than males
    - Females have greater fat stores than the male – some 15 kg as opposed to the male's 7.5 kg
    - Diet, genetic factors and sex hormones determine fat stores
- Subcutaneous fat forms an energy reserve, which can be called upon in starvation
- When fat is catabolised, considerable metabolic water is produced – a factor of importance to humans in starvation.

Brown fat

- Brown fat tissue is more vascular and the cells contain many small droplets of fat and so form a more readily and rapidly available energy supply and are capable of an increased rate of metabolism
- Brown fat has an important role in the neonate as it provides an easily mobilised energy source:
    - The neonate has a large body surface area relative to its weight and it is also unable to shiver
    - The newborn baby therefore has the potential problem of inability to conserve body heat and a propensity to lose too much heat
    - The neonate uses the brown fat stored around the back of its neck and kidneys, free fatty acids being liberated from this in response to cold, noradrenaline and glucagon
    - It loses its importance in thermal regulation as the child develops muscular control and hence uses muscular activity and shivering as a method of heat production
    - It is possible that some individuals may retain their stores of brown fat into adulthood, and such individuals may be less prone to obesity and be able to lose weight more easily.

Appendages of the skin

Along with the skin, the integumentary system includes extensions or appendages including the hair follicles, hair, nails, sweat glands and sebaceous (oil) glands. Each plays a major role in maintaining body homeostasis.

Hair

Hair is formed largely by keratin and its function is to protect the skin from ultraviolet light, extremes of temperature and also from trauma; the total number of hairs decreases with age.

- Hair follicles lie in the dermis, surrounded by its blood and nerve supply. The shaft of the hair projects beyond the surface of the skin.

The lower end of the shaft in the dermis is distended to form the bulb. If a hair is sharply pulled out of the scalp, the bulb at the end can be seen quite clearly. Cell division occurs in the bulb and hence cytotoxic drugs affect this area. Human hair is of 3 types:

- Lanugo is fine, long, silky non-pigmented hair present in the first 7–8 months of foetal life, after which time it is shed in utero
- Vellus is short colourless hair, forms the child's body hair and remains on the adult female's face
- Terminal hair is the hair found on the adult head and pubis. When, as a result of disease such as Cushing's syndrome, a person becomes hirsute, it is terminal hair that appears on the face. This is much more noticeable and may cause distress

- Hair production is influenced by hormones such as androgens (e.g. testosterone), and genetics in relation to colour, texture and balding
  - Hair tends to grow in cycles of activity, and at any one time about 85% of scalp hairs are in an actively growing stage, which lasts for about 2 years. This active period is followed by a period of rest, then regression. About 70–100 scalp hairs are lost daily out of the total of about 100,000 scalp follicles
  - The rate of hair loss is influenced by such factors as severe illness, very low calorie diets, exposure to radiation and childbirth.

Nails

- These are protective keratinised plates resting on the stratified squamous epithelium that forms the highly sensitive and vascular nail beds
- The nails protect the tips of the fingers and toes from injury
- The nail root extends deeply into the dermis
- Nails can give an indication of certain diseases to the observer. This will be discussed under assessment of the skin.

Sweat glands

Sweat glands have a cholinergic sympathetic innervation. There are 2 types of sweat gland (sometimes known as sudoriferous glands) in the skin, each of which has a separate function:

- Eccrine glands – there are between 3 and 4 million sweat glands, not all active at the same time:
  - Distribution throughout the body is uneven:
    - 400/cm^2 on the hands and feet
    - 70/cm^2 on the back

    - Formed as coiled tubular down-growths from the epidermis, each having its own blood supply and innervation from cholinergic sympathetic fibres (see Figure 16.1)
- Apocrine glands – sweat secretion from these glands has a distinctive odour, and used for the recognition of mates and territory:
    - Present in the areas of the pubis, genitalia, areola, axillae, umbilicus and external auditory canals
    - 10 times larger than the eccrine glands
    - Become functional at puberty when they begin actively to secrete and thus appear to be affected by the sex hormones
    - Secretion increases in stress and there may be some sympathetic nervous influence
    - Secretion is scanty and sticky, odourless when first secreted, but quickly acted upon by bacteria, which gives rise to a distinctive, rather unpleasant, smell
        - Deodorants work on a bactericidal principle and also attempt, with perfumes, to mask any odour produced
        - Antiperspirants act by plugging the openings of the ducts, usually with metal salts such as those of aluminium
- Sebaceous glands – formed as outgrowths of the developing hair follicles (see Figure 16.1):
    - Activity:
        - Low in childhood, and a child has very small and few sebaceous glands, hence babies and children are prone to chapping of the skin on exposure to damp conditions, predisposing to nappy rash
        - Increases during puberty
        - In old age, the number of sebaceous glands diminishes, with resulting potential skin care problems
    - Found:
        - Plentiful over the scalp and face where there may be up to 900/cm^2, and also over the middle of the back, the auditory canal and genitalia
        - Few sebaceous glands on the hands and feet and in some individuals over the forehead
    - More than 2 g of slightly acid sebum may be produced each week.

Sweat

Sweat glands produce sweat when the skin surface temperature rises above 35°C. They have a minor role in ridding the body of some waste substances and a more important role in helping to bring about heat loss.

- Composition:
  - 99% water, with a small amount of sodium chloride, urea, lactic acid and potassium in solution
  - Hypotonic with reference to plasma, containing fewer electrolytes and very little glucose
- It is usually acid in reaction
- The specific gravity of sweat is normally about 1.004, but this varies with the rate of secretion, aldosterone levels in the blood and acclimatisation to extreme heat
- Sweat forms a minor excretory route for some drugs, allergens and substances such as garlic
- There is always some slight activity, with a resultant insensible loss of some 400–500 ml per day. This loss is not all via the sweat glands; the skin does allow some loss through diffusion and osmosis
- Sweat production:
  - In a temperate climate, approximately 500 ml of sweat each day is produced in addition to the insensible loss
  - This amount varies with the degree of activity and the environmental temperature
  - Can rise in very hot climates
  - Secretion increases in response to:
    - Spicy foods
    - In stressful and emotional states. This forms the basis for lie-detector machines (polygraphs) which measure galvanic skin response
- Heat loss:
  - The evaporation of sweat from the skin surface requires latent heat from the surface of the skin and is thus a method of heat loss
  - The areas which are most active in this thermoregulatory sweating are the face, trunk, axillae, palms and soles
  - The evaporation of 1 litre of sweat from the skin requires 2400 kJ (580 kcal) of heat, and it is the evaporation of sweat that causes heat to be lost (not simply the production of sweat)
  - Sweat will not evaporate if the environment is already laden with water vapour.

Sebum

Sebum is a mixture of triglycerides, waxes, paraffins and cholesterol. The function of sebum is to:

- Waterproof the skin
- Protects from fungal and bacterial infections: athlete's foot, for instance, occurs in an area between the toes where there are no or

very few sebaceous glands and a damp environment. The skin forms a dry barrier and pathogenic bacteria on its surface often die simply through desiccation
- Sebum production is stimulated by a rise in temperature and by androgens; it is inhibited by oestrogen.

The functions of the skin

Protection

- The skin as the outer covering protects the body from trauma, undue entry of bacteria, the loss or gain of water and from sunlight
- It is also protection from all the minor mechanical blows that the environment deals, for example pressure and friction
- When intact, the skin is virtually impermeable to microorganisms, and gives rise to protection in four different ways:
  - The physical skin barrier:
    - Protects us from all minor mechanical blows that the environment deals for example pressure and friction
  - The chemical skin barriers – the skin secretions and melanin provide these:
    - The low pH of skin secretions (acid mantle) retards the multiplication of bacteria
    - Many bacteria are killed outright by bactericidal substances in sebum
    - The skin cells secrete a natural antibiotic called human defensin that punches holes in bacteria
    - The melanin produced within the skin gives protection from ultraviolet radiation
    - Protects us from chemicals (weak acids, alkalines) and most gases (although some gases developed for use in chemical warfare can be absorbed through the skin. The skin also protects against some forms of radiation such as:
      - Alpha-rays (cannot penetrate skin at all)
      - Beta-rays (can penetrate a few millimetres of skin but are unable to reach the underlying organs)
  - Biological skin barriers
    - The Langerhans cells of the epidermis, which are active elements of the immune system, present the foreign substance or antigens to the lymphocytes to activate the immune response
    - The macrophages in the dermis dispose of viruses and bacteria that have managed to penetrate the epidermis.

Absorption

- Certain substances can be absorbed through the skin:
  - Oestrogens
  - Fat-soluble vitamins (A, D, E and K)
  - Steroids
  - Methyl salicylate alcohol skin preparation e.g. surgical spirit
  - Drugs such as glyceryl trinitrate (GTN)
- Such substances can be administered as either ointments, gels or transdermally via slow-release skin patches. The patches should be applied to clean, non-hairy skin to facilitate absorption, which will depend on the site and its blood flow.

Cutaneous sensation

The skin forms the largest sensory organ of the body and is richly supplied with cutaneous sensory receptors (part of the nervous system).

- Nerve endings are found in the dermis, and are more concentrated in certain areas (for example the fingertips and lips)
- They are classified as exteroceptors because they respond to stimuli arising outside the body. These include:
  - Meissner's corpuscles (in the dermal papillae) – allow awareness of a caress or the feel of our clothing against our skin
  - Pacinian receptors (in the deeper dermis or hypodermis) – give awareness to bumps or contacts involving deep pressure
  - Root hair plexuses – wind blowing through our hair and a playful tug at an arm or leg
  - Painful stimuli (irritating chemicals, extreme heat or cold, touch) – are sensed by bare nerve endings that meander throughout the skin
- In addition, skin hairs are supplied by nerve endings sensitive to touch. Through the awareness of these sensations appropriate action can be taken.

Temperature regulation

- The maintenance of a constant core temperature is a major function of the skin, and is controlled by the hypothalamus
- Losing the heat produced by metabolism
- Homeostasis is achieved via conduction, convection and radiation of heat from the skin surface
- Dilation or constriction of the blood vessels, which supply the skin, so increasing or decreasing its blood flow, can vary this heat loss
- Heat is also lost by the evaporation of sweat

- The skin protects the body from excessive heat loss in cold weather, by a decrease in both the blood supplies to the skin surface and the production of sweat
- The organs lying deeper in the body are further insulated from the environment by subcutaneous connective tissue and fat.

Excretion

- There is a very small amount of gas exchange through the skin, a negligible amount of carbon dioxide being lost in this way – about 0.5% of that lost through the lungs
- The skin also serves as a minor excretory route for urea, ammonia and uric acid in body sweat, although, most of these substances (wastes) are excreted in urine
- Profuse sweating is an important avenue for water and salt (sodium chloride) loss.

Vitamin D synthesis

- Vitamin D is obtained through our diet from fish-liver oils and dairy produce; synthesised when ultraviolet light falls on uncovered skin and acts on the 7-dehydrocholecalciferol present in the dermis, converting it to pre-vitamin D_3
- This is then slowly converted into vitamin D
- This process indirectly promotes calcium absorption from the gut. However, in the UK, dietary intake usually provides an adequate supply of vitamin D and, in this situation, the production of vitamin D by the skin is not essential for health. A full discussion of calcium metabolism can be found in chapter 4.

Energy and water reserve

- The skin forms a reserve of energy and water for use in emergencies
- In order to restore a fall in blood volume (e.g. in haemorrhage), fluid can be withdrawn from the dermis via capillary dynamics.

The healing process

Following tissue injury the ideal situation would be primary healing with minimal scarring Complications may ensue, leading to secondary healing with poor cosmetic result. The healing process (Figure 16.2) is a normal reaction to injury. The best results of healing are found in healthy individuals, but this may not always be the case as patients with wounds may have multiple other problems or conditions.

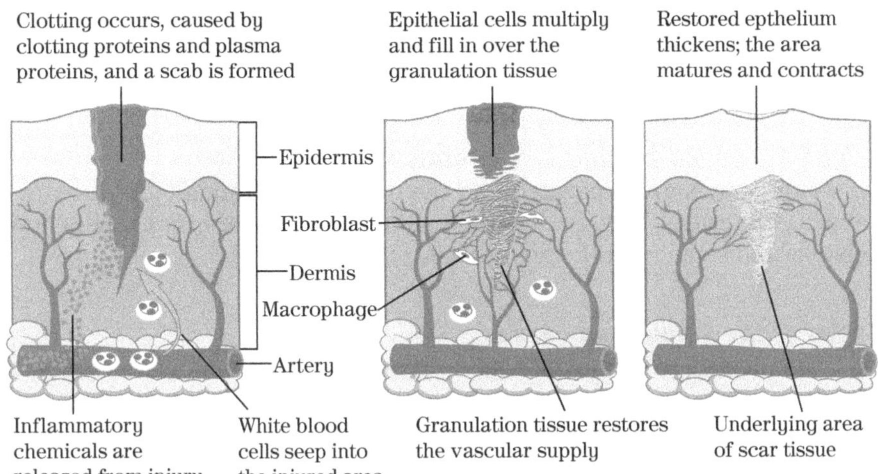

Figure 16.2 The healing process

- Intentional wounds:
  - Surgical excision, incisions and skin grafting
  - Usually heal by primary intention, the wound is sutured together
- Accidental wounds
  - Lacerations, stab wounds, gunshot, shrapnel, burns, bite and any traumatic injury which breaks the skin, e.g. pressure ulcers and leg ulcers
  - Where tissue has been lost skin grafting may be necessary
  - Usually heal by secondary intention
- Categories of wounds
  - Clean, bacterially contaminated, infected, complicated, open.

Wound healing is a homeostatic response aimed at replacing damaged tissue and restoring function. Wound healing occurs in all connective soft tissues in a uniform process, which involves the formation of new epithelium and contraction of healthy granulation tissue beneath, to form a scar.

Primary wound healing (1st intention) (Figure 16.2)

In primary wound healing the wound edges are held together by mechanical aids, such as sutures or clips. This should be achieved in all incised surgical wounds or primarily sutured traumatic lacerations. The wound should heal quickly because there is no tissue loss and no mobility at the wound edges. There should be prevention from external contamination and observation for changes that indicate deeper problems e.g. secondary haemorrhage, inflammation, fistula formation, because the only part of the wound visible is the suture line.

Secondary wound healing (2nd intention)

The wound edges are separated and the defect will gradually be filled with granulation tissue. This is observed in pressure ulcers, leg ulcers, open excisions and some full thickness burns.

Stages of the healing process

It is convenient to describe the healing process of a wound in five stages, but in reality it is a continuous process with one stage merging into the next:

- Inflammatory stage (0–5 days)
  - When tissue is disrupted, blood vessels are injured and they bleed into the space created
  - Damaged cells release histamine, causing vasodilation of surrounding capillaries and exudation of serum and white blood cells into damaged areas
  - The increased blood supply, oedema and engorgement account for the inflammatory appearance
  - Coagulation system and platelets cause the blood to clot. Injured vessels thrombose and bleeding stops
  - Red blood cells entangle into a fibrin mesh, which helps to prevent further blood loss and invasion of micro-organisms
  - The fibrin mesh holds the clot in place
  - As it dries it becomes a scab
  - Local blood vessels dilate and the circulation slows down
  - Polymorphs and macrophages arrive to defend against bacteria, ingest debris and begin the process of repair
- Destructive/migratory stage (1–6 days)
  - White cells congregate on the wall of the blood vessels, ready to break down invading bacteria
  - Blood vessels near the wound edge become porous, allowing moisture to escape
  - Macrophages engulf and digest bacteria and dead tissue and stimulate the formation and multiplication of fibroblasts
  - New blood vessels grow into the wound edge and fibroblasts follow
  - Enzymatic breakdown of unwanted fibrin increases capillary osmosis and localised oedema
- Proliferation/granulation stage (3–24 days)

  - Begins 2–3 days following injury with the replacement of damaged and lost tissue
  - With the appearance of new blood vessels and multiplication of fibroblasts this stage commences
  - Fibroblasts form collagen fibrils in a structure that has none of the organisation of normal tissue
  - Tensile strength increases with collagen synthesis. Collagen is a protein produced by fibroblasts, which forms scar tissue at the wound site and gives strength to the scar tissue
    - In wounds healing by primary intention collagen formation reaches a peak in around 6–7 days
    - In wounds healing by secondary intention wound cavity must fill up with granulation tissue and collagen
  - This fibrous network traps blood cells, which go on to form new blood vessels (angioneogenesis). The new blood vessels form within 36 hours of tissue damage, leading to granulation tissue. Healthy granulation tissue is bright red and has a moist, shiny appearance, but it is very fragile and easily damaged
    - The cellular and chemical activity results in the tissue, which consists of new fragile capillary loops supported in a scaffold of collagen fibres
    - There is a rapid increase in tensile strength of the wound
    - Signs of inflammation subside, but the wound remains red and raised
    - The process of contraction begins:
- Maturation stage (24 days–1 year):
  - When the wound bed is filled with granulation tissue, collagen fibres start to pull in the wound
  - The wound space becomes smaller, vascularity decreases, fibroblasts shrink and collagen fibres change red granulation tissues to avascular tissue as epithelium migrates inward
- Epithelialisation:
  - Epithelial cells migrate and proliferate from the wound edge and hair follicle remnants
  - They can only migrate over viable tissue until similar cells from the opposite edge are met. This results in closure of the wound by a new layer of epidermis, which gradually gains strength during the maturation stage
  - Migrating cells differentiate and lose their ability to divide
  - When migration is complete the epithelium thins. Hair follicles are not replaced.

Optimal wound healing occurs in a moist wound environment.

PATHOPHYSIOLOGY OF THE SKIN

Disease states in body cells and specific organs can reveal themselves on the skin.

- A great deal of information can be obtained by observing and monitoring the skin (Richards and Edwards, 2012):
  - Nutritional status
  - Fluid balance
  - Circulation
  - Emotional state and age
- The skin can provide evidence important in both nursing and medical care:
  - The diagnosis of patients' problems
  - An evaluation of the effectiveness of the patient's treatment and/or interventions
  - Can help to determine deterioration or improvement in patients' condition.

Assessment of the skin

Age

- With increases in age the skin tends to develop a drier and/or more wrinkled appearance
- Older adults suffering from disease may not be able to spend time grooming the skin, giving clues to their physical and mental state:
  - Neglect of toe- and fingernails which may become lengthy and dirty, as is it difficult for the patient to reach them
  - Offensive odours as the patient cannot wash themselves adequately, bath or shower
  - Loss of weight
  - Change in the colour of the skin
  - Temperature of the skin.

Observation of the skin

Observation of the skin can indicate signs of shock, anaemia, high or low temperatures, reduced oxygen or a particular disease or condition (Richards and Edwards, 2012):

- Skin colour is of great importance in assessment of a patient:
  - Pallor is when blood flow is reduced; it will occur due to the vasoconstriction in response to neurological stimulus and the release of noradrenaline

    - Occurs in conditions whereby the body is maintaining homeostasis, such as hypovolaemia, fluid overload and myocardial infarction (MI)
    - Exposure to a cold environment
    - Anxiety and pain may also lead to the appearance of pallor
    - Anaemia when the haemoglobin concentration of the blood is low:
        - In anaemia oxygen saturation monitor reading is not a good estimate as a normal reading will be obtained, as all haemoglobin present in the blood will be fully saturated
        - A better estimate of the severity of the condition is to look at the mucous membranes, e.g. inside the lips or lower eyelid; this is because blood vessels in these areas lie nearer the surface, so colour can be observed
- Flushing:
    - An increase in blood flow to the surface of the skin gives it a red appearance and it will be hot to touch
    - This occurs when a patient is suffering a high temperature, or in hot weather, as vessels will dilate to facilitate heat loss through the surface of the skin
    - May be localised to a specific area of inflammation due to pressure ulcer, surgical wound, vasodilation occurs over the affected area, and redness is a characteristic feature
- Cyanosis:
    - Occurs in individuals suffering from diseases, which lead to a reduction in oxygen carried by the blood (hypoxaemia) Cyanosis can be:
        - Central cyanosis and occur over the face or lips
        - Peripheral cyanosis is when the extremities become affected indicating a slow or reduced blood flow to the peripheral tissues
        - Cyanosis can be difficult to assess in black patients, as their skin pigments can obscure the condition. A better indication of the condition is to look on the inside of the lips, palms of the hands and soles of the feet (Richards and Edwards, 2012)
- Jaundice:
    - An abnormal yellow discolouration of the skin, and is often a sign of liver disease e.g. gall stones, alcohol – induced liver disease
    - The liver cannot excrete sufficient amounts of bilirubin through the gall bladder into the bowel and out into the faeces, leading to an accumulation of bilirubin in the blood

    - Any excess is excreted in the urine or deposited in body tissues, giving the skin a yellow discolouration
    - Early diagnosis of jaundice is a simple urine test for the presence of bilirubin, which should not normally appear in the urine
- Scars:
  - The presence of scars, striae, purpura and bruising on the skin can indicate conditions such as previous history of bleeding disorders, sepsis, and abuse and can be very significant
  - Injection marks on the:
    - Upper arms, legs or abdomen may give a clue to type 1 diabetes
    - If marks appear just on the arms drug abuse may be suspected
    - If conditions requiring prophylactic medication less often, by single injection, such as pernicious anaemia or blood transfusions for haemophilia.

Palpation of the skin

The feel of the skin can give information about the patient's state of health:

- Moderate and severe dehydration can be assessed by pinching up a fold of skin firmly on the back of the hand or on the inner forearm:
  - In a hydrated person, the skin will immediately return to its normal position
  - In a patient who is dehydrated, the fold of skin can stay like this for up to 30 seconds
- Oedema is a collection of fluid in the tissues or interstitial fluid space; it is recognised by pressing firmly over a bony prominence such as the medial malleolus of the ankle for about 5 seconds – waterlogged tissue retains the imprint of the finger (pitting oedema) The causes of oedema are:
  - Tight-fitting clothes and shoes
  - Limited movement of an affected area
  - Symptoms associated with an underlying pathological condition e.g. heart failure, renal failure
- Obesity is an increase in body fat mass or can be due to a metabolic disorder:
  - Body fat mass is increasing nationally and is an energy imbalance, with energy intake exceeding energy expenditure (Hignett and Griffiths, 2009), and is a major risk factor for:
    - Cardiovascular disease
    - Type 2 diabetes

    - Cancer (colon, breast, prostate, kidney and oesophagus)
    - Hypertension
    - Gall stones
    - Stroke
    - Osteoarthritis
  - Metabolic abnormalities that contribute to obesity are:
    - Cushing's syndrome and disease
    - Polycystic ovary syndrome
    - Hypothyroidism
    - Hypothalamic injury
- Temperature
  - An estimation of body temperature can be obtained by feeling the skin, which is determined by placing the back of the hand to an area of the skin:
    - Pyrexia – the skin will feel hot to the touch, and may be in conjunction with flushing of the face
    - Hypothermia – the skin will feel cold to the touch, and may look pale as in the case study outlined below:

Case study 16.1

Henry is a 62-year-old man who lives on the street and is well known to the ambulance service as he is regularly found intoxicated on the streets of London. It had been a cold winter night of –2°C. A man walking his dog found Henry early in the morning. He was very pale, unconscious and cold to touch. There was blood on his forehead and on the floor where he was lying. There was also a wet patch on his trousers and a puddle of urine close by. It was thought that he may have been beaten or sustained an injury when he fell. Henry is admitted to your ward for re-warming, re-hydration and observations of his vital signs.

  - In addition to this, the skin is a powerful observational tool when assessing the critically ill patient, but requires experience and knowledge of the nurse undertaking it:
    - If the skin is cold it can indicate hypothermia (as mentioned above), however, it may be noted that the patient is peripherally shut down, possibly due to the body maintaining homeostasis for a worsening/deteriorating condition.

If the skin is warm to the touch such as a high temperature, in conjunction with other observations, such as a purpura on the skin, the patient could be developing a worsening condition such as sepsis.

Changes in pigmentation

Changes in pigmentation of the skin can occur, which can be used as an aid to diagnosis:

- In pregnancy:
  - Pigmentation is affected by oestrogen production, which causes the marked darkening of the nipple, the surrounding areola and linea nigra in pregnancy
  - It occasionally causes patchy brown pigmentation of the face in pregnancy, which can be upsetting for those affected; this phenomenon is sometimes referred to as the 'mask of pregnancy'
- Albinism:
  - An autosomal recessive hereditary condition characterised by a lack of ability to synthesise melanin in the skin, hair and eyes due to lack of the ability to synthesise the precursor enzyme tyrosinase
  - The albino skin is pink, the hair pale or white
  - Sufferers have no protection from ultraviolet light and, unless precautions are taken such as constant wearing of dark glasses, retinal problems may develop.

Vitamin D deficiency

- Problems of vitamin D_3 deficiency (rickets in children and osteomalacia in adults) can occur when:
  - Dietary intake is insufficient (i.e. below 2.5 g per day for adults and 10 g per day for children and pregnant women)
  - Dietary intake is usually adequate, but deficiencies can occur
- Deficiencies can also occur when:
  - The body is deprived of sunlight, for example if sunlight is prevented from reaching the body.

Organic solvents and heavy metals

Organic solvents such as acetone, dry-cleaning fluid, paint thinner and heavy metals such as lead, mercury and nickel can be absorbed through the skin. They should therefore never be handled with bare hands. If this occurs the effects of lead poisoning can be quite subtle at first but can be lethal:

- Absorption of organic solvents through the skin into the blood can cause the kidneys to shut down and can also cause brain damage
- Absorption of lead results in anaemia and neurological defects.

Burns

Widespread burns can be a devastating threat to the body primarily because of their effects on the skin.

Pathology

- Tissue damage inflicted by intense heat, from:
  - Blazing fire
  - Electricity
  - Radiation
  - Chemicals
- All of which denature cell proteins and cause cell death in the affected areas
- The immediate threat to life resulting from severe burns is a catastrophic loss of body fluids containing proteins and electrolytes
- As fluid seeps from the burned surfaces, dehydration and electrolyte imbalance result
- These lead to renal shut down, and circulatory shock due to inadequate blood circulation due to reduced blood volume (Edwards 1998).

Clinical features

Burns are classified according to their severity (depth):

- Superficial burn injury, first degree burns:
  - Only the epidermis is damaged
  - Localised redness, minimal swelling and discomfort rather than pain
  - Heals quickly in 2 to 3 days without special attention; includes sunburn
- Superficial partial-thickness burns, superficial second degree burns:
  - The epidermis and superficial region of the dermis are damaged
  - Observed in scalding injuries
  - Symptoms of superficial burns, but blisters also appear
  - Regeneration occurs with little or no scaring within 3 to 4 weeks
- Deep partial-thickness burns, deep second degree burns
  - Involves the epidermis and most of the dermis
  - Less sensitive to touch
- Full-thickness burns, third degree burns:
  - Involves epidermis, all layers of the dermis, extends into the subcutaneous tissue
  - The nerve endings are destroyed and the burned area is not painful

  - Usually requires skin grafting, as healing takes too long
- Full thickness burns, fourth degree burns:
  - Extend to the muscles or bone
  - Usually due to electric shock or serious injury from fire
- Burns are considered critical if any of the following conditions exist:
  - Over 25% of the body has second degree burns
  - Over 10% of the body has third degree burns
  - There are third degree burns of the face (possible burns to the respiratory passageways, which can swell and cause suffocation), hands or feet.

Treatment

- Fluids lost must be replaced immediately
  - In adults estimated by calculating the percentage of body surface burned using the rule of nines
  - This method divides the body into 11 areas, each accounting for 9% of total body areas
  - An additional area surrounding the genitals accounting for 1% of body surface area (Figure 16.2)
- Nutrition – an increase in calories daily to replace lost proteins and allow tissue repair
- Prevention of infection as this becomes the main threat and is the leading cause of death in burn victims. Bacteria, fungi and other pathogens easily invade areas where the skin barrier is destroyed, and they multiply rapidly in the nutrient-rich environment of dead tissues and protein-containing fluid
- Appropriate wound management (see below).

Wounds

A wound according to Clancy and McVicar (2009) is 'interruption to the continuity of the external surface of the body.'

Aetiology

- Puncture to the skin e.g. by a bullet or stab wound, compound fracture
- Pressure ulcer (see above)
- Burn (see above)
- Incised wounds as in surgery, which is a clean-cut wound
- Fungating wound e.g. cancer growth from bowel or breast (palliative care)

- Drain site following surgery or aspiration (ascites, pleural effusion)
- Tracheostomy
- Leg ulcer (arterial or venous).

Clinical features

- Breakdown in skin integrity
- Inflammation – redness, swelling, pain, heat.

Investigations

- Assessment of the wound(s) e.g. size, colour, exudate, appearance, smell to determine state of healing
- Wound swab to determine the presence of infection.

Treatment/drug therapy

- Promote healing e.g. cleansing the wound(s), selection of dressings appropriate to different types of wounds, optimal wound environment to allow healing to take place
- Additional therapies such as the vacuum assisted wound closure (VAC) system, which uses negative pressure (Richards and Edwards, 2012):
    - Improves circulation to the wound and encourages growth of new blood capillaries (angiogenesis)
    - Removes excessive exudate, which reduces oedema and haematoma formation
- Prevention of infection, diet/nutrition, appropriate moving and handling, pain management
- Antibiotics may be required if wound becomes infected – determined by swab results
- Consideration of patients age, other underlying pathologies, drugs, circulation, nutrition.

Pressure ulcer formation

The skin can break down, ulcerate, leading to death of the cells and tissues due to interference with blood supply.

Aetiology

- The blood flow to an area of superficial skin tissue ceases due to:
    - Increased pressure occluding or collapsing the capillaries and small blood vessels
    - Sliding and shearing against resistant surface vessels.

Pathology

- The lack of blood supply to an area of the skin leads to:
  - Cessation of blood flow to an area of skin
  - The insufficient delivery of oxygen and nutrients to the cells with the resultant ischaemia, cell death and tissue necrosis (Figure 2.2)
  - Blood flow falls below a certain level and cell viability is unable to be maintained (Edwards, 2002)
  - The interrupted supply of oxygenated blood to cells results in:
    - Anaerobic metabolism – tissue perfusion is insufficient, there is a reduction in oxygen, the cell resorts to anaerobic metabolic pathways for energy production
    - Glycolysis diminishes and adenosine triphosphate (ATP) stores are rapidly used up, producing lactic acid and nitric oxide, which can rapidly build up in high concentrations
    - The loss of ATP – leads to a reduction in energy for cellular work (Edwards, 2002) and the plasma membrane of the cell can no longer maintain normal ionic gradients across the cell membranes and the sodium/potassium, and calcium pumps can no longer function
    - Without intervention oxygen deprivation will be accompanied by cellular membrane disruption leading to electrolyte disturbance and cellular skin death and necrosis
- Skin death and pressure ulcer formation
  - When a pressure ulcer forms the first stage is redness due to inflammation (Figure 2.1)
  - A severely debilitated patient can experience cellular death in the affected area of the skin after the first half-hour of unrelieved pressure
  - The dermal – epidermal junction is sheared apart and deeper blood vessels are damaged
  - In severe cases necrosis may occur in the deeper tissues while the surface skin initially appears normal, but eventually results in a deep pressure sore
  - A pressure sore usually occurs over bony prominence, such as the bottom, hip or heel, because body weight is concentrated on a smaller area of skin and so the degree of tissue compression is greater (see Figure 16.2)
  - Pressure ulcers are potentially an avoidable complication of bed rest and decreased mobility as outlined in case study 16.2 below:

> **Case study 16.2**
>
> Mandy is an 80-year-old woman who was brought from her own home (a bungalow) to your ward with a sacral pressure ulcer. She is clinically obese and has severely reduced mobility due to this, and spends much of her time in an armchair. Her daughter lives with her, works full time and is unable to give her mother 24-hour care. On admission the pressure ulcer was examined and found to be a grade 3 ulcer, with an offensive smelling discharge. Mandy's vital signs were:
>
> Heart rate 104 bpm
> Blood pressure 145/80 mmHg
> Temperature 38.2°C
> Respiratory rate 24 bpm
>
> Her dressings need changing on a regular basis and Mandy finds this very painful, so is prescribed 1 g of paracetamol 30 minutes prior to the procedure.

Clinical features

- Immobilisation – patients are more likely to experience tissue damage as a result of sustained pressure and need help to move and so redistribute their weight
  - Thin and obese patients are equally at risk of pressure ulcer formation
    - Thin patients due to exposed bony areas, susceptible to damage quickly by constant pressure
    - Obese patients as they may be unable to easily shift their body weight and fat cells readily break down when subjected to pressure
  - Elderly adults due to multi-pathological basis of their degenerative illnesses and the loss of elasticity of their skin tend to be particularly vulnerable
  - Paralysed or unconscious patients
  - Patients in pain, too weak, too obese or who are heavily sedated
  - Patients who have musculo-skeletal mobility problems
  - Patients with restricted movement due to constraints such as intravenous lines, traction or other equipment
  - Poorly nourished or dehydrated patients – often thin and in negative nitrogen balance, with skin that is already in a poor condition; this can reduce wound healing, enhance the

breakdown of the skin and quickly lead to the development of infection, due to:
  - Vitamin deficiency (especially of vitamin C) leads to poor healing
  - A reduced protein will reduce the ability of cells to divide and reduce the skin's white blood cell population residing in the deep tissues of the skin
- Patients subjected to mechanical injury due to shearing forces and friction:
  - Shearing forces
    - When strapping or dressing tape is removed roughly
    - Hard support surfaces, such as operating tables, commodes, trolleys
    - A too-tight plaster cast
    - Crumbs in the bed
    - Wrinkles in the sheet
    - Hard lavatory paper
    - Damage from the nurse's sharp finger-nails, watch or rings
    - Poor moving techniques
    - Incontinent or oedematous patients
    - Produced during slipping down the bed

Practice point

It is important when moving and handling patients that an assessment is first undertaken using the TILEE acronym e.g. task, individual, load, environment and equipment. This takes into account any possible harm during the process such as shearing forces.

  - Friction when 2 moist body surfaces are juxtaposed and subjected to friction:
    - Under heavy breasts and between obese thighs
    - Clothing which is slippery and non-absorbent and causes the patient to sweat (for example nylon)
- Patients suffering from:
  - Skin infections or generalised sepsis increase the risk of tissue damage as a result of pressure
  - Febrile conditions increase the body's metabolic rate and therefore oxygen demand in an area that is already potentially hypoxic

- Patients who already have circulatory problems, for example anaemia, atherosclerosis or hypoxaemic conditions
- Patients with malignant disease are similarly susceptible to skin death and pressure area problems
- Shock, with its associated peripheral circulatory failure, can predispose to rapid cellular death.

Investigations

- Wound assessment
- Nutritional assessment e.g. BMI, anthropometric measurements
- Blood tests for serum albumin, serum transferrin, serum haemoglobin
- Urine test for ketones
- Regular examination of the skin areas prone to pressure ulcer formation e.g. elbows, buttocks, hips, heels and back of the head.

Treatment/drug therapies

- Frequent moving/turning of patient
- Wound dressings (see wounds)
- Pressure-relieving equipment
- Vitamins and minerals, iron tablets
- Adequate feeding and nutrition may require enteral feeding
- Maintain continence e.g. faeces and urine, a catheter may be required if contributing to the development of pressure ulcers.

Drains

- This is an abnormal opening on to the surface of the skin that removes excess exudate or fluid caused by disease, trauma or surgery. Can be used as a method of prophylactic treatment either:
  - Therapeutic to relieve symptoms
  - To prevent complications such as pressure on other organs or blood vessels
- There are different types of drains (Richards and Edwards, 2012):
  - Corrugated strips of rubber or plastic
  - Tubes or catheters
  - Suction drainage systems.

Stomas

A stoma is an artificial opening of a tube e.g. the colon or ileum (bowel) or ureters (urine) that can be brought to the surface of the abdomen as a colostomy (large intestine), ileostomy (small intestine) or illeoconduit (ureters) to allow drainage of faeces or urine.

- Performed when the bowel is diseased and non-functioning
  - Cancer of the colon
  - Diverticular disease
  - Severe inflammatory bowel disease
  - Familial polyposis coli
- Performed for cancer of the bladder, trauma or intractable incontinence
- Types of stomas:
  - Colostomy – an opening onto the skin of the large bowel e.g. colon:
    - Temporary/reversible – emergency due to obstruction in the distal part of the colon to rest or heal the bowel. Some (usually elderly patients) decide to keep the temporary colostomy as it functions and do not want to undergo another major operation
    - Permanent – performed for cancer when there is no distal bowel left following previous resection
    - Usually a Hartmann's procedure is performed – the proximal part of the bowel is made into a colostomy and the distal part is closed leaving no rectal functioning
  - Ileostomy – an opening onto the skin of the small bowel e.g. the ileum
    - Parks' pouch may be made – total colectomy, terminal ileum joined to anus, continence maintained
  - Ileoconduit – an opening onto the skin of the ureters from the kidneys
- The faeces or urine is collected in a removable plastic bag attached to the abdominal skin by adhesive
- Early complications of stoma:
  - Sloughing or necrosis due to ischaemia
  - Obstruction due to oedema or faeces
  - Leakage due to badly fitted appliances
- Complications of major abdominal surgery:
  - Infection
  - Pelvic or subphrenic abscess
  - Breakdown or leakage of anastomosis (connection between two channels)
  - Diarrhoea (bowel)
  - Impotence in men
  - Bowel obstruction due to adhesions.

Skin cancer

Basal cell and squamous cell carcinomas are the most common (McCance and Huether, 2010).

Aetiology

- Exposure to:
  - Ultraviolet (UV) solar radiation causes most skin cancers, areas exposed the most to the sun's rays such as the face, hands and neck are the most vulnerable for such lesions
  - Coal tar, creosote, arsenic compounds and radium usually in the workplace
  - Papillomavirus and human immunodeficiency virus
- Fair skin or complexion.

Pathology

- Basal cell carcinoma:
  - Found on surface of the skin, originating from germination cells of the skin
  - Is the most common type of skin cancer
  - Small cancers may not be clinically significant
  - Usually caused by exposure to UV rays
  - Common in people who live in areas with a high level of intense sunlight
- Squamous cell carcinoma:
  - A tumour of the epidermis
  - Found in areas where arsenic is found in higher rates in drinking water (McCance and Huether, 2010)
  - Gamma rays and X-rays, and patients who are immunosuppressed are associated with this type of carcinoma
- Melanoma:
  - A malignant tumour of the skin originating from melanocytes (cells that synthesise the pigment melanin)
  - Can originate from a mole or naevus.

Clinical features

- Basal cell carcinoma:
  - Skin lesion or nodules, pearly or ivory in colour and slightly elevated above the skin surface
  - Ulcerating lesion, that can become firm to touch
- Squamous cell carcinoma:

    - Actinic keratosis – white, scaly lesions on exposed areas of the body
    - Bowen disease – flat, reddish, scaly patches on unexposed areas of the body
    - Both types rarely metastasise to other areas
- Malignant melanoma
    - Suspicious of changes in colour, size, irregularity of margin, itching, bleeding or oozing to a mole or nevi.

Investigations

- Early recognition through history taking identifying any changes in skin e.g. moles or pigmented growth or spot
- Biopsy – a histological examination of tissue to determine diagnosis e.g. cancer benign, malignant, differential diagnosis.

Treatment/drug therapies

- Surgical excision and removal
- Electro-desiccation (destruction of tumour by heat)
- Radiation therapy
- Cryosurgery (destruction of the tumour by freezing).

Practice point

Healthcare professionals can encourage regular checking of changes to the skin e.g. moles or spots as early detection and prompt diagnosis can affect outcomes.

CONCLUSION

The skin has 3 main layers but several important functions. When the skin is intact it protects, contributes to maintaining homeostasis, ensuring a constant supply of sensory information to the brain, can absorb and excrete substances and is a source of stored energy and water. The skin can be an early indicator of disease elsewhere in the body. When seriously damaged it can affect nearly all body systems, not forgetting the psychological and physiological scars left behind following skin injury.

SELF-ASSESSMENT QUESTIONS

1. List the tissue types that consist of the dermis and the epidermis of the skin.
2. Consider at least 5 different functions of the skin.
3. What physical changes occur to the skin when disease is present in the body?
4. List several changes to the skin anatomy and physiology that may occur.

REFERENCES

Clancy, J. and McVicar, A. (2009) *Physiology and Anatomy for Nurses and Healthcare Practitioners,* 3rd edn, London: Hodder Arnold.

Edwards, S. (1998) Hypovolaemia: pathophysiology and management options, *Nursing in Critical Care*, 3(2), 73–82.

Edwards, S. (2002) Physiological insult/injury: pathophysiology and consequences, *British Journal of Nursing*, 11(4), 263–274.

Hignett, S.M. and Griffiths, P.L. (2009) Manual handling risks in the bariatric (obese) patient pathway in acute, community and ambulance care and treatment, *Journal of Prevention, Assessment and Rehabilitation*, 33(2), 175–180.

McCance, K.L. and Huether, S.E. (2010) *Pathophysiology: The Biologic Basis for Disease in Adults and Children,* 6th edn, Missouri: Mosby Elsevier.

Marieb, E. (2012) *Essentials of Human Anatomy and Physiology,* 9th edn, San Francisco, CA: Benjamin Cummings.

Richards, A. and Edwards, S. (2012) *A Nurse's Survival Guide to the Ward,* 3rd edn, Edinburgh: Churchill Livingstone, Elsevier.

Index